Communication in the Nursing Context

Communication in the Nursing Context

Jean C. Bradley, R.N., Ph.D.
Assistant Professor
University of Illinois
College of Nursing
Peoria, Illinois

Mark A. Edinberg, Ph.D.
Associate Professor
Center for the Study of Aging
College of Health Sciences
University of Bridgeport
Bridgeport, Connecticut

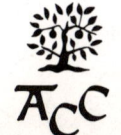

Appleton-Century-Crofts/New York

Copyright © 1982 by APPLETON-CENTURY-CROFTS
A Publishing Division of Prentice-Hall, Inc.

All rights reserved. This book, or any parts thereof, may not be used or reproduced in any manner without written permission. For information, address Appleton-Century-Crofts, 292 Madison Avenue, New York, N.Y. 10017.

82 83 84 85 86/10 9 8 7 6 5 4 3 2 1

Prentice-Hall International, Inc., London
Prentice-Hall of Australia, Pty. Ltd., Sydney
Prentice-Hall of India Private Limited, New Delhi
Prentice-Hall of Japan, Inc., Tokyo
Prentice-Hall of Southeast Asia (Pte.) Ltd., Singapore
Whitehall Books Ltd., Wellington, New Zealand

Library of Congress Cataloging in Publication Data

Bradley, Jean, 1927-
Communication in the nursing context.

    Includes index.
    1. Communication in nursing. I. Edinberg, Mark A., 1947–   . II. Title. [DNLM: 1. Communication—Nursing texts. WY 87 B811c]
RT23.B7   011.54'2'024613   81-12698
ISBN 0-8385-1180-5   AACR2

Text Design and Production: Judith Warm Steinig
Cover Design: Gloria Moyer
Illustrator: Bob Jackson

PRINTED IN THE UNITED STATES OF AMERICA

To our spouses and children:
Barbara and Daniel Edinberg
and
Arthur, Bill, John, Betsy, and "K.C." Bradley

Contents

Preface/xi

I. COMMUNICATION COMPETENCIES........................... 1

1. Communication and Nursing Models • 3

   Communication Models/5; One-Way and Two-Way Communication/9; The Nursing Process/12; Nursing Actions/14; Degrees of Visibility/15; Conclusion/20; Bibliography/21

2. Communication Channels • 23

   Communication in Three Primary Channels/25; The Use of Language, Channels, and Communication/37; Putting It Together/47; Conclusion/51; Bibliography/51

3. Communication Styles • 53

   Communication Styles; Satir's Categories/61 Conclusion/80; Bibliography/80

4. Communication Skills • 81

   The Development of Trust/82; Therapeutic Use of Self/84; Therapeutic Communication Skills/86; Techniques Related to Trust and Therapeutic Use of Self/95; New Areas of Health Care Based on Touch/104; Therapeutic Communication Skills and a Plan of Care/105; Conclusion/106 Bibliography/107

5. Information Gathering Techniques • 109

   The Interview: An Assessment Tool/110; Pitfalls of Interviewing: Common Ways of Hindering Communication/124; Integrating the Skills with Avoidance of Pitfalls—An Exercise/139; Conclusion/144; Bibliography/144

II. COMMUNICATION AND ROLE RELATIONSHIPS 145

6. Nurse/Client Dyads • 149

The Changing Role of the Nurse/150; The Changing Role of the Client/154; The Changing Aspects of the Illness Role/156; Conclusion/162; Bibliography/162

7. Nurse/Co-worker Dyads • 165

Nurse/Co-worker Relationships/166; Communication with Other Health Professionals/178; Conclusion/186; Bibliography/186

8. Nurse/Nurse Dyads • 189

Personal and Professional Identity/190; Student-Student Communication/193; Student-Nurse Relationships/194; Nurse-Nurse Relationships/199; Conclusion/202; Bibliography/202

III. COMMUNICATION AND THE PRACTICE SETTING 205

9. Communication in Secondary Nursing Practice • 211

Secondary Nursing Practice/212; The Secondary Practice Setting and Communication/222; Conclusion/230; Bibliography/230

10. Communication in Tertiary Nursing Practice • 233

The Client in the Tertiary Care Setting/235; Channels of Communication in Tertiary Care Settings/238; The Nurse in the Tertiary Care Setting/241; Conclusion/247; Bibliography/248

11. Communication in Primary Nursing Practice • 249

Primary Nursing Practice/249; Conclusion/268; Bibliography/268

IV. COMMUNICATION IN INTERDISCIPLINARY TEAMS AND GROUPS 271

12. Interdisciplinary Teams and Communication •275

Definition, History, and Rationale of Teams/276; Communication in Teams/278; Team Dynamics/297; Effective Communication Skills for Teams/300; Conclusion/306; Bibliography/306

13. Communication and Groups • 309

Reasons for Group Work and Cautions to Consider/310; Group Development, Processes, and Communication/316; The Nurse Leader's Communication with the Group/323; Types of Groups/325; Conclusion/331; Bibliography/332

Glossary • 335

Index • 347

Preface

The purpose of this book is twofold: to present a base of knowledge and skills in all areas of communication and to allow nurses the opportunity to develop an awareness of how these skills can be effectively utilized in clinical settings. The authors, having collaboratively taught the communication component of a "bridge course" for registered nurses in a baccalaureate nursing curriculum, found that even though students have had adequate exposure to communication and related counseling theorists, they have difficulty applying the concepts to clinical settings, such as medical and surgical hospital units, intensive care units, or nursing homes. Conversely, while many practicing nurses are "hospitalwise" in terms of how they handle themselves in their particular type of setting both with the client and with other professionals, they have difficulty finding useful concepts to accurately describe systematic communication problems in the setting.

This book addresses both of these gaps, namely the gap between communication theory and clinical application, as well as the lack of a systematic framework to examine communication in the clinical context. The book is not intended to take the place of primary source materials, such as the work of Rogers, Jourard, Watzlawick et al, and others in counseling areas. The book is also not intended to take the place of Birdwhistle, Hall, Sommers and others in nonverbal communication. At a baccalaureate level, students are able to read primary source materials as theoretical contributions. The authors have cited these authors and trust that a course instructor will integrate this book with appropriate primary source materials.

The book is written from the vantage point of the neophyte nurse, as opposed to a formal presentation of theories relating to nursing communication. (One exception is Section IV, which covers Groups and Teams.) This direction was taken because it is both "true to reality" and is often missing in other texts. There is an emphasis on exercises and discussion as well as didactic content. Exercises are placed within the chapters after the presentation of concepts. Ideally, students would read, take part in the exercises, have clinical experiences, and be able to process their experience in light of the exercises and concepts from the text, as well as from more theoretical readings. The authors believe that the concurrent presentation of both didactic and exercise content enables nurses to develop self confidence and self worth through the use of this text before they go into the clinical setting.

The book includes the work of Bandler and Grinder, which is relatively new and has not, to date, been adapted to a nursing context. An adaptation of Satir's communication styles to nursing environments is also new. The discussion of interprofessional relationships including nurse–nurse and nurse/co-worker issues, while not necessarily new, is a beginning step in the consideration of how nursing relates to other emerging professionals in the health field.

The references in the book are primarily nursing, psychology and counseling references. The content of the book is interwoven in a nursing framework that is based upon several nursing theories, for example Hays and Larson, and Yura and Walsh. The book continually relates material to nursing and specific problems nurses experience in different settings. The "Curriculum Project" undertaken by the Southern Regional Educational Board in 1975 provides the theoretical background for the different working roles and contexts found in Sections II and III.

The text is divided into four sections: Section I presents communication concepts and skills which are essential for nurses in any context. We envision that this section of the book could be used in a beginning "Fundamentals of Nursing" course. It also could be used for "bridge" courses for registered nurse students. Section II introduces the three dyads that are most often experienced by student nurses: the nurse–client dyad, the nurse/co-worker dyad and the nurse–nurse dyad. The uniqueness of each dyad is highlighted as well as some of the communication barriers that are present within each dyadic interaction. Section III builds on the two previous sections of the text: that is, the nurse is seen utilizing dyadic communication skills and knowledge about role relationships within three different settings of nursing practice: secondary, tertiary and primary. The secondary setting is presented first as it constitutes the setting in which over 85% of nurses choose to practice upon graduation today. Both Sections II and III should also be useful in "Fundamentals of Nursing" courses.

Section IV introduces concepts which are in part a forecast of the future: communication in groups and interdisciplinary health teams. While group work is commonly taught at the baccalaureate level, we also felt that, based on one of the authors' experience in working with baccalaureate nursing students in an interdisciplinary team training project, the students at the baccalaureate level would benefit from an introduction to these materials, even though they

Preface — xiii

might not be working on teams during their training. Section IV should best be utilized in Leadership or Group Process courses.

On a more personal level, we have found the writing of the text a rewarding experience. We learned from each other as well as from the materials we read and re-read to pull this together. We even found ourselves using some of the materials to help us work out our own communication problems. We also appreciate the help we have received from friends, spouses and colleagues who have helped with revisions.

Special thanks go to Allison Bailey, Elizabeth Bastis, Phillis Beveridge, Steffi Bloch, Art Bradley, Ruth Canty, Evalyn Carruthers, Barbara Edinberg, Grace Eckelberry, Jean Gala, Mary Lou Jansen, and Libby Zagorin for their input and comments on drafts of the book. We also appreciate the work and efforts of Charles Bollinger, Acquisitions Editor, Judith Warm Steinig, Associate Managing Editor, and Gloria Moyer, Art Director to help us publish this book. Finally, we have a special message of appreciation for Lorry Goorevich, Linnet Graze, Aberta Guise, and Carol Mason for their diligent typing of what must have been endless revisions of endless chapters.

SECTION I

COMMUNICATION COMPETENCIES

The first section of this book presents communication competencies and the relationship of these competencies to the conceptual framework of the nursing process. In looking at the way in which the nurse and client become actively involved in each of the four phases of the nursing process—*assessment, plan, implementation,* and *evaluation*—we see that communication is the common thread tying these phases together. To communicate is to understand both verbal and nonverbal messages; it is the ability to share experiences with another and to set mutually chosen goals with the client. Communication implies not only understanding the unique needs of each client, but interacting with other health care professionals as well.

The purpose of Section I is to provide a foundation of knowledge on which effective communication skills can then be developed. Chapters 1 through 3 provide the student with a fundamental knowledge of individual dynamics in the communication process. Chapter 4 is designed to give the student a beginning comprehension of the techniques for interviewing. And Chapter 5 presents information designed to help students gain an increase in their capacity for self-understanding and for their "professional use of self."

Chapter 1

Communication and nursing models

BEHAVIORAL OBJECTIVES

By reading this chapter and participating in the exercises, students will be able to:

1. Describe the five elements of a generic communication model
2. Demonstrate an understanding of the basic principles of communication (as proposed by Watzlawick et al.)
3. Describe the differences between one-way and two-way communication
4. Identify three clusters of nursing actions and relate them to the nursing process
5. Explain the concept of "degrees of visibility" in relation to nursing actions.

A nurse working on a surgical unit in a hospital is assigned the following client:

> Mary Cole, a 32-year-old mother of two children had a mastectomy two days ago. She has had a rapid physical recovery, and as the nurse assists her to sit up on the side of the bed prior to ambulation, Mary states: "I'm really worried about what caused this illness.

I don't think it was the smoking. Anyway, I don't intend to stop that now. What do you think?"

What should the nurse say or do in this situation? It is important to have several questions answered before venturing a response to what is obviously not a simple question. The nurse who is taking care of Mary would want to know how much she has been told about her condition by others, including her physician. He or she would also want to know Mary's reactions to her diagnosis and operation to date and what physical progress she has been making in relation to her operation. He or she might even want to know what Mary's disposition has been for the last 24 hours.

Even with all that information, the nurse would still have many options for responding. Several that seem appropriate include:

Taking her hand, sitting next to her and asking, "What is your concern?"
Asking, "What would you like to know about smoking?"
Pulling up a chair and waiting for her to continue.

Are there any other responses that seem appropriate and fitting?

There are also several responses that do *not* seem appropriate:

Walking away and pretending one doesn't hear her.
Saying, "You look so healthy! Don't worry!"
Saying, "Oh, you'll have to ask the doctor that," and moving away.

Are there others that would be inappropriate?

Nurses meet many Marys and find themselves in many situations where the "right" response is not automatically obvious. They need more information than is available; they will have to make educated guesses about what is meant and then "instantaneously" make a response to the situation.

As soon as the nurse makes a response, Mary, or anyone else, will say or do something that requires another response from the nurse. This series of "situations" and "responses" can be called a communication sequence. Each response depends on the "situation" that preceded it. Furthermore, the nurse's response becomes the "situation" or "stimulus" to which Mary will respond. Any communication can be thought of as "interactive," that is, each piece of information is partly affected by the previous communication. So what the nurse says or does depends on what Mary said, as well as the communication skills and knowledge utilized in the particular situation.

After the nurse has figured out *what* to say, *how* might it be said? What tone of voice should be used? What specific words would be best? How would the nurse position arms, stand or sit? How would he or she speak, or what facial expression would he or she use? Do nurses think about any of these questions or do they respond automatically?

Needless to say, if nurses went through the above list of questions and figured out answers to each of them before a response was made, it would take three to five minutes before they could say anything to Mary, who would, by that time, be thinking that something was wrong with the nurse! Nursing responses should be "automatic" *and* appropriate for the particular client. While the dissection of communication that is made in this book may tend to overanalyze the pieces, learnings ultimately have to become so integrated that the message sent will automatically reflect a nurse's knowledge of body language, communication channels, communication skills, communication styles, and role relationships. The student's responsibility as a learner is to try out the pieces and exercises presented in this book so that effective communication skills become part of his or her nursing repertoire.

How effectively nurses communicate with others is certainly one of the most, if not *the* most, important components of nursing practice. Research evidence indicates that, on the average, Americans spend about 70 percent of their active hours communicating verbally, listening, speaking, reading, and writing, in that order (Berlo, 1960). When we consider how often these communication skills are utilized in a practicing profession such as nursing, we realize that nursing *is* communicating in the fullest sense—seeing, listening, and feeling.

In the course of this book some theoretical concepts, ideas, and specific strategies will be presented in order to make students more effective as nurse communicators. An active involvement as a thinking human being is necessary in order to use anything presented in these pages. While the theoretical materials are important for thinking, the skills and exercises are perhaps even more important for clinical experience. "Good" communication requires practice as well as the development of several styles or types of responses so that one will be able to respond appropriately to what is seen, felt, and heard in all nursing experiences.

COMMUNICATION MODELS

Researchers and authors have broken up the communication sequence into smaller parts; these are often called elements or components. At other times, the pieces are more or less observations about aspects of communication. Communication becomes more complicated the more it is examined. Also, there is not necessarily one "correct" way to analyze communication, but each view can add its own understanding and, hopefully, expand our thinking and awareness about communication and nursing. Looking at "models" enables one to delineate the elements or components of communication. Consider the basic

FIGURE 1-1. Laswell's communication model. (Based on data from Laswell, H.D., The structure and function of communication in society, in *The Communication of Ideas,* Bryson L., ed. Copyright 1948 by the Institute for Religious and Social Studies. Reprinted by permission of Harper & Row, Publishers, Inc.)

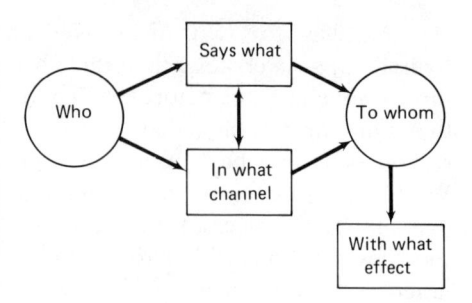

communication model in Figure 1–1, which consists of essential questions that can be asked about a communication process.

Who? The Sender. The individual who generates or sends the message is also referred to as the "source-encoder." The source is an idea, event, or situation. Encoding involves the selection of specific signs or symbols (codes) used in transmitting the message, such as the use of language.

For example, when the nurse asks the client, "Do you have pain?" The nurse is the sender. The idea that the client has pain is the source, and the use of language as well as placing a hand on the client's shoulder constitute encoding.

Says What? The Message. The message consists of stimuli (verbal and nonverbal) that are generated by the source and responded to (or not responded to) by the receiver. Messages consist of words spoken (content) and nonverbal cues, for example, gestures, posture, tone of voice.

In Which Channel? The Channel. The channel refers to the medium through which the message is transmitted. The three primary channels, which will be covered in Chapter 2, are visual (seeing), auditory (hearing), and kinesthetic (feeling).

To Whom? The Receiver. The individual who receives the message is also referred to as the "decoder." The receiver perceives what the sender intended (through the sensations of seeing, hearing, and feeling) and then analyzes the information (through interpretation of what is thought to be seen, heard, or felt). When we use language, our primary concern is with interpretation of the message. Since communication involves at least two people who are sending and receiving messages, each communicator in the process can be thought of as *both* a sender and receiver.

For example, the client (receiver) responds to the nurse's (sender) question "Do you have pain?" by saying, "Yes, I feel terrible." The client thus becomes the sender and the nurse the receiver of the message.

Communication and Nursing Models

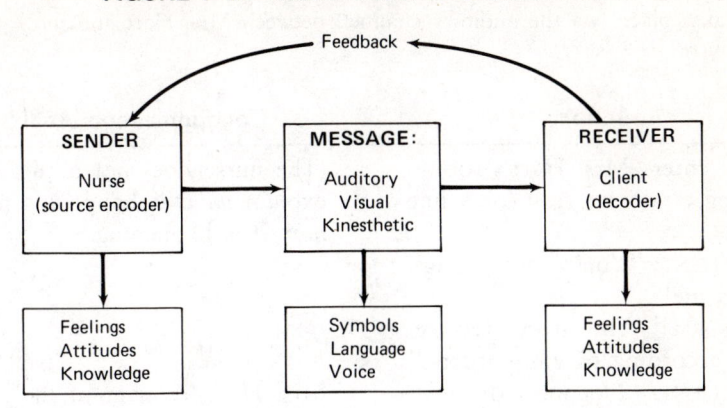

FIGURE 1-2. Ross's model of communication.

```
                          Feedback
              ┌─────────────────────────────┐
              │                             ↓
      ┌──────────────┐   ┌──────────────┐   ┌──────────────┐
      │   SENDER     │   │  MESSAGE:    │   │  RECEIVER    │
      │              │ → │   Auditory   │ → │              │
      │    Nurse     │   │    Visual    │   │    Client    │
      │(source encoder)│ │  Kinesthetic │   │  (decoder)   │
      └──────┬───────┘   └──────┬───────┘   └──────┬───────┘
             ↓                  ↓                  ↓
      ┌──────────────┐   ┌──────────────┐   ┌──────────────┐
      │   Feelings   │   │   Symbols    │   │   Feelings   │
      │   Attitudes  │   │   Language   │   │   Attitudes  │
      │   Knowledge  │   │    Voice     │   │   Knowledge  │
      └──────────────┘   └──────────────┘   └──────────────┘
```

With What Effect? Feedback. Feedback constitutes the information the sender receives about the receiver's reaction to the message that has been generated. Feedback is effective when the two communicators are sensitive to each other's message and modify their behavior accordingly. Changes in the sender's behavior that are reactions to the feedback that has been received are part of the total feedback process. The nurse receives the feedback and administers a pain medication.

A second model, illustrated in Figure 1–2, and adapted from Ross (1965) is more complex but is closely related to the elements presented in the Laswell model.

The five elements of communication are present in this model. However, the model also illustrates that the communication process is affected by feelings, attitudes, and knowledge of the sender (source-encoder) and receiver (decoder). In addition, the communication process is affected by the setting in which it occurs. Both the Laswell and the Ross models are developed and used as a reference in the succeeding chapters of this book.

Each step in the communication sequence constitutes a place in which information and meaning can be added or lost. If the sender does not accurately transmit the message, and the receiver does not accurately decode the message, then the message received will have little to do with the message sent. The following incident serves as an example:

> Mrs. Hart is scheduled to have an abdominal perineal resection and a colostomy. Her tests indicate cancer of the sigmoid colon. The oncology nurse (Miss Peck) has visited Mrs. Hart and explained exactly what is involved in the operation and what the colostomy will mean in terms of her life style postoperatively. On the evening before the operation, the nurse is expecting to give Mrs. Hart "saline enemas

until clear." The dialogue that follows records the interaction that takes place (via the auditory channel) between Mrs. Hart and the nurse:

Action	Communication Analysis
(Nurse enters Mrs. Hart's room carrying treatment tray for saline enemas.)	(The nurse does not accurately explain *what* is happening and *why* it is happening.)
CLIENT: "You're not giving that to me!"	
NURSE: "You are to receive saline according to your orders."	
CLIENT: "Not me, you've made an error!"	Mrs. Hart (receiver of the message) does not accurately perceive what was happening. Assumes nurse makes an error.
NURSE: "Mrs. Hart, you seem upset! It's not easy for you."	Message sent interpreted by nurse.
CLIENT (distraught): "Miss Peck told me I would have irrigations to regulate the colostomy *after* the operation, not before."	Sender (client) encodes message; sends to receiver (nurse) who decodes. The receiver (nurse) then sends or encodes message back to client. The client and the nurse transform roles from sender to receiver to sender and so on.
NURSE: "I think I understand where the confusion is—let me explain why the saline enemas were ordered."	

This interaction shows how communication is a continuous, changing process in which the sending and receiving of messages occurs over a period of time. Each message sent affects the receiver. Both participants in the interaction continuously respond to each other, having been affected by the previous message sent.

The following three principles of communication are also useful in conceptualizing the communication process (Watzlawick et al., 1967):

1. "One cannot NOT communicate" (p. 48). No matter what happens in any communication interaction, some form of communication is taking place.

Activity, inactivity, or even silence can convey a message. Thus, clients who do not respond are conveying a message. Not only is it impossible *not* to communicate, one cannot *un*communicate (Pluckham, 1978). That is, once the message is sent, it is impossible to retract it.

2. "Every communication has a content and a relationship aspect such that the latter classifies the former and is therefore a metacommunication" (p. 51). Communication not only conveys information (content), but it also imposes behavior (relationship). In other words, how we communicate depends not only on *what* we say, but how we *relate* to the person we are communicating with. This relationship aspect is one feature of "communication about the communication" (metacommunication) and will be explained in greater detail in the following chapters.

3. "A series of communications can be viewed as an uninterrupted sequence of exchanges" (p. 54). Communication is a continuous, circular process. It is a dynamic process in which messages are sent and received. The content of the message sometimes becomes less important than keeping the channels open and the communication continuous and uninterrupted.

Exercise in Communication (Watzlawick's Principles)

Break up into pairs and have a conversation about school, your families, or any other topic. After a few minutes, ask yourselves the following questions:

1. Can you accurately report what the other person has said? (content)
2. Are you aware of how it was said? (relationship)
3. Can you describe your partner's gestures, facial expressions and posture? (relationship)
4. Did you encourage further communication from your partner? How? Did your partner encourage further communication from you?
5. Did you ask questions when you did not understand what the person was trying to communicate both in content and feeling?
6. Did you interrupt when your partner was talking? If you did, what led you to do so?
7. Did your talking together bring a positive feeling between you?

ONE-WAY AND TWO-WAY COMMUNICATION

Although, as was mentioned earlier, almost all communication is interactive and dependent on the sender and receiver responses, people can act *as if* there is no feedback or response to whatever they are communicating. Thus, the flow of information is in one direction. This kind of communication is called "one-way."

One-way communication is quick, uncomplicated, and easy for the communicator to accomplish. Examples of one-way communication include public speeches, memos, and many university lectures. The communicator is in control of the situation; she or he can present information in an organized manner and usually can outline his or her talk or communication before it takes place.

Television and radio are the two most common forms of public one-way communication in our culture. Think for a moment what happens to you as the "recipient" or "spectator" to these forms of one-way communication. Do you understand everything that is said? If not, how can you find out the answers to your confusion? What is your level or type of involvement with one-way media? How is it different from a discussion with a friend?

In the health professions, people find themselves using one-way communication often and in a variety of settings. Written memos, announcements over the public address system, physicians' and nurses' orders, and even client education can be done in a one-way communication manner. Again, this method is quick, easy, and gives control to the communicator.

There are times, however, when the one-way communication model is self-defeating. That is, the purpose of the communication may be to teach others how to perform a procedure, to understand their illness, or to know which clients need which medication. The one-way model does not allow the communicator to know if the message has been accurately understood. Also, it tends to inhibit questions from the recipient until the very end of the communication instead of when the questions occur, which in turn may mean that the questions are forgotten.

As an example of the difficulties in one-way communication, consider the problems teachers encounter in large lecture classes. At the end of 40 minutes of speaking, they may ask, "Are there any questions?" By that time the students have, understandably, forgotten the questions or uncertainties they had the first 20 or 30 minutes and their attention is not as focused as it was in the beginning of the class. No hands are raised, and teachers can (incorrectly) assume the students understood everything that was said.

But to ensure that there is understanding, teachers use the only way they know to find out how much was understood—a test the next week. However, once the test is given and corrected, teachers are faced with more problems. Now that they know what people got wrong, should they (again) review the material for the class or go on with the syllabus? It is also possible that teachers begin to feel isolated from the students and that the students begin to regard teachers solely as evaluators, not as people who are there to facilitate their learning.

The situation just described is analogous to how some clients view their health providers. Often, clients with ongoing medical problems will need to monitor their own physical changes or take medication as part of a treatment

Chart 1-1
Comparison of One-Way and Two-Way Communication

	One-Way	Two-Way
Ease	Easy	Difficult
Control	Sender	Sender and receiver
Feedback	None	Maximum
Flexibility	None required	Sender needs to be able to change according to receiver's feedback
Role of nurse	Teacher, evaluator	Therapeutic, corrective
Ways of determining understanding	Tests, long-term	Immediate

plan. One of the most difficult issues in health care today is compliance in these areas. If the client education on self-monitoring, medication, or expected progress of the illness is given in a one-way fashion, nurses will not *really* know how much clients understand. A client may say "yes" when asked if he or she understood something only to find out the next day he or she did not understand it to the point of being able to remember it. Also, clients are likely to view nurses as evaluators who judge whether they are complying with their health regimens. Thus, a client may choose to wait until the next appointment (one-way), rather than providing feedback by calling in and reporting to the nurse when an untoward reaction occurs (two-way).

The alternative to one-way communication is two-way communication, in which the "recipient" becomes actively involved in the communication process, giving responses immediately to the message sender, who in turn can modify the next message based on the other's response (or "feedback"). The two-way process may be slower than one-way, it requires listening and flexibility on the part of the message sender, and it may be difficult to accomplish: A comparison of one-way and two-way communication is shown in Chart 1-1.

Although in functioning as two-way communicators, nurses are able to maintain their roles as health providers, new opportunities are opening up for them to be therapeutic communicators—individuals who are able to find out what clients are hearing and understanding. These tasks require more time and effort, but they also can save needless suffering by both clients and nurses.

Two-way communication is generally more effective than one-way communication. Yet many nurses who understand this principle continue to perform many communication tasks as one-way communicators.

What follows is a list of reasons why nurses may use one-way communication even though they believe in a two-way model.

1. The communicator controls one-way communication.
2. One-way communication can take place more easily while doing something else. Full attention to the recipient is not always necessary.
3. Nurses feel under pressure to do a lot of tasks. Two-way communication may take away from other important aspects of client care.

Can you think of others?

Exercise in One-Way and Two-Way Communication

Pair up. One partner will be A, the other will be B.

1. Both A and B will (individually) think of two "nursing procedures" (or anything else) that have five steps.
2. Both A and B then write down their own two procedures without showing them to each other.
3. A then reads the five steps in procedure one to B two times without any questions from B. (one way).
4. B then tells A what the steps are to the best of B's memory.
5. A then reads each step in procedure two to B and asks for questions or feedback after each step (two-way).
6. B then tells A the steps in procedure two to the best of B's memory.
7. Switch "roles" and re-do steps 3–6.
8. Discuss differences between the one-way and two-way communication sequences for both the "sender" and "receiver."

Two-way communication is not always better than one-way communication. There are circumstances under which one-way communication is appropriate (like telling people the building is on fire). Furthermore, it may not, in certain circumstances, be possible to have immediate feedback and two-way communication, as in the case of a comatose client. Another alternative which falls in between one-way and two-way communication is called "limited two-way communication" or "one-way communication with a feedback loop." In such a communication sequence there are specified limits or methods for feedback, such as question-and-answer periods. However, in many situations, the nurse can have a strong influence in facilitating two-way communication.

THE NURSING PROCESS

All nursing actions are carried out through a systematic methodology similar to the scientific method called the nursing process. The nursing process provides the foundation for nursing practice. It is a step-by-step method of selecting an action or actions to reach a desired goal. The major common thread throughout the nursing process is communication; it is the primary tool through which the nursing process is applied. The nursing process can be subdivided into four phases: assessment, plan, implementation, and evaluation.

Assessment

The assessment phase of the nursing process begins with the nursing history (Yura and Walsh, 1978). The purpose of this phase of the nursing process is to gain information about the client in order to formulate goals and a nursing diagnosis. In Chapter 5, the information-gathering skills necessary for the interview, as well as some pitfalls in interviews, are discussed.

Plan

The second phase of the nursing process includes setting priorities and goals for the client, and it encompasses relationships with other health care workers as well as written communication. The planning phase provides a means of communication between the nurse and other nurses caring for the client; between the nurses and other members in related health disciplines; and between the nurse and the client. In other words, the planning phase of the nursing process is a means of enabling the nurse to communicate with all other members in the health care system (Vasey, 1979).

Implementation

Implementation is the action phase of the nursing process. This phase draws heavily on interpersonal and communication skills. Effective use of these skills enhances the success of the action. These communication skills may be utilized with the client, co-worker, and other nurses. While the focus is action, this action may be intellectual and interpersonal as well as technical (Yura and Walsh, 1978).

Evaluation

The fourth phase of the nursing process is evaluation, in which the nurse considers how well the client responded to the planned action. Were the goals accomplished? If the client, for example, received a pain medication, is the pain alleviated? Nurse-client interaction is necessary for ongoing evaluation;

however, observation of nonverbal behavior is important as well. In some settings, interacting with the client includes the client's family as well.

NURSING ACTIONS

All nursing actions can be grouped into three major clusters: physiological, psychological, and socioeconomic (Brown and Fowler, 1971). These three clusters (Fig. 1–3) represent the totality of nursing behaviors required to meet the needs of the client, as depicted in the model.

Physiological nursing actions include attending to the most obvious physical needs of the client. They relate to Maslow's (1970) basic needs: oxygen, food, elimination, sex, sleep, and comfort. Examples of physiological nursing actions are attending to physical comfort, bathing the client, monitoring nutritional intake, and administering medication, as well as performing other nursing procedures.

The physiological nursing actions are generally easily observed and quantified; that is, an outsider could come on the unit and count how many medications have been administered, how many clients have been bathed, and (using predetermined criteria) how well the physiological nursing actions have been carried out.

Psychological nursing actions include any and all activities that affect (and aid) the emotional well-being of the client. Such activities are consolation, showing empathy, giving a back rub to reduce client anxiety, or even psychotherapy.

Almost any nursing activity can have a psychological function in that the nurse can influence client concern, anxiety, and self-worth in almost any instance. The same could be said about physiological nursing actions in that any

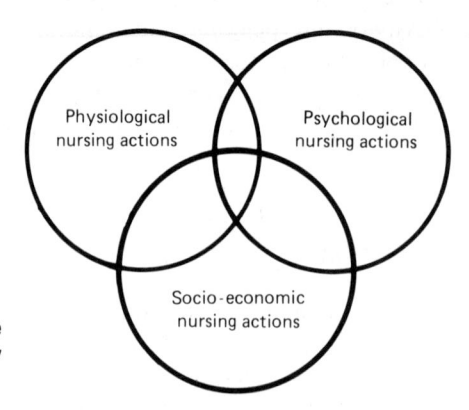

FIGURE 1–3. Representation of the three spheres of nursing action and how they overlap.

nursing intervention will cause some slight change in physiological functioning. In the model in Figure 1–3, the three circles are not independent. They overlap, which means that, conceptually, one specific action by a nurse can represent a physiological action, a socioeconomic action, a psychological action, two of the nursing actions, or even all three nursing actions.

Socioeconomic nursing actions relate to those nursing activities which address the client as a total person within the environment. Such actions include discharge planning, health education of the client and/or family members, and referrals to any of the numerous health-related or social agencies that exist within the hospital or in the community. Knowledge of the client's cultural background is necessary; for example, consider what it means to be an observant Jew in terms of diet planning. Who is this client? Where does he or she live, and what are some of the socioeconomic influences such as ability to pay for the hospitalization versus other demands on his or her salary, that will relate to the nursing care actions needed by this client?

Socioeconomic nursing actions often involve work with people other than the client, such as welfare agencies, the Social Security system, or family members. When such actions involve the client, the client is an immediate source of information with a long-term need as opposed to simply an organism with a physiological need to be met through the nurse's physiological actions. It is sometimes more difficult to observe and quantify nurses' performance of socioeconomic actions than their physiological actions. The results of socioeconomic actions are less tangible and more difficult to measure. For example, a nurse might contact a health agency for a client referral, but the agency might resist the request or even refuse to provide any assistance.

Of the three areas of nursing actions, psychological nursing actions are the most difficult to observe and measure. It is not easy to determine if what a nurse is saying has a therapeutic value for the client. For a moment, consider the case of Mary in the beginning of the chapter. How would you know from her reaction whether or not the nurse had *definitely* said the right thing?

DEGREES OF VISIBILITY

One way of thinking about the three areas of nursing actions is to examine each in light of degree of visibility (Brown and Fowler, 1971), that is, what aspects of each area are most easily seen by others? As noted earlier, those actions related to the patient's physiological needs are most easily defined as specific tasks and are most visible, while those related to psychological actions are the least visible. The latter are also most "person-oriented."

A nurse who is administering a tube feeding to a client is performing a nursing action related to a physiological need—maintenance of adequate nutritional status. This nursing action has a high degree of visibility. A nurse who is communicating with a client in a caring manner is performing a nursing action related to a psychological need. This nursing action has a low degree of visibility. That is, one cannot easily observe the outcome or the methods used to communicate in a caring manner. The assumption might be made by someone observing these nurses that the nurse administering a tube feeding is performing a nursing action to maintain the client's adequate nutritional status and that the nurse who is standing at the bedside talking to the client has finished with client care and wants to catch her or his breath before proceeding to the next client.

Chart 1–2 summarizes the characteristics of high- and low-visibility actions (Brown and Fowler, 1971).

High-visibility tasks are easily seen by others, and are usually related to physiological functions. They can easily be broken down into steps, and require a high degree of psychomotor manual skill. At a less obvious level, they are easily routinized and are staff-centered. That is, high-visibility tasks focus on a nurse's activities and can therefore be controlled, monitored, and standardized. Similarly, the control and evaluation of these tasks is administered by power figures in the system, such as supervisors. Finally, high-visibility tasks have traditionally been the basis for reward (promotion, pay raises, and evaluation) in the hospital setting, which means that there has been a tendency to overvalue these tasks.

Chart 1–2
Nursing Actions

High Visibility (Task Oriented)	Low Visibility (Person Oriented)
Easily seen by others	Not easily seen by others
Require a high degree of psycho-motor manual skill	Require high degree of cognitive/affective skill
Usually related to biological functions and processes of the individual	Usually related to psychological functions of the individual
Non-verbal	Verbal and non-verbal
Easily routinized—staff-centered	Not easily routinized—patient centered
Can be easily broken down into steps—easy to teach	Cannot easily be broken down into steps that are identifiable and are difficult to teach
Controlled by power figures—supervisors	Less easily controlled by high-status personnel
Traditionally highly rewarded in hospital settings	Traditionally not highly rewarded in hospital settings

On the other hand, low-visibility tasks are not easily seen by others, are usually related to psychological actions, require cognitive or affective skills as opposed to psychomotor skills, and cannot usually be broken down into identifiable steps. Because these tasks are highly interactive and dependent on immediate changes in the client, they cannot be routinized easily. They are also "client-oriented" for the same reason and are therefore less easily controlled by power figures, including supervisors.

A further point about low-visibility tasks is that their successful completion has not traditionally been rewarded or valued in the hospital setting. In part, the lack of reward follows from the difficulty of determining if a "good" job is, in fact, being done. At another level, the lack of reward is also due to the value judgment and philosophical orientation that stresses meeting the immediate physical needs of the client. Thus, areas such as counseling and health and family education are relatively recent arrivals in nursing curriculum. The growing evidence and research that points to the importance of less obvious activities (low-visibility tasks) in client care signal a change in nursing orientation that will strongly affect how nurses of the future function.

Exercise in Task Visibility

Which of the following are high-visibility tasks? Which are low-visibility tasks? Which are both? Why?

1. Giving a bath.
2. Counseling a client who is depressed.
3. Showing a client how to administer insulin to himself.
4. Talking to the client about her impending surgery.
5. Taking a nursing history.
6. Changing a dressing.
7. Referring a "discharge patient" to the visiting nurse.
8. Teaching a client crutch walking.

Communication: High- and Low-Visibility Tasks

It is now obvious how communication relates to low-visibility and high-visibility tasks. Counseling, talking, and all such psychosocial activities require good communication, but what about fundamental nursing procedures? If you hold with the traditional value that high-visibility tasks are the only relevant ones for nursing, you might find no use for this book. However, before closing the book forever, stop and think a minute. Put yourself in the client's place. Imagine yourself receiving care from a nurse. There are many ways in which the nurse communicates something to you. To put it another way, is it really possible for the nurse to *not* communicate?

Communication and High-Visibility Tasks. High-visibility tasks, as was pointed out earlier, are marked by use of psychomotor skills, are usually related to physiologic actions, and can be nonverbal. The communicative aspects of high-visibility tasks are not necessarily obvious but may have dramatic impact on the client, the nurse, and task completion *because* of their "hidden" or covert nature. Consider the following situation:

> A nurse was told to administer an intramuscular medication of vitamin K to a client. The medication was ordered to be given in the upper outer quadrant of the client's buttocks. The client, who had undergone surgery the week before, was uncertain what his status was. He thought the surgeons might want to operate on him again, but he wanted a second opinion before they "put him under." He remembers from the previous operation he had had a "preop" medication.
>
> The nurse came in and, thinking this was a simple physiologic (high-visibility) task, started to turn the client over. The client saw the needle and physically resisted turning over. He also started to yell, "You're not going to give that to me!"

Clearly, a few words of explanation and reassurance (low-visibility tasks) would have made the procedure more acceptable to the client. Many nursing procedures for high-visibility tasks involve specific steps that include communication; namely telling what is going to happen and why. These steps are designed to prevent the problems the nurse encountered in the above example. How the message is delivered, and what the client's physical, emotional, and verbal response is are important aspects of the communication process in high-visibility tasks.

There is also some communication in how the task itself is performed. For example, the nurse who is physically abrupt in turning a client over gives a very different message than one who is firm yet gentle. The response to the abrupt message will not always be obvious at that moment in time. However, you can be sure that the client's attitude toward the abrupt nurse will be different from that toward the firm yet gentle nurse, with a variety of possible effects, including differences in compliance, demands, and personal anxiety.

Another area of high-visibility tasks that directly involves communication is history taking. Even though there may be a standard set of questions or data the nurse wishes to obtain, how the nurse asks the questions or communicates the questions will influence how much the client shares, how much concern is voiced, and even the client's mood. While history taking is primarily fact finding, communication and rapport building go on as well.

Communication and Low-Visibility Tasks. Low-visibility tasks generally focus on psychological functions. They are verbal and therefore have an "obvious" relationship to communication or how the message (information) is transmitted. At the same time, nurses, as well as other health professionals, often forget the impact even a small gesture, phrase, or motion can have on a client. The client is in a vulnerable, high-anxiety situation, either in a hospital, clinic, or at home, and will be affected strongly by almost everything the nurse says or does. This type of client interaction is described in more detail in Chapter 6.

Some authors go so far as to state that all psychological disturbances can be considered to be problems in communication (Watzlawick et al., 1967). While this may or may not be true, the role of communication in both understanding and alleviating psychological distress is crucial. The term "therapeutic communication," discussed in greater detail in Chapter 4, is used to denote or point out communication sequences in which the purpose of the communication is to alleviate psychological distress. Ideally, the manner in which the communication is performed is caring, concerned, and empathic. While the specific knowledge needed to carry out therapeutic communication with severely disturbed clients is beyond the focus of this book, some of the basic skills covered in Chapters 2 to 4 will help in expressing care and concern for others more effectively.

A New Nursing Perspective and Communication. Today, nurses are shifting their emphasis from high-visibility tasks to an integrated approach that combines low-visibility skills with high-visibility skills. Qualified nurses do not perform a set of nursing tasks to the exclusion of the client's personal concerns. Nurses are finding out that often the best therapeutic communication can be carried out while they are performing high-visibility tasks.

> One of the authors was recently talking to a neighborhood child, Michael, a 10-year-old. Michael had hurt his arm at school while playing football. He had an ace bandage put on his arm by the school nurse. The author, who was working on the book, asked Mike if he had any advice for nurses on how he likes to be treated. His first answer was "Be nice." When asked how the school nurse was nice to him, he replied, "She talked to me while she was putting on the medicine. She told me what would hurt and what she was going to do."

Although we were not at the "scene of the communication," we can speculate that the nurse used appropriate tones of voice, body gestures, and words to assure Michael that he would be all right. What the school nurse was in all likelihood doing was providing therapeutic communication (low-visibility, psychological action) *along with* administering first aid (high-visibility, physiological action) plus giving Michael health education information (low-visibility, socioeconomic and physiological action). The nurse, by combining high-visibility physiological tasks and low-visibility therapeutic communication did a good job with an upset 10-year-old. The ability to integrate the two areas is one we hope nursing students will develop in their nursing education and careers.

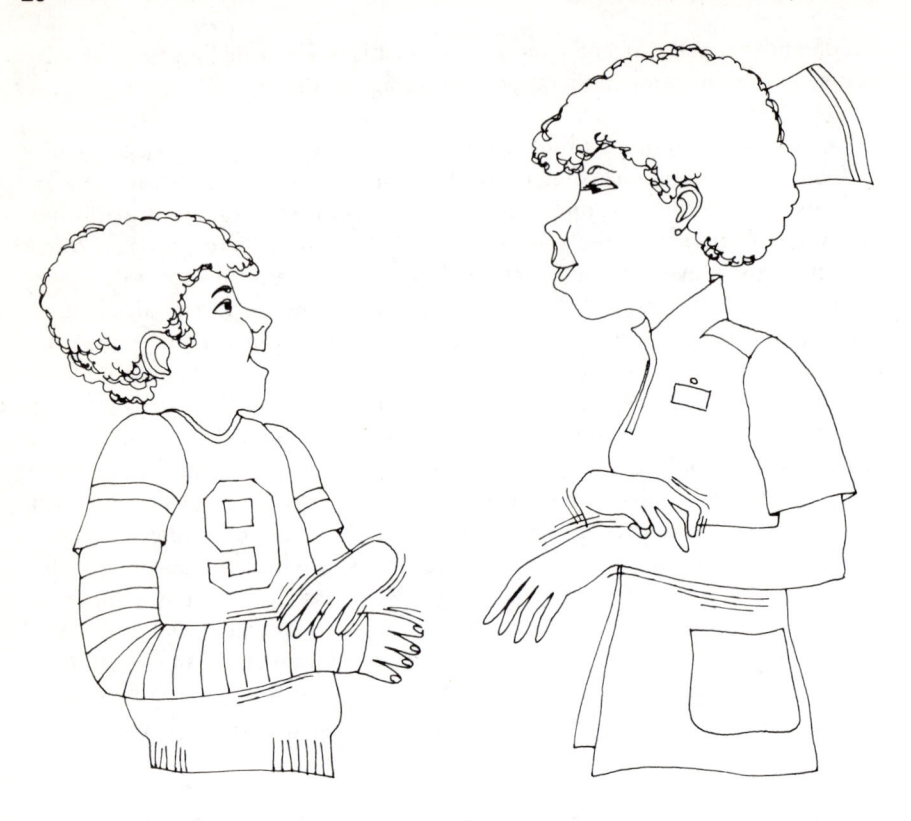

CONCLUSION

The purpose of this chapter has been to present a conceptual framework in order that nurses can begin to integrate a basic knowledge of communication skills into their roles as health professionals. Communication models depicting the basic components of communication, as well as how these components interact in nurse-client relationships, are described. To enhance their effectiveness as communicators, nurses must also begin to be aware of the content, as well as the relationship aspects of the message, and to know the advantages of feedback in order to encourage two-way communication.

Nurse-client interactions do not occur in a vacuum; they occur in a health arena in which nurses are utilizing the nursing process to carry out their actions. These nursing actions can be contrasted, in terms of visibility, with highly technical nursing actions at one end of the spectrum and communication interactions at the other end.

The unique role of the nurse is one that combines both high- and low-visibility actions; it is a role in which nurses minister to clients' physical and psychological needs. This is not an easy role, and much of the material presented in this chapter and those that follow is designed to help students meet the challenge of assuming the demands of this professional nursing role.

BIBLIOGRAPHY

Berlo, D. *The process of communication*. New York: Holt, Rinehart, and Winston, 1960.
Brown, M. and Fowler, G.R. *Psychodynamic Nursing*. Philadelphia: W.B. Saunders, 1971.
DeChow, G. Our greatest need. In Reitt, B. (ed), *To serve the future hour: An anthology on new directions for nursing, Pathways to Practice* (Vol. 2). Atlanta: Southern Regional Education Board, 1974.
Henderson, V. and Nite, G. *Principles and practice of nursing*, 6th ed. New York: Macmillan, 1978.
Laswell, H. The structure and function of communication in society. In Bryson, L. (ed), *The communication of ideas*. New York: Harper & Row, 1948.
Maslow, A. *Motivation and personality*, 2nd ed. New York: Harper & Row, 1970.
Mundinger, M. *Autonomy in nursing*. Germantown, Md: Aspen Systems Corp., 1980.
Pluckham, M. *Human communication: the matrix of nursing*. New York: McGraw-Hill, 1978.
Ross, R. *Speech communication—fundamentals and practice*. Englewood Cliffs, N.J.: Prentice-Hall, 1965.
Vasey, E. Writing your patient's care plan...efficiently. *Nursing 79*, April 1979, 9, 67.
Watzlawick, P., Beavin, J. and Jackson, D. *Pragmatics of human communication*. New York: W.W. Norton, 1967.
Yura, H. and Walsh, M. *The nursing process—assessing, planning, implementing, evaluation*, 3rd ed. New York: Appleton-Century-Crofts, 1978.

Chapter 2
Communication channels

BEHAVIORAL OBJECTIVES

By reading this chapter and participating in the exercises, students will be able to:

1. Categorize aspects of communication into visual, auditory, and kinesthetic components
2. Demonstrate an understanding of the three levels of integration within each of the three channels
3. Explain how thought relates to the major communication channels
4. Describe how language use relates symbolically to the major communication channels.

Look at the following situation:

    A physician, nurse, and client were in the client's room: The physician was looking at the chart, the nurse was listening to the P.A. system, and the client was feeling some pain. The client moaned.
    "What did you say?" the nurse asked, turning to the client.
    "What seems to be the problem?" asked the physician.
    "I have pain !" stated the client, silently wondering why the physician and nurse were insensitive.

While the above incident is not dramatic, the communication between physician, nurse, and client was not totally effective. Messages "sent" were not received. One way of analyzing the miscommunication is to examine the channels that each person in the communication sequence used. Channels "couple" or link the source of the message with the receiver. It is not always possible to isolate one channel from the others; however, the more channels utilized, the better understood the message. Nurses knowledgeable about channel use can detect systematic miscommunication and develop ways to improve communication with clients and co-workers.

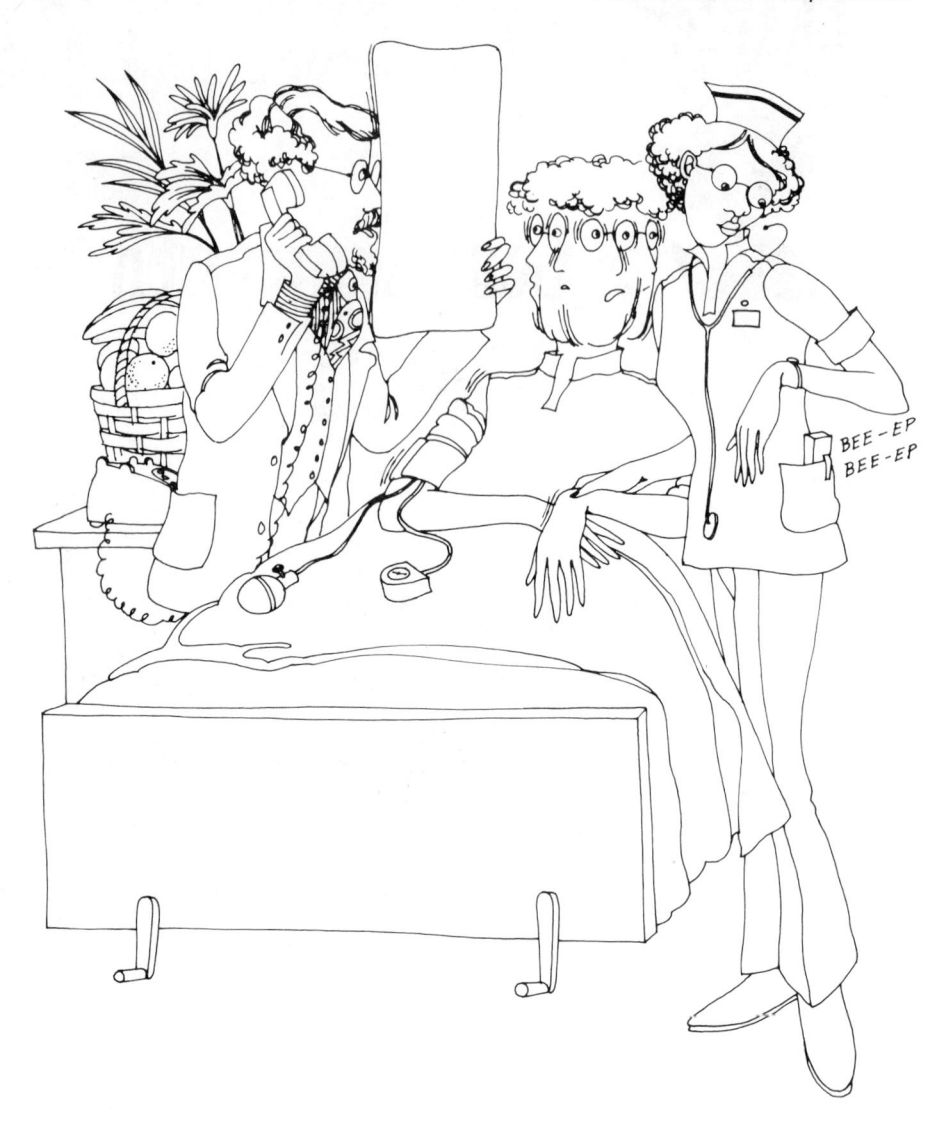

COMMUNICATION IN THREE PRIMARY CHANNELS

One of the many interlocking components of the communication process is the channel or medium through which the message is conveyed. In communicating with a client, a nurse can notice the client's looks, clothes, manner of sitting, choice of words, tone of voice, voice volume, how the nurse responds to the client, how it feels to touch the client, and even how the client smells. These are only a few of the possible things that could be experienced during a single communication!

One way of organizing all of this input is to categorize it into three general categories or channels: seeing (visual), hearing, (auditory), and feeling (kinesthetic). These three represent major senses that all normal functioning human beings have to one degree or another. The content of a message may be important, irrelevant, immaterial, subliminal (that is, the communicator is not aware of it), overlooked, or whatever, but in every nursing communication, there is visual, auditory, and kinesthetic input.

Within each channel, there are different levels of integration. That is, information that is seen, heard, or felt may be reported as it actually was seen, heard, or touched (Level I). The information may be reported in terms of observations, what the nurse got by really listening, or the nurse's feelings about a client (Level II). A third level integrates data from all three channels into the nurse's perceptions about the client (Level III). Level III builds on the information which was first sensed and was then integrated into one higher "full channel" level through the utilization of sensory input from all three lower channels (Levels I and II). Perception then includes attending to what has been sensed (Level I), giving order and structure to the sensed data through one channel (Level II), and finally making associations from all three channels by interpretation of the data from Levels I and II. It is apparent that perception is the most complex cognitive activity of all our behavior (Pluckham, 1978). The three levels are presented in Figure 2–1.

The remainder of this chapter will focus on Levels I and II, since they are the most relevant to specific channel communication.

Many persons are unaware of the differences between these levels of integration. Our past experience has often been to state what we see, hear, and feel without observing, listening, and feeling. It is essential that nurses clearly separate these levels of integration so as to be able to assess the client's behavior, as well as to record findings accurately and to communicate effectively with clients. Imagine the following situation:

> A nursing student was asked by a nursing instructor to report on the condition of a client's wound:

"It's ghastly," the student said. "Also, it's oozing and the client is upset."

"How you feel is not relevant in this instance," replied the instructor. "Let's see if we can find out some information about the dimensions of the wound, the degree of infection, and the client's state of mind."

In this instance, the nursing student had to separate personal feelings from what was observed (Level II), as well as to categorize additional Level II data clearly; that is, the size of the wound and the degree of infection from how the client felt.

It takes practice to learn how to see and observe; to hear and listen; and to feel and react to clients or others in the environment. A good beginning is to master Level I; then move on to Levels II and III. An important point to emphasize is that functioning accurately at Level I (seeing, hearing, feeling) is as difficult as using Levels II or III. Persons selectively attend to a limited amount of information, usually in one channel.

The following sections examine the kinds of information to which nurses have access within each channel, as well as the ways they sense, perceive, and interpret this information.

The Visual Channel

Take a look around the room or place where you are now. What do you see? The office in which this chapter is being written has a phone, a desk, a desk lamp, tall bookcases with books, a pink elephant (a toy one), a lamp, a cluttered desk, some messages taped to the wall, a file cabinet, a window, some books on the floor, three chairs, an overhead light that is not on, and an open door. The more one looks, the more one will notice, such as the colors of the books, their titles, the kind of print on their bindings.

In nursing communication, visual data can be interpreted rapidly to be given meaning. So, a shrug of the client's shoulders could mean "I don't know,"

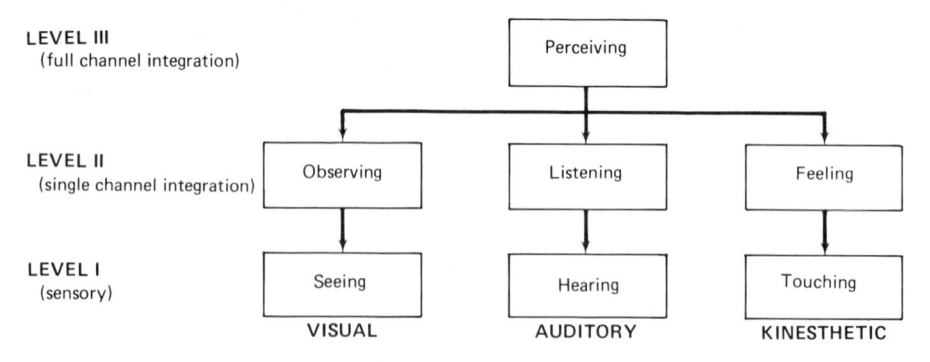

LEVEL III (full channel integration) — Perceiving

LEVEL II (single channel integration) — Observing | Listening | Feeling

LEVEL I (sensory) — Seeing | Hearing | Touching

VISUAL | AUDITORY | KINESTHETIC

FIGURE 2–1. Communication levels.

Communication Channels ——————————————————— **27**

a clenched fist may mean "I'm angry," and a man pacing back and forth in the waiting room of a surgical floor may mean "I'm anxious about the outcome of someone's surgery." One way of looking at visual information is to separate it into three levels: (a) what you *see;* (b) what you *observe;* and (c) what you *perceive.*

Seeing. Seeing is the least judgmental visual level. It is the closest nurses come to being a camera. Nurses are not, of course, merely cameras. They interpret what they see continuously without realizing it. For example, picture the room in which you ordinarily sleep. In one sense it is simply all of the hundreds of items that are found together (like a bed, blankets, floor, ceiling, light switch, dresser, and so forth). Another way of seeing it is to view it as "my bedroom."

In communication, it is extremely important and difficult to be able to see things as they are. People are so prone to interpret visual information that a good deal of time is wasted being angry, upset, and so on over what is an "imagined" event.

One example of misinterpreting what is seen is given in the following story:

> While a nurse was changing a dressing on Mr. Kennedy's leg, she kept glancing at her watch. Mr. Kennedy was to go to the x-ray department in a half-hour and she did not want him to be late.
>
> "Why does she keep looking at her watch?" Mr. Kennedy asked himself. "She must be in a hurry to get the dressing changed so she can go have a coffee break with her friends."

Nurses sometimes find it difficult to report accurately what they have seen. The following exercise will help you begin to sharpen your "seeing powers."

Exercise in Seeing

1. Pair up.
2. Sit across from your partner. Each of you will look carefully at your partner. Form a mental picture of your partner.
3. With your eyes closed describe your partner's face, body, body position, and clothing.
4. Listen carefully as your partner tells you what you look like.
5. Describe how it felt to try carefully seeing another person, as well as to be carefully seen.

Observing. Observing what a client does is an important part of nursing. The term "observing" implies that the nurse is operating at a higher conceptual level than just "seeing." The nurse is now making sophisticated interpretations about the client.

For example, a common observation found in nursing notes is that the "patient slept well." The nurse does not literally see a client "sleeping well." Rather, during her shift the nurse *sees* the client asleep without tossing, turning, or disruptions and then *interprets* this seeing into an observation of "sleeping well."

Observing Body Language. The major focus of nursing observation is the clients' body language. The use of body language, often referred to as kinesic behavior, is how one communicates through body actions. Body language may either accompany, modify, or even substitute for verbal actions. Such actions include how one stands and moves, a drooped or erect posture, the way the head is held, facial expressions, eye contact, and how one looks with the eyes while talking. Body language may portray the emotions in an accurate way. In some instances, however, body language may even contradict the emotions that are felt (Key, 1975).

The body language of clients assumes importance because it is often the mechanism through which clients express their emotions.

There are a number of ways persons can express themselves through the use of body language. For the purpose of our discussion we have chosen three specific areas of body language behavior through which clients can communicate their inner feelings; facial expression, posture and body movements, and appearance.

FACIAL EXPRESSION. The facial expressions of clients can be the most important indicator of the emotions they experience. Ekman and Friesen's (1975) studies on the "universality of facial expressions" through photographs concluded that six emotions can be accurately described through observation of facial expression alone. For example, clients who are sad, have a feeling of hopelessness, or have suffered a loss might display the following facial characteristics: the inner corners of the eyebrows are drawn up; the corners of the lips are drawn down or the lips are trembling, and the chin is quivering (Ekman and Freisen, 1975). Facial expressions for the emotions of surprise, fear, disgust, anger, and happiness can also be described and pictured. A fixed smile might indicate that the client is anxious to please, or it might be used to mask depression and fight off a desire to weep (Enelow and Swisher, 1979).

EYE CONTACT. Eye contact provides a unique and special form of communication. Whether one avoids or maintains eye contact is significant. The eye can send and receive messages simultaneously (Smith and Willamson, 1977). Avoidance of eye contact may express shame, fear, or low self-worth. Eye contact can be a highly sensitive form of communication, as shown in the following example:

> Mrs. Bigley, a new postoperative client, was to receive her first colostomy irrigation. As the nurse proceeded to explain the procedure, Mrs. Bigley was observed to avoid eye contact consistently. Because of her inability to establish eye contact, the teaching approach to Mrs. Bigley's colostomy care was not emphasized by the nurse, and the colostomy was irrigated without detailed explanation. The nurse's perception was that Mrs. Bigley was not yet ready to accept the teaching because of the psychological trauma of accepting the newly created defecatory exit. The nurse waited until Mrs. Bigley seemed ready to accept instruction at a later time.

Avoidance of eye contact was used in this situation to maintain distance and prevent direct confrontation. The nurse, perceiving this behavior, changed the client care approach.

POSTURE. There is always ample opportunity for nurses to observe facial features and other aspects of body language in clients. One aspect that is sometimes neglected is the postures of clients; how they position themselves in the bed. Are they curled up, rigid and tense, huddled under the blankets. Client's postures in a sitting position can also indicate their overall feelings. Are they slouched over, or are they sitting rigidly or loosely?

Along with tips on specific problems, such as a sprained ankle or Parkinson's disease, clients' posture can give valuable information about how they feel about themselves. If you stop for a moment and think about your own posture and gait when you are feeling "up" or happy, it is probably quite different from when you are feeling "down," "blue," or depressed.

The posture of clients not only indicates self-worth, but how they feel physically (Key, 1975). Experienced nurses are expert in recognizing the characteristic slouched, shuffling, uneasy gait of the client in pain. Clients often can even maintain this gait after the pain has subsided because they fear that the pain will return.

APPEARANCE. A client's general appearance can also give obvious clues as to how he or she feels. Men who are unshaven or women whose hair is uncombed may be communicating that they do not care or do not possess enough energy to care about their general appearance. A sudden change in appearance is worth observing as a sign of health status change.

It should be noted that when some clients or other people speak, their body language does not always match their speech. An example is the client who sits with his head down, slumped over, looking at the floor and says, "I feel real happy today." Rather than trying to figure out which is the "real" message, one can consider that both messages are, in part, "real" to the person communicating them. Effective nurse communicators make note of the messages and skillfully interpret them or have the client do so (see Chapter 4.)

Exercise 1 in Observing Body Language

1. Pair up. Let one partner be *A*, the other *B*.
2. *A* picks one of the following emotions without telling *B* which one and expresses it by his or her facial expressions:

   Anger   Joy
   Fear   Boredom
   Surprise   Impatience
3. *B* guesses which one *A* picked, and *A* then tells whether *B* is right or wrong. If wrong, tell the correct answer.
4. Repeat steps 2 and 3 three times.
5. Repeat the exercise but switch so *B* gets to express the emotion.
6. After the exercise is over, talk about it. Were there any expressions you could not "read" until you were told what they were? Did you notice any patterns in your partner's expressions of which he/she was not aware? You can also ask yourself, "What did I *see* that gave me the clue to observe that my partner was feeling anger, joy, or whatever?"

Exercise 2 in Body Language Skill

(This exercise is intended for in-class use and requires preparation.)

1. Pair up. One partner will be *A*, the other *B*.
2. *A* randomly picks one topic from the list below and one body stance from the list below:

   Topics
   a. The happiest moment of my life
   b. The time I was scared
   c. How to be a good communicator
   d. Christmas with the family
   e. Being nervous for an exam
   f. Falling in love
   g. Falling out of love

   Body Language
   a. Arms folded, legs crossed, look above partner's head while talking
   b. Lean forward, arms/legs uncrossed
   c. Lots of gestures, smile
   d. Frown, no gestures
   e. Lean back, make no eye contact
   f. Turn half away from partner, touch hand to chin
   g. Legs crossed, arms open, grimace

3. *A* talks to *B* about the topic for a minute using the body language guide somewhere during the minute (this may not be easy to do!).

4. At the end of the minute *B* reports back to *A* what *A* talked about, the body language *A* used, and where the body language fit or did not fit the content.
5. Switch roles and repeat.

The Auditory Mode

One way of thinking about all of the auditory aspects of communication is to imagine yourself sitting in a totally dark room talking to a person you cannot touch. Whatever goes on between the two of you will be completely auditory! Auditory aspects would include the words that are spoken as well as the volume, tone, pitch, rhythm, and speed of speech.

One way of organizing auditory input is to distinguish the content of words that are used (digital communication) from the tone, pitch, and speed of speech (analogical communication).

Nuances in auditory communication are often overlooked by nurses, as well as by others. The following exercise is designed to help you sharpen your awareness of how all of the analogical qualities of a message (tone, volume, pitch, rapidity of speech, and so forth) can influence the impact of the message on the receiver.

Exercise in Auditory Awareness

1. Pair up. One partner will be *A*, the other *B*.
2. *A* will say something that would normally be said to a client, such as, "How are you today?" *B* listens with eyes closed.
3. *B* then describes what *A* said in terms of the following:
    a. Speed of speech
    b. Volume (loudness)
    c. Pitch (how high, low the voice is)
    d. Inflection (how sing-song or "up and down" the words are)
    e. Rhythm of the words
4. Repeat steps 2–3 with roles reversed.

Hearing. The same way that the first level of visual communication is seeing, the first level of auditory communication is *hearing*. Being able to identify accurately what you hear is a crucial step in nursing communication. It is also important to hear all aspects, not simply the words that are said.

Exercise 1 in Hearing

1. Pair up. One partner will be *A*, the other *B*.
2. *A* says something *A* believes is true.
3. *B* mimics (tries to sound just like *A* did) the statement, reproducing *A*'s speed of speech, inflection, pitch, volume, and rhythm.
4. Discuss how easy or difficult it is to mimic another.

Exercise 2 in Hearing

1. Pair up. One partner will be *A*, the other *B*.
2. *A* says a simple statement.
3. *B* mimics *A*, but exaggerates *one* of the following:
   a. Speed of speech
   b. Volume
   c. Pitch
   d. Inflection
   e. Rhythm
4. Repeat steps 2–3 with reversed roles.
5. Discuss how easy or difficult it was.

The above exercise is difficult and demonstrates that how the message is delivered has a tremendous impact on others. An awareness of one's own speech, as well as that of others, can be increased through practice in this exercise with a friend or with a tape recorder.

Listening. The next level in organizing auditory information (Level III) is *listening*. Listening means both accurately hearing what is said and making meaning out of what is said. We are always putting pieces of the verbal and auditory communication of others together. A nurse continually listens to the client to detect unspoken concerns, fears, or misunderstandings. The next exercise will sharpen your listening awareness.

Exercise in Listening

1. Record a conversation with a partner for 5 minutes using a tape recorder. The topic should be: "My own health habits."
2. Force yourself to listen to the *qualities* of the other's speech, that is, tone, speed, inflection, mannerisms, and so forth, as well as what is said.
3. Answer the following questions for yourself:
   a. When does the person's content (what they say) fit with how they say it? When does it not fit?

b. What are the most striking aspect(s) of the other's speech? How does it (or they) effect you?
c. Can you figure out any *patterns* in the other's speech? (For example, is there a rhythmic sequence that indicates anxiety, a certain inflection to emphasize words and so forth?)

One of the mistakes often made in nursing communication is that meaning is assumed to be understood. That is, because two people are both nurses, they assume they know exactly what each other means by "care," "compliance," "following orders," or almost anything else. The following *true* story shows how a misinterpretation can occur in nursing communication.

> Some beginning student nurses were working in a newborn unit. One of the infants had hydrocephalus, a condition in which the child's head is enlarged. The nurse in charge told the students, "Be sure to weigh and measure the head each day." To her surprise she returned to find the students trying to put the infant's head on a scale. What she had meant was "weigh *the baby* and measure the circumference of the head."

Rather than assume that all nurses should understand everything they hear, the effective nurse communicator has to work hard and listen carefully to "make meaning" or understand what others communicate.

Exercise in Making Meaning

1. Pair up. One partner will be *A*, the other *B*.
2. *A* then makes a statement.
3. *B* then asks, "Do you mean...?" and finishes the question with *B*'s guess as to some of the underlying meanings behind *A*'s statement. For example, if *A* says, yawning, "I think it's late," *B* could ask, "Do you mean you're tired?"
4. *A* then replies, using only one of the following answers:
   Yes
   No
   Partially
   (*A* may be surprised by what *B* says in that it is a "yes" even though *A* was not aware of it in making the initial statement.)
5. *B* then asks, again, "Do you mean...?" until such time as one of the following happen:
   B gets a total of 3 "yes" answers or
   B gets so frustrated that she or he says to *A*, "What *did* you mean?" *A* then tells *B*.
6. Switch roles and repeat.
7. When the exercise is over, think or discuss how meaning can be misinterpreted and how there can be more meaning in what you say than you realize when you say it.

The Kinesthetic Modality

The third major modality or communication channel is the kinesthetic channel. The term "kinesthetic" refers to all aspects of communication relating to feelings. Touch and physiological responses to the environment can be considered at the first level of integration (Level I). However, when the physiological reactions are given a descriptive label or are called "feelings," they are at the second level of integration (Level II). It is important to realize that what are commonly called "feelings" have a cognitive as well as emotional component.

Touch. The major form of communication in the kinesthetic channel involves touch. What gets communicated through touch? A partial list might include affection, pain, emotional support, physical support, giving direction, playfulness, and getting someone's attention.

When we touch another person we use an "immediate" receptor, rather than a "distance" receptor (eyes, ears, or nose). In other words, we examine the world close up rather than from a distance (Hall, 1969). In this regard, touch is the most personally experienced of all sensations.

Many of us, as a result of our American cultural upbringing, have been taught not to touch each other, especially strangers. When we do, we usually excuse ourselves. Some cultures have a much higher tolerance for touching, for example, the Japanese and Arab cultures (Hall, 1969).

Much of our culturally learned behavior changes in nurse-client relationships. Physical contact with clients is allowed and even required; touch is an essential part of the nursing process. Nurses communicate with clients through baths, backrubs, and dressings, for example. This change in behavior with reference to the use of touch can be difficult for nurses. To assimilate the use of touch into a professional role requires taking risks. A touching gesture might appear "forward" to a group of clients; on the other hand, some clients like to be touched and interpret it as caring on the part of the nurse. Touch can be the key to unlocking a client's feelings. The following situation represents a true story:

> Cathy, a beginning student nurse, was assigned to Mr. Moore, a 38-year-old male client with a diagnosis of severely advanced arteriosclerotic heart disease. Mr. Moore had a coronary bypass operation but was still immobilized and could not even sit in a chair without experiencing severe anginal pain. He was receiving pain medication p.r.n. While Cathy was assisting Mr. Moore with his A.M. care, she felt a sense of frustration in not being able to communicate effectively with this man about his illness.
>
> After Cathy finished with Mr. Moore's bath and was about to leave the room, she stood by the head of his bed for a few minutes and placed her hand on his shoulder. After a few moments of silence, Mr. Moore began to

Communication Channels 35

share his feelings about his family, his loss of his job, and his hospitalization. As Cathy stated later, the act of touching seemed to break down the last barrier to communication and close the distance between them.

An unplanned effective use of touch to which the client responded was utilized in the above situation. The use of touch as a therapeutic tool is covered in Chapter 4.

The following exercise is designed to sensitize you to the ways nurses can communicate through touch.

Exercise in Touch Communication

1. Pair up. One partner will be *A*, the other *B*.
2. Sit so you can touch each other.
3. *A* then picks one of the following messages to communicate through touch (*don't tell B*).
   a. "I'm angry with you."
   b. "I'm anxious about touching you."
   c. "I care (have empathy) for you."
4. *A* then touches *B* on the hand, arm, shoulder, or some other part of the body, and
   a. communicates the "touch message" *A* has picked *while*
   b. *A* says, "Hello _____, how are you today?"
5. *B* guesses what *A* was communicating through the touch (*A* tells *B* what the answer was).
6. *A* tries two more touches with the same verbal message: "How are you today?"
7. Switch so *B* can try some touch messages.
8. Discuss what you learned *or* are unsure of.

Some of you will find this exercise easier to do with your eyes closed. When you talk about the exercise, answer the following questions:

1. How much did you think about your touch messages?
2. How aware are you of your own or other people's touch messages?
3. How do you and others respond when two different messages are given verbally and by touch?

Physiological Reactions. Physiological reactions are specific body reactions to external events. There has been some interesting research about how people's bodies express (or symbolize) emotional states. A whole branch of medicine/psychiatry/psychology is devoted to the most dramatic forms of body communication of emotional problems. This field is called psychosomatic medicine. An example of how the mind (psyche) and body (soma) are interrelated is demonstrated by Norman Cousins (1980) in his book *Anatomy of an Illness.* He tells of his critical illness, one in which physicians gave him a slim chance of recovery and how he used his own creative ability to help cure himself. It is obvious that there are illnesses which do not always respond to one's own attitude, but the use of humor or a decrease in excessive amounts of medication (as in Cousin's case), might help in some situations to alter the course of illness. Cousins states that the client's most powerful weapon is the "will to live," which he saw not as a "theoretical abstract but a physiologic reality with therapeutic characteristics" (Cousins, 1976, p. 1462).

Real physical ailments, such as ulcers, hives, and certain skin conditions, can be related directly to emotional functioning. The following exercise will help you become more aware of how your body expresses (and communicates) feelings. This is related to the earlier discussion of body language.

Exercise in Feelings and Physiological Reactions

1. Sit with your eyes closed.
2. Imagine a time when you felt *very* happy.
3. Think how your body felt at that time (and how it feels now remembering that time).
4. Write down *your* body's "happy reactions."
5. Do the same for each of the following feelings:
   a. sad
   b. loving
   c. afraid
   d. anxious
6. Share these in a large group. Do any commonalities or differences come up? Note them. Each person may have different ways of experiencing different feelings.

When you think about it, there are not many different "feelings." There are, however, an infinite amount of *kinds* of one feeling, such as love. A fairly complete list of feelings includes:

loneliness	sadness
hurt	disappointment
love	frustration
sexiness	fear
happiness	anxiety

While feelings are experienced by the individual, often the nurse responds to the client's feelings by having similar reactions. This sense of being in the "other's shoes" is called empathy and is an important tool in therapeutic communication, which is discussed further in Chapter 4.

THE USE OF LANGUAGE, CHANNELS, AND COMMUNICATION

The concept of communication channels has a wide range of applications (see Bandler and Grinder, 1975, and Grinder and Bandler, 1976, for a therapeutic system based on principles of channel use; the following discussion is in part based on their system. All communication can be analyzed by the three major channels. We can even break down how we think, how we feel, what we say, and the kinds of activities we like to do into visual, auditory, and kinesthetic components. For example, listening to the radio is obviously an auditory activity, although we may visualize images based on what we hear. Playing tennis or many other sports are a combination of visual and kinesthetic activities (if we have ever played doubles and our partner got angry with us for a mistake, we may have also found an auditory component as well).

Nursing communication is similar to all other communication in that all nursing communication can be broken down and analyzed by auditory, visual, and kinesthetic components. Imagine the following case:

> You are given an assignment by your head nurse. Your instructions are to help pass out meals. The meals arrive, you read the names on the plates, and give the trays to the appropriate clients. Feeling you have done this quite well, you wait until all are finished, then quickly collect and stack up the trays. As you are stacking them up, something drops out onto the floor. You look at a set of dentures and go immediately to the head nurse, dentures in hand. "Don't worry," she tells you, "you see we know this happens. If you look inside the dentures you will find the client's name on them. Many older people don't eat with their dentures in. They place them on the tray. We have to be careful to watch after the client has finished, as well as before, to make sure they don't lose their dentures."

There are many ways to examine what happened in this imaginary series of communications and activities. From the communication channel view, a partial breakdown would be as follows:

1. Auditory—you were *told* directions.
2. Visual—you successfully *saw* the names on the trays and matched them to the clients
3. Kinesthetic—you *gave* the meals to the clients
4. Kinesthetic—you *felt good* about doing the job, which may have lowered your level of watchfulness after the meals were passed out

5. Visual—you *saw* the dentures fall out but did not *see* the name in the dentures
6. Auditory—you *spoke* to the head nurse
7. Auditory—the head nurse *told* you information and a visual strategy to watch carefully *after* the meal for future use
8. Kinesthetic—you *gave* the dentures to the client

It should be stressed that this analysis is extremely basic. One could go even deeper and examine how you interpreted the instructions (did you repeat them to yourself or make a picture?), how you went about matching the trays to the clients, how you used the "feeling good" to relax your watchfulness after the meal, and how you processed the final information from the head nurse. All of this could have been done through the channels concept. It is thus possible to examine thinking, use of language, and many aspects of nursing process and communication through the concept of channels.

Thinking in the Three Major Channels

People rarely pay attention to how they think. They can usually tell you what's on their mind, what their secret hopes are, or what they want for Christmas, but most of them are not aware of *how* they think. By "how," we are talking about visual, auditory, and kinesthetic thinking, as well as the steps people go through to decide what they want for Christmas, what is on their mind, or, in the case of client-nurse communication, what the presenting complaint is. It can be quite important to understand how (not what) a client thinks, because the *process* of thinking and speaking may overlook important information that is essential to the client's care. An example will help clarify the last statement.

> Suppose you are the nurse for a postoperative client. You come by and ask him, "How do you feel?" He thinks for a second and says, "Lousy." You pursue the point and discover that the client, when asked "How do you feel?" uses visual thoughts (he pictures himself) to decide how he feels. Furthermore, because it is difficult to "picture how you feel," he quickly (without being aware of it) pictures himself in bed, groggy eyed, in a hospital, and then compares this picture to one of himself playing golf on a golf course and says "Lousy."

Visual Thinking. When we think visually, we create pictures. If we imagine for a moment what our house or apartment looks like, we begin to get some sort of a picture of a building or rooms in our mind's eye. People who are very good visual thinkers can make mental lists of tasks to do, can picture each

Communication Channels 39

step in a nursing procedure, or can imagine how a certain size client will fit a certain size wheelchair.

These last examples show us some of the advantages of visual thinking (picturing). Visual imaging can also be useful in interpreting what a client or staff member is saying. In the case of the falling dentures, we could make a picture of ourselves looking at the trays after the meal and use that picture to remind ourselves to do it.

Information from hearing or feeling channels can also be visualized. If we have trouble listening or being responsive to feelings at a moment in time, this can help our understanding and communication. One way to visualize what a client is saying is literally to make the words go across our mind's eye like a typewriter. That way, we can "see" what is being said. If there are many "feelings" coming out, we can make pictures in our mind's eye of someone feeling those feelings. That way, we can "see what they mean."

Ideally, all nurses develop abilities to communicate and think in all channels. The following exercise is a simple way of sharpening our visual thinking processes.

Exercise in Visual Thinking

1. Pair up. One partner will be *A*, the other *B*.
2. *A* then slowly describes a nursing procedure to *B*. The procedure should have between three and five steps. (Procedures like how to take a temperature, ambulate a client, or give a bed bath are fine.)
3. As each step is described, *B* pictures performing the procedure.
4. At the end of the description, *B* tells *A* how to do the procedure by thinking of each picture and describing what is there.
5. Repeat steps 2–4 with roles reversed.
6. Optional: Repeat steps 2–5 with a nine-step procedure.

Thinking in the Auditory Channel. In the same way that some people picture their thoughts, others think in auditory mode, primarily by subliminally talking to themselves.

Visual and kinesthetic information can be thought about in an auditory way simply by using words to describe the information. For example, when a nurse writes "patient slept well" on a chart, these nursing notes represent auditory thinking about what was observed. The nurse received the information through the visual channel and thought of appropriate words to use.

As nurses, we are aware of the extreme importance of being able to describe accurately or to find the right words for behavior and symptoms.

Mistakes in auditory thinking can lead to confusion for both the client and the nurse. For example, a common nursing procedure is to obtain a "clean catch" urine specimen. Because of the nature of this specimen collection, the procedure must be explained (auditory channel) to the client and the client must "collect" the specimen. The client is instructed to wash thoroughly before voiding and then, while emptying the bladder, to "catch" the midstream portion of the voiding in a sterile container. This is sent to the laboratory for examination of microorganisms present in the urine. In order for the client not to contaminate the specimen, instructions are given to void the first and last parts of the urinary stream into the urinal or bedpan. As is obvious even in the explanation here, this is not an easy procedure to explain. Clients will often void the entire specimen into the bedpan because they did not "hear" the nurse, and the procedure must be re-explained and performed again. It might be far easier in this instance to demonstrate by a chart (visual channel), but many hospital procedures do not lend themselves to visual demonstrations.

Thinking Kinesthetically. Although most people tend to use visual or auditory channels, some do think kinesthetically. Usually "feeling" thoughts are triggered by "feeling" words. If we began to think about the last time we felt really sad about something, we might find ourselves feeling sad: our breathing might change and our stomach might "feel a little sad." We could also be seeing the scene and hearing the words that were said, but because we are assessing kinesthetically, we will be feeling "feelings" or body responses.

Exercise in Kinesthetic Thinking

1. Say each of the following emotion words to yourself or out loud with "feeling":

anger	joy
silly	rude
crazy	sentimental
sad	happy
sexy	

2. Think about how each "feels."

It is also possible to think through the sense of smell. While we do not usually think in this mode, odors are often related to strong emotional experiences in the past.

Speaking in the Channels

Along with thinking in the modes, people's use of language can be related to channels. According to Bandler and Grinder (1975), who have developed a system of psychotherapy and have stated the use of modalities in communication most eloquently, the majority of people have a predominant mode; that is, they are primarily visual, auditory, kinesthetic, and occasionally olfactory in their use of language. For example, some people use a lot of phrases like "I see what you mean," "I need a clear picture," or "My view is." The key words here are *see, picture,* and *view*. They are all visual terms. The person using them can be considered a visual person.

Another person may habitually use phrases like "I hear you," "Let's talk about," and "Listen to what I have to say." The key words for this person's major channel are *hear, talk, listen,* and *say*. These words are all auditory, that is, they relate to hearing. A person using predominantly phrases like these is likely to be an "auditory" person.

A third possibility is the person who uses phrases like "My feeling is," "I'm in touch with," or "I can't grasp his meaning." The key words in this instance are *feeling, touch,* and *grasp*. All of these words are kinesthetic. They all relate to "feeling." A person who uses phrases like these will be referred to as a "kinesthetic" person.

According to Grinder and Bandler (1976), many people use primarily one channel for communication. That is, they use either visual, auditory, or kinesthetic terms to express themselves. In addition, they are likely to appreciate communication from others in their own channel. What this suggests is that the effective nurse communicator needs to be "fluent" in all channels and capable of switching to the client or other health professional's channel to be understood, as well as to create empathy and rapport. The following section is designed to facilitate the development of channel-specific language.

Visual language. Several "visual" terms have been given above. A good list of visual terms includes:

television	appear
see	look
clear	seemingly
picture	clearly
view	focus
perspective	watch
demonstrate	reflect

show
design
chart
map
graph
viewer
read
review

visionary
overview
clairvoyant
preview
seem
appearance
vision

Many people have some familiarity with these words. Often, these words appear in phrases like "I read your mind," "look out," "I see where you're at," and "show off." They can all be used to convey or make meaning. Some people (low-visualizers) rarely use them to describe their experiences. Others (high-visualizers) may use them exclusively. The following exercise is designed to help develop and recognize the abilities we have as a speaker of visual images. "See" how you do.

Exercise in Making Visual Meaning

1. Read the first nursing-related statement in list 1 below.
2. Then, say the *same* thing, only use a *visual* image to convey your meaning.
3. Compare your answer to the statement in list 2 to see if you matched or were close to the one we give. (There are more options than the ones in list 2. The ones we give are simply to help you if you cannot come up with one of your own.)
4. Continue down the rest of the list, comparing your answers with ours.

List 1

1. I need to know more about your health history.
2. Where is the pain?
3. I understand you.
4. I do not understand you.
5. I hope you are comfortable here.
6. What is your problem?
7. Did the doctor communicate what is wrong?
8. How are you feeling today?
9. I need some information about your family?

List 2

1. Let's *focus* a bit more on your health history.
2. *Show* me where the pain is.
3. I *see* what you're saying.
4. I don't *see* what you mean.
5. I hope everything *seems* well.

Communication Channels

6. What *seems* to be the problem?
7. Did the doctor *review* your diagnosis?
8. How does everything *seem* today?
9. Give me a *picture* of what your family is like.

The more we practice statements such as those listed above, the more likely we are to communicate clearly with a visualizer. In a very important way, being able to speak in the other person's channels is like talking in Spanish to a resident of Mexico. We stand the best chances of being understood when we speak the client's language. If we *see* the meaning and will *review* this point several times, we will be more effective visual communicators.

Auditory language. All auditory language relates to hearing. A good list of auditory terms is:

auditory	say
hearing	tell
hear	ear
read	aural
speak	record
music	concert
perform	melody
radio	spoken
words	roar
blast	whistle
thunder	sound
resound	soft
speaker	sing
singing	noise
loud	

Many of these words are part of phrases or slang that are commonly used in American culture. "I hear you," "sounding board," "tell him off," and "speak your mind" are only a few. As was the case for visual expressions, each conveys its own special meaning. They will be particularly useful if the person with whom we are speaking is a "high-auditory," that is, the person uses a lot of auditory words and is sensitive to the nuances of auditory communication.

As was the case for visual language, auditory language can be used to make meaning out of language in other channels (sentences using seeing or feeling words), as well as language without a specified channel. One example from common nursing communication is as follows. Suppose you went to a client's bedside and wanted to ask about the operation. In a visual channel you might say, "What was your *view* of the operation?" An auditory translation would be

"*Tell* me how the operation went." It is surprising how some clients will respond to one of these more easily than the other. (Some clients will respond best to a "kinesthetically phrased" question—see below.)

The following nursing-related statements are similar to those translated into visual language earlier. This time, translate them into auditory language that gives the same meaning as the original statement. After you have made your translation, compare your answer to the ones on the right side of the page.

List 1	List 2
1. I need to know more about your health history.	1. *Tell* me more about your health history.
2. Show me where the pain is.	2. *Tell* me where the pain is.
3. I understand you.	3. I *hear* what you are saying.
4. I do not see what you mean.	4. I can't *tell* what you mean.
5. Are you comfortable?	5. How would you *say* you feel?
6. What seems to be the problem?	6. *Tell* me what the problem is.
7. Did the doctor communicate what is wrong?	7. Did the doctor *say* what the problem is?
8. How are you feeling today?	8. *Say*, how are things here today?
9. Give me a picture of what your family life is like.	9. I'd like to *speak* to you about your family. How does that *sound*?

Kinesthetic language. Kinesthetic words and phrases refer to feeling, touch, and other aspects of kinesthetic senses. They are often combined with visual or auditory connotations. A list of kinesthetic terms would include the following:

sadness	glad
touch	move (also visual)
feel	blast (also visual or auditory)
hostility	touchy
grasp	felt
handle	fear
rough	smooth
hard	soft (also auditory)
itch	scratch
pain	painful
anger	hurt
joy	love

Communication Channels

Many slang expressions use feeling words. Some familiar ones include "go with the *feelings*," "it's *hard* to tell," "caught between a rock and a *hard* place," and "on the *run*." Several of these are combined with terms from other modalities.

Along with high-visualizers and people who are primarily auditory in language use, some people have a great deal of skill in using kinesthetic language. While one may hesitate to call them the "feelers" because of how that can be misinterpreted, they can be considered as high-kinesthetics.

The following exercise is similar to the previous translation exercises. Translate the nursing communication in list 1 on the left of the page into kinesthetic sentences. Compare your answers to those in list 2 on the right side. Remember, there is more than one way to say something in a "feeling manner."

List 1	List 2
1. I need to know more about your health history.	1. I need to get a *feel* for your health history.
2. Show me where you think the pain is.	2. Where do you *feel* the *pain* is?
3. I hear what you are saying.	3. I *feel* I *grasp* your meaning.
4. I do not understand you.	4. I am not in *touch* with your meaning.
5. I hope that everything seems right.	5. I hope you *feel comfortable*.
6. What is the problem?	6. What do you *feel* is wrong?
7. Did the doctor tell you the diagnosis?	7. Did the doctor tell you what he *felt* was wrong?
8. How does everything seem today?	8. How are you *feeling*?
9. I need some information about your family history.	9. I need some *hard* facts about your family.

Some of these statements might be *hard* to say. You are encouraged to practice them as a challenge.

Olfactory Language. Few if any of the readers of this book will use olfactory words as their major channel of communication. However, words that suggest smell or taste (the two are closely related) can quickly remind us of emotions. The following is a list of olfactory and taste-related words:

smell	odor
scent	tangy
taste	bitter
spit	salty

sweet	sugary
pungent	aroma
aromatic	smelling
stuffy	moldy
mildew	acidic
baking	perfumed
fumigate	odorless
tasteless	sniff

Olfactory terms are also commonly used in the folowing expressions. As an exercise, translate each into the channel noted at the end of each statement. Compare your answers to those we have supplied in list 2.

List 1
1. Something smells fishy. (make it visual)
2. The food is bland. (make it auditory)
3. She sure is saccharine sweet. (make it feeling)
4. This is bitter medicine to swallow. (make it visual)
5. What's cooking? (make it auditory)
6. That joke is so old it's moldy. (make it feeling)
7. That was a tasteless comment. (make it visual)
8. I'm just sniffing around. (make it auditory)
9. Spit it out! (make it feeling)

List 2
1. Things do not *look* right. (visual)
2. I *hear* the food stinks. (auditory)
3. It is *hard* to believe that she's that nice. (kinesthetic)
4. This *seems* awful to accept. (visual)
5. What's the good *word*? (auditory)
6. That joke is so old it *feels* corny. (kinesthetic)
7. In my *view*, that comment was inappropriate. (visual)
8. I'm just *listening* to what everyone is saying. (auditory)
9. Say what you *feel* about the matter. (kinesthetic)

Channel-Specific and Channel-Nonspecific Language

So far, much of the discussion has focused on language that suggests a channel. For example, "see" suggests the visual channel, "hear" the auditory channel, and "feel" the kinesthetic channel. However, not all words suggest a channel.

Communication Channels — 47

That is, there are many words that are not specific to any channel. They are good to use when one is not sure "what channel" the other person is on. A partial list of verbs or action words *without* a specified or implied channel is as follows:

think   distinguish
decide   wonder
sense   like
conclude   understand

As you think about it, you can *think, decide, wonder,* or do any of the above terms in *any* of the channels if you put your mind to it. The important distinction here is to separate words that imply one channel from words that do not directly indicate any particular channel.

PUTTING IT TOGETHER

We deal now with the importance of channels and language to you as a nurse communicator. This section will explain how all of the channels come together in a single communication sequence and how to use the skills you are developing in channel awareness to make you a more effective nurse communicator. As an initial step, do the following exercise, which could take up to a half-hour to complete.

Exercise in Channel Sorting

1. Pair up. One partner will be *A*, the other *B*.
2. *A* states three things *A* thinks are true about *B*.
3. *B* then writes down the following:
   a. What *A* said, underlining words that are visual, auditory, and kinesthetic
   b. What *B* saw *A* do (body language)
   c. What *B* noticed about *A*'s voice tone, pitch, loudness, and rhythm of words
   d. How *B* felt hearing *A*'s statements
4. After writing all of this, *B* will then determine which aspects of *A*'s communication made the most impact:
   a. The choice of words used
   b. Body language
   c. The tone, pitch, loudness, or rhythm of *A*'s statements
   d. How the combined aspects affected *B*'s response to *A*'s statements
5. Reverse roles and repeat steps 2–4.

6. Think about how you "ordinarily" sort and interpret messages from different channels.
7. Discuss your "findings" about yourself and about sorting out channels with your partner with the rest of the class.

What should have come out in the previous exercise is that different people are influenced by various combinations of channel messages. With a little practice, you can determine your own major channel(s) *and* those of others. The easiest way to do this is to listen to or picture or get a feel for the language they use. If, in addition, you also want to know in which styles they think, ask them the following questions:

1. Do you make pictures in your mind's eye a lot? (A "yes" indicates a visual thinker.)
2. Do you talk things over with yourself? (A "yes" would indicate an auditory thinker.)
3. Do you "go with" your feelings? (A "yes" here would mean a kinesthetic thinker.)

Once you have established the other person's major thinking system, you can translate what you have to say into words he or she can understand. And, by understanding *how* others relate to the world, you will become more empathic and more able to relate to others.

The tools of channel identification are important in establishing therapeutic relationships and good lines of communication with clients and co-workers. Sometimes, misunderstandings can come about as a result of mixed channel messages, as the following scenario demonstrates.

> An auditory nurse once had a visual supervisor. The two never quite hit it off. The supervisor kept complaining that the nurse did not *look* (visual!) professional. The nurse complained that the supervisor could not *listen* (auditory!) to reason. They called in a social worker, who was kinesthetic, to help them settle their differences. "The problem," the social worker intoned, "is that neither of you is in *touch* (kinesthetic) with your true feelings."

How often have you been in situations like the one above, where there is no attempt to understand the other's position? In this case, all three participants are "right." What would help the most would be some channel learning. That is, the nurse could begin to try to "look" professional after finding out the specifics of the supervisor's complaints, the supervisor could learn to *listen* more closely to staff, and the social worker could learn to develop the use of both auditory and visual channels. Similarly, both nurses *might* find a way to communicate through feelings, so in that sense, the social worker was correct. In general, when two people's channels are not matching, good options for improving communi-

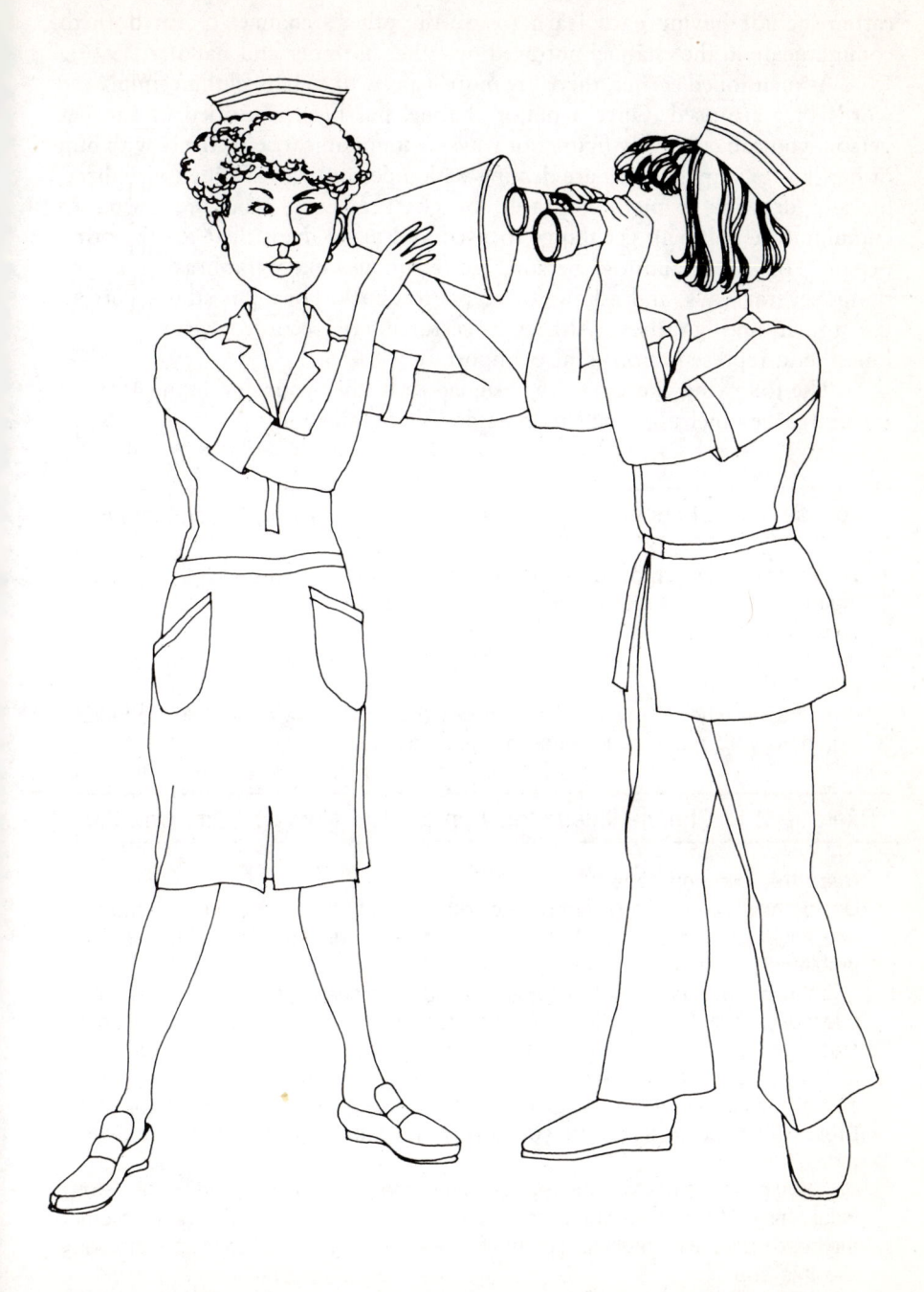

Communication Channels — 49

cation include having each learn to use the other's channel *or* for both to communicate in the channel not used by either (Grinder and Bandler, 1976).

As mentioned earlier, there are more aspects to a channel than simply the words that are used. Once a major channel has been identified in another person, you can creatively figure out ways to communicate effectively with him or her. For example, if you are dealing with a person who is a high-visualizer, literally drawing a picture, graph, or chart of what you are trying to communicate will help get things focused and make them clear for the other person. For a high-auditory person, use techniques like paraphrasing, saying things several ways, and asking for verbal feedback. For a kinesthetic person, use touch and gestures. Although gestures are recorded visually, their kinesthetic representation is also important.

The following exercises are designed to further your development of an integrated channel approach to nursing communication.

Exercise 1 in Channel-Integrated Approach to Nursing Communication

1. Think of a nursing procedure that should be explained to a client.
2. Figure out how you would explain the procedure to:
   a. a visualizer
   b. an auditory
   c. a kinesthetic
   d. someone who you weren't sure about (hint: to be safe, use all channels)
3. Compare your answers to those given by others.

Exercise 2 in Channel-Integrated Approach to Nursing Communication

1. Read the following case.
2. Decide how you would communicate with each of the parties involved and what you might do in the way of channel use to solve some of the communication problems.

   You are a "float nurse" in a hospital and have been assigned to a new unit for a few days. You notice a client, Mr. Brown, age 46, who appears withdrawn, quiet, and depressed. He rarely speaks to anyone. From a review of his chart, you see he is in for a prostate operation. You realize that men often have concerns about sexual functioning with such an operation. However, when you try to talk to Mr. Brown, all he says is: "Nurse, you're very nice but I don't want to talk to anyone today."

   You go to the doctor, who replies: "I don't see what kind of problem Mr. Brown would have. It is a clear and simple operation." You then mention the problem to the head nurse, who replies: "I do not feel we should get involved in hard problems like this one."

3. Discuss some options and strategies in a large group. Include the possibilities of:
   a. talking with Mr. Brown's wife
   b. making each person more aware of the problem *in their own channel.*

CONCLUSION

The purpose of this chapter has been to highlight the differences inherent in the three major communication channels. The relationship among the channels of communication when we think, speak, and feel has been presented. Channel preferences and the utilization of one major, predominant channel have been emphasized throughout.

BIBLIOGRAPHY

Bandler, R. & Grinder, J. *The structure of magic I.* Palo Alto, California: Science and Behavior Books, 1975.
Cousins, N. Anatomy of an illness (as perceived by the patient). *New England Journal of Medicine,* 1976, *295,* 1458–1463.
Cousins, N. *Anatomy of an Illness.* Boston: G.K. Hall, 1980.
Edinberg, M.A., Edinberg, B.S. & Baldwin, D.C. Jr. *A viewer's guide for Virginia Satir's communication tape 1.* Palo Alto, California, Science and Behavior Books, 1976.
Ekman, P. & Friesen, W. *Unmasking the face.* Englewood Cliffs, N.J.: Prentice-Hall, 1975.
Enelow, A. & Swisher, S. *Interviewing and patient care.* New York: Oxford University Press, 1979.
Grinder, J. & Bandler, R. *The structure of magic II.* Palo Alto, Cal.: Science and Behavior Books, 1976.
Hall, E. *The hidden dimension.* Garden City, N.Y.: Anchor Books, 1969.
Key, M.R. *Paralanguage and kinesics (nonverbal communication).* Metuchen, N.J.: Scarecrow Press, 1975.
Pluckham, M. *Human communication: the matrix of nursing.* New York: McGraw-Hill, 1978.
Smith, D.R. & Williamson, L.K., *Interpersonal communication—roles, rules, strategies, and games.* Dubuque, Iowa: W.C. Brown, 1977.

Chapter 3 Communication styles

BEHAVIORAL OBJECTIVES

By reading this chapter and participating in the exercises, students will be able to:
1. Identify the following aspects of communication styles: openness, person-task orientation, self-disclosure, acceptance, defensiveness, and congruence
2. Understand the concepts of self-worth and stress
3. Contrast the communication styles of blaming, placating, super-reasonableness, irrelevance, and congruence
4. Translate incongruent communication into congruent responses.

All human interactions include some form of communication. In addition, these interactions are characterized by unique communication styles utilized by individuals in the process of sending and receiving messages. What exactly is a communication style? In one sense we all have our own style of communicating; each of us is unique, with different ways of communicating and interpreting the same message. If we stop to think about it, we could no doubt describe the way we communicate in so many words or phrases. The following words or phrases have been used to describe the communication styles of different people at various moments in time:

talks too fast   talks slowly
gestures a lot   undemonstrative
dominates discussion   submissive
kids around   serious
passive   aggressive
scattered   straightforward
open   closed
listens   doesn't listen

Communication styles can vary in an individual depending on the situation. For example, some nurses may be submissive with a physician and then turn around and be dominant with a client. Clearly, style is a function of abilities and strategies, as well as the context in which the communication takes place.

One way to think about our own communication style is to examine it in light of several concepts or dimensions. Six dimensions have been selected for the purposes of our discussion of communication styles: openness, person-task orientation, self-disclosure, acceptance, defensiveness, and congruence. By placing ourselves on an imaginary line along a continuum for each dimension, we might gain clues to our own personality make-up. It should be emphasized at this point that there is no magic formula relative to these dimensions that constitutes a "healthy" style of communication. If one is open, accepting, or able to self-disclose with another person, this might indicate a more positive communication style. However, which styles should be used in specific situations depends to a great extent on the person and the context.

Openness

The concept of openness is commonly used to describe communication styles. We often hear another person described as "really open." Similarly, the other end of the openness dimension is characterized by the statement, "He's pretty closed to praise or criticism." Openness is related to the ability to listen, understand, and accept differences and criticism.

A formal definition of communication openness is "the extent to which messages can be modified once the communication process has been initiated" (Katz and Kahn, 1966). That is, whether or not new information can be added to an existing communication system will determine its openness.

At a practical level, the idea of openness is not clear. In order to adequately understand another's "openness," it is necessary to ask the following questions—"Open to what?" and "Open to whom?"

"Open to what?" refers to kinds of messages you, as a nurse, are open to receive. A short list of types of messages includes:

Information (e.g., how to perform a procedure)
Praise (e.g., a compliment)
Criticism (e.g., a complaint)
Inquiry (questions)
Corrective feedback (criticism and suggestion)

To which of these are you most open? That is, which are easiest for you to listen to and accurately understand about yourself? Which are the most difficult for you?

"Open to whom?" refers to the role relationship in which nurses and the other person exist. Some examples include: physician-nurse, nurse-nurse, nurse-aide, nurse-client, and nurse-family member. (See Chapter 7 for a much more extensive explanation of roles and nursing communication.) Although individuals differ, people in general respond differently in terms of openness to communication from superiors, peers, or subordinates. For example, students react differently to criticism from a teacher (superior), a classmate (peer), or someone in the class behind them (subordinate). In thinking about how open we are to various kinds of messages, we can examine our reaction to the source (superior, peer, or subordinate).

Person-task Orientation

Another way of describing a person's communication style is person-task orientation (Blake and Mouton, 1969). The idea is that people vary in their focus on the person and the task. A common description for some people is "totally task-oriented." Others may be highly person-oriented. People can be high on both, low on both, or high on one and low on the other. The person-task orientation can also change depending on the situation. Although not technically a style, your person and task orientation will affect how you communicate and what information you attend to in communicating with others.

Exercise in Rating Your Person-Task Orientation

1. Pair up with a partner.
2. First rate yourself in general as low, medium, or high on the following two dimensions:

Person	Task
Low: Little or no attention to other's emotions, feelings	Little or no concern about work being done well or on time

Medium: Some attention paid to other's emotions, feelings
High: Much attention paid to other's emotions, feelings

Moderate concern that work is being done well and on time
High concern that work is being done well and on time

3. Discuss the following questions with your partner:
   a. What made me rate myself as I did?
   b. What are the advantages *and* disadvantages of a task orientation in nursing communication?

Self-disclosure

Jourard (1971) is one of the best-known proponents of self-disclosure in communication. By self-disclosure, he means that the therapist is willing and able to talk about his or her own feelings and perceptions honestly and directly to the client. According to Jourard, one of the goals of psychotherapy is for the client to learn how to self-disclose. Egan (1977) points out that people can be overly self-disclosing or not self-disclosing enough. An example of being overly self-disclosing is the nurse who tells everyone everything he or she is feeling all the time. Some of the nurses who work with this person will find the "nonstop" self-disclosure inappropriate or boring. On the other hand, the nurse who is totally non-self-disclosing shares few feelings or views and may well be perceived by his or her co-workers as "distant."

An additional aspect of self-disclosure is timing or appropriateness. It is possible to be self-disclosing too early in a relationship or at an inappropriate moment. Sensitivity to the client is necessary in order to determine the timing and appropriateness of self-disclosure. One way to assess your own communication style in terms of self-disclosure is with the exercise that follows.

Exercise in Assessing Self-Disclosure

1. Rate yourself as "high," "medium," or "low" in self-disclosure when communicating with a supervisor, friend, and client about each of the following topics:
   a. Your personal life
   b. One of your personal problems
   c. Giving a big compliment
   d. Giving criticism.
2. Compare your answers with those of others in the class.
3. Discuss some of the differences and similarities you find.
4. How "OK" do you think it is for nurses to be self-disclosing? What are the risks and payoffs?

Acceptance

Another dimension that is related to openness and self-disclosure is acceptance. Acceptance of others is a key concept in Rogers' client-centered therapy system (1951). Acceptance of both self and others is a crucial part of the therapeutic process.

What exactly is acceptance? Acceptance does not depend on one's approval of another. Some people think that acceptance means that one never gets angry or has criticism of another's actions. Needless to say, with that kind of definition, acceptance would be seen as a weakness or a trap, especially if one had to believe everything told by another person.

A working definition of acceptance is understanding that (1) what others believe or feel is their true belief, (2) others have the right to believe or feel that way, and (3) there is no need to blame others for anything they do, even if the behavior is wrong or has to be changed to protect the individual or society. The key to acceptance is allowing another the freedom to feel and think. It is only through separating the acceptance of another as a person with rights and feelings from "going along with" whatever is said or done that acceptance is a desirable and useful attribute.

How do people show that they are "accepting"? Generally, they respond to others without judging them. Thus, the nurse who can listen to a client complain about not being able to smoke in the hospital room and can respond to the client's sense of frustration and (perhaps silently) disagree with the *content* of the complaints, will come across as accepting. Some of the body language the nurse might show includes head nods and a caring pat on the shoulder.

Acceptance of others is not always easy. There are few, if any, people who accept everyone all of the time. The possibility always exists that one's feelings *can* be hurt by something that is said. Frustration and disappointment can quickly turn into blame and anger. A beginning step to improve our own acceptance of others is to accept ourselves as being human, capable of mistakes and able to learn and grow from them.

Self-acceptance is like acceptance of others—we do not have to like everything we do. We may want desperately to change some things. Acceptance of ourselves involves acknowledging that, in some way, we are doing the best we can at a certain moment in time.

Exercise in Acceptance of Others

1. For each of the following, rate yourself as accepting or not accepting of a supervisor, another nurse, or a client when they exhibit the following behavior or quality:
   a. belligerence

b. tardiness
   c. complaining
   d. sloppiness
   e. affection
   f. confusion
   g. lying
   h. honesty
   i. criticism
2. Answer the following questions either in pairs or in a large group:
   a. Am I more accepting with some types of people than with others?
   b. Where do I get "hung up" accepting others?
   c. What happens to my communication when I am not accepting of others?
   d. Do I confuse accepting with "going along" or denying my own feelings/reactions?
   e. What are some ways I can begin to be more accepting?
   f. What are the advantages of being accepting in communicating with clients, aides, other nurses, and physicians? Are there any disadvantages?

Defensiveness

Defensiveness is a term that is usually used to describe a person's behavior in specific situations such as the nurse who responds to criticism by saying "That's your problem." There are two overlapping meanings to the term as it is commonly used. The first meaning is that the other person is "on the defensive," being hostile, aggressive, not listening, but rather responding as if she or he were being attacked.

A second and somewhat more general definition is that the defensive person is responding by using a defense mechanism, one of several ways of defending against anxiety. Some of the major defense mechanisms include *denial,* the negation of an uncomfortable impulse or truth; *projection,* placing one's inner conflicts on others; *rationalization,* making up excuses or reasons to "cover" behavior; *reaction formation,* acting the opposite of how one feels; and *repression,* "forgetting" or putting uncomfortable thoughts or feelings out of awareness. Many books have been written that discuss defense mechanisms in more depth than this brief description (e.g., Altrocchi, 1980). It is important to remember that defense mechanisms are used unconsciously.

Both definitions of defensiveness have certain things in common. When persons are defensive, they are not fully able to understand the messages from others. That is, often the message is unconsciously perceived to be an attack on self-worth. The resulting response is an attempt to "save the self" but will, in all probability, mean little to another individual.

> Two nurses were working at a station when a nurse from another shift came by. One of the nurses looked up, saw her and said, "Hi! We haven't

Communication Styles

seen *you* for a long time." The nurse, who had been feeling guilty about being late three days in a row, replied, rather defensively, "Look, I work just as hard as anyone else around here!"

"What's eating her?" they wondered as she left.

There are times when almost anyone acts defensively. Fatigue, hard work loads, changes in work, or personal problems can all contribute to a defensive communication style. Do any of the following areas make you feel defensive?

Being insulted
Being praised
Talking about your love life
Talking about your relationship with family members
Having your school or professional work criticized
Being audited by Internal Revenue Service

Exercise in Self-Defensiveness Identification

---

1. On a piece of paper, write down three specific situations in which you have been defensive in the last two weeks. Include what "triggered" this reaction and what you did that was defensive.
2. Exchange lists with one other person in the class. Discuss what it is like to be "open about being defensive" with them. Share your experience in the large group or class.

One question that arises around the issue of defensiveness is how to deal with others' defensiveness. Commenting about the situation is one way to work on another's defensiveness. The following story is an example of how commenting about the situation can ease another's defensiveness.

> A nurse was assigned Mr. Bartowski, a 76-year-old postoperative patient who was described in the nursing notes as being "abusive and angry." The nurse went over to his bed and said "Good morning, Mr. Bartowski, how are you feeling?" "Get away from me," Mr. B. snarled. "Mr. Bartowski," the nurse replied, "you seem upset. Is something bothering you?" She then pulled a chair over to his bedside. Mr. Bartowski looked at her a minute, and then tears started to form in his eyes. "Am I going to be well again?" he asked.

In this story, the key statement was the nurse's saying, "You seem upset." She was able to comment on the situation. Comments about a situation are, in technical terms, called "meta-comments." Meta-comments allow the communicators to talk *about* what they see, hear, or feel the other is feeling. While meta-communicating is not a sure-fire success for another's defensiveness (after all, Mr. Bartowski could have responded, "Nothing's bothering me, now get out of here."), it opens up a new set of options for the nurse communicator by commenting about how the other is communicating rather than simply responding to the content of what is being said.

Congruence

Another way of describing a communication style is to assess its congruence. By congruence, we mean how well the words, body language, tone of voice, and all other aspects of the communication fit together. For example, the client who bends over, grimaces, holds his hands to his stomach and says, "I feel just wonderful," is not communicating congruently. His body language, gestures, facial expression, and probably his voice quality all say "I am feeling sick," while his words say just the opposite.

Satir (1972) has added further meaning to the term "congruency" by noting that the message sent should be consistent with the internal feelings and beliefs of the message sender. Although some people are able to lie in a congruent way, the concept of the fit between how one feels and how one communicates is important to consider.

Does this expanded definition mean that the goal of congruency is to be perfectly honest all of the time? Fortunately, this is not the case. The question of appropriateness must also be answered in trying to be congruent. One issue in considering congruence is how to be congruent when it is *not* appropriate to share inner feelings, as in the following story:

> A nurse was talking to a young mother in an outpatient clinic about care for her 12-month-old baby. The baby was with her. As the session progressed, the nurse began to notice that any time the child moved away from the mother, the mother would smile apologetically at the nurse, turn to the child, sternly say, "Stop that," and grab the child by the arm or leg. The baby eventually whimpered softly and seemed listless. The nurse became quite concerned about the interaction but knew from previous history that the woman had stopped coming into the clinic when confronted about potential child abuse by another nurse.

What would you say in this case? While there are no obvious perfect answers, several you might consider are:

1. Commenting that the child seems to be healthy and active, waiting for the mother to respond to the statement, and then talking about how hard it must be to be a mother with an active child.
2. Describing what the nurse sees, being very careful not to imply that the mother is wrong: "I notice that you have to tell your child to keep still often."
3. Placing yourself in the other's shoes: "If I had to keep an eye on a child all the time, I'd be worn out and irritated at the end of the day."

None of the above options involve the nurse's denying his or her own feelings. (All of the options are congruent.) Meta-commenting is the general strategy employed. The nurse in all three situations has a goal of attempting to help the woman verbalize parenting problems.

Instances like potential child abuse, alcoholism, and other substance abuse can be very difficult for a nurse to handle, especially when the nurse decides that direct confrontation is inappropriate and not useful for the client.

Even in less dramatic circumstances, questions can still be raised as to how to be congruent when an open statement of feelings or beliefs is too costly, for example, in a situation where you could lose your job. One guiding concept is: given the range of choices for communicating (including doing nothing!), what can you do that does not violate your feelings, beliefs, or standards?

COMMUNICATION STYLES: SATIR'S CATEGORIES

Another way of looking at communication styles is to categorize them, that is, to imagine common patterns in the way we communicate. Several authors have devised methods of categorizing communication styles. One that the authors of this book have found to be quite useful in understanding nursing communication is the system devised by Virginia Satir. We recommend her books, *Peoplemaking* (1972) and *Making Contact* (1976), to those readers who are interested in finding out more about communication styles. The explanation that follows is a shortened version of the Satir communication model with specific examples related to nursing.

There are two concepts that are important to understand before examining Satir's communication styles. They are the concepts of *self-worth* and *stress*.

Self-worth

In Satir's system, self-worth is a major influence on all communication. Self-worth is the positive value we place on ourselves as individuals. It can be our greatest asset in human interactions (Smith and Bass, 1979, p. 6). An understanding of one's own self-worth is essential in being able to communicate effectively with others. This is true for nursing as well as other professions.

We depend to a large extent on the reactions of others to determine who we really are. These reactions provide a reflection for us to view ourselves. All of us would like to have a positive regard for ourselves, to view ourselves as mature people. We also try not to judge others more harshly than ourselves. But self-worth often gets in the way of praise, blame, criticism, and fairly routine exchanges, even though message senders are not evaluating or judging the other person; only their behavior. It is easy for nurses in leadership roles to forget how easily self-worth becomes involved in evaluations of another's work or in normal informational exchanges. Students have difficulty separating self-worth from their performance as nurses. We all equate high levels of performance with self-worth. Self-worth can also interfere with how we perceive the actions of others. This is shown in the following example:

> Two nurses were comparing notes about a head nurse. The first one said, "She's great. She takes time to show me how to do procedures I don't understand and makes sure I do things right." The second looked at her with surprise on his face. "What do you mean?" he retorted. "She's always telling me what to do. She tries to control everything. She must think we're pretty stupid."

It is possible that the second nurse is allowing his feelings of "low" self-worth to influence his perception of the head nurse's motives. In reality, the head nurse is really trying to help him. His lowered self-image contributes to not only his dislike for himself, but to thinking others, who in this case are trying to help him, dislike him as well.

Sometimes we form unconscious links between our degree of self-worth and certain feelings. That is, self-worth is often low because of a self-inflicted rule that says, "I am a bad person because I feel angry, sad, incompetent, crazy, stupid, upset, or anything else." For example, nurses might feel low self-worth if they are "mad" at a client or if they cannot solve another client's problem. These two examples represent instances of feeling low self-worth because of a feeling (anger) or a rule (only feeling self-worth when a client's problems are solved). There is no reason that self-worth has to be lowered due to a feeling or to failing in a task. In fact, keeping one's sense of high self-worth can help us in changing undesired behavior. "Self-assessment," in which one uncovers the unconscious links between self-worth and feelings or behavior, is one important step towards the growth of the adult individual, as well as promoting understanding.

Stress

In Satir's system, stress, which is closely related to self-worth, is felt whenever self-worth is threatened. This means that we tend to feel stress whenever we unconsciously link feelings or the behavior or words of others with a lowering of our own sense of self-worth. The link may be uncalled for, but it is made. Stress is felt when self-worth is endangered.

People respond to stress in many ways. Consider the following situation:

Communication Styles

Kim (nurse 1) was talking to her friend John (nurse 2) about a "problem client" with whom she had had no success in terms of adherance to medical orders. The client, who was supposed to be staying in bed, was always getting up and walking around. "I finally had someone else talk to him," she stated. "Why didn't you confront him?" John asked.

At this point, Kim, if she interprets the question (unconsciously or consciously) as an attack on her self-worth, may respond in one of the following defensive ways:

BLAMING: That's none of your business. You always question me!
PLACATING: You're right. I was wrong, it was my fault. I'm so sorry I did my job badly.
SUPERREASONABLE: Studies have shown that in 75 percent of cases similar to these, a different nurse has more success. Thus, I decided to utilize the research data in coming to the problem solution.
IRRELEVANT: He wasn't good-looking enough to be worth the trouble.

There is also the possibility that Kim could respond congruently:

CONGRUENT: I decided to let someone else try. I was having no success and felt frustrated.

The first four responses represent noncongruent responses. That is, they are as much responses to internal stress as they are to the question. Furthermore, they are not particularly useful in helping the nurses talk about how they feel *or* how they feel about what their feelings are (meta-commenting about self-worth). The fifth response, the congruent response, was one in which feelings were accurately verbalized, and self-worth was separated from behavior. In this way, John's question was treated as an inquiry rather than as an attack and the question that was asked was answered.

This simple scenario points out the complexity of any communication. The major aspects are:

1. Nurse 1's behavior
2. Nurse 1's feelings about what was done
3. Nurse 1's self-worth about what was done
4. Nurse 2's question
5. Nurse 2's feelings or reactions to nurse 1 at that moment in time
6. Nurse 2's feelings of self-worth at that moment in time
7. Nurse 1's response to nurse 2's question
8. Nurse 1's feelings upon hearing the question
9. Nurse 1's feelings of self-worth about her own feelings from hearing the question

For the sake of presentation, it was assumed that nurse 2's comment was congruent and not presented in a stressful manner. Imagine the potential confusion, miscommunication, and hurt feelings that might have ensued if both nurses had their self-worth involved where it didn't belong!

The nine actions in the example just presented can be grouped into three general aspects of a communication; the self, the other, and the context.

Satir represents them as shown in Figure 3-1. *Self* refers to one's feelings, perception, and self-worth in a given communication. *Other* refers to the other person's feelings, perceptions, and self-worth in the communication. *Context* refers to both the context in which the communication takes place and the specific content of the communication.

One of the major attributes of noncongruent communication styles is that each partner ignores at least one aspect of the self-other-context configuration. Another disadvantage of noncongruent styles is that they do not successfully alleviate stress. They do not allow meta-commenting, talking about feelings of what is going on. They are often misunderstood and are not a free choice as a response. When people act in a noncongruent way (blaming, placating, being superreasonable or irrelevant), they are not consciously choosing that response category. They are simply trying (unsuccessfully) to protect their self-worth; to say, "I count; I am OK."

Each of the noncongruent response styles has its own characteristics, physical postures (body language), language uses, and effects on others. By reading about and practicing the noncongruent responses, we can begin to identify them in our own nursing communication, as well as begin to discover them in others. This, in turn, should help us become more congruent and effective nurse communicators.

Blaming

The first response Kim gave to John in the earlier example was, "That's none of your business. You always question me." In this response, while Kim is

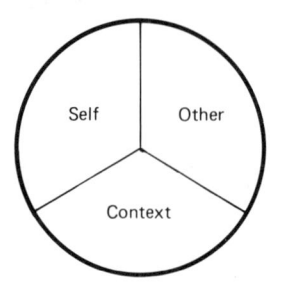

FIGURE 3-1. The three general aspects of communication according to Satir's model.

Communication Styles

responding to her own needs and the content of John's question, she is not taking John's feelings into account. At the same time, John is given responsibility for the blamer's behavior (*"you* always question me"). A diagram of the blaming response is represented in Figure 3–2. When someone blames, while he or she defends the self and pays attention to the issues, the other person is attacked. The blamer frequently disagrees.

The language used in blaming includes the frequent occurrence of the following words and phrases:

you always	never
should	you made me
no	it's your fault

These words are usually said in a hostile manner, although we all know some subtle blamers who seem to "make" us feel guilty, depressed, or put down even though they do not seem to be very hostile.

The body language of the blamer is most easily characterized by the "blaming finger." There is tremendous power in finger pointing. One can most readily observe the "blaming finger" in supermarkets. Adults are able to immobilize a child at 30 paces without speaking a word.

Other parts of the body language of blaming include tight arm and neck muscles, clenching the teeth, and tightening of facial muscles. A caricature of the blamer would be a person standing, one foot in front of the other, leaning forward, and glaring, with one hand on the hip, and the other hand extended and pointing at the person with whom the blamer is "communicating."

People respond to blame in many ways. What usually happens is that people who are blamed feel guilty, hurt, angry, put down, and occasionally blame in return. Usually all that is seen is the blaming finger, not the scared self-worth hiding behind it. One thing is certain; blaming does not foster effective communication. The following exercise is designed to have you *consciously* practice blame.

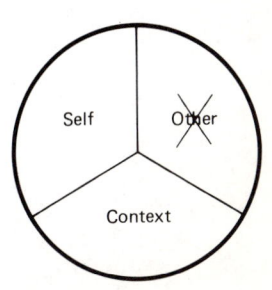

FIGURE 3–2. Representation of the blamer's denial of the aspect of the "other."

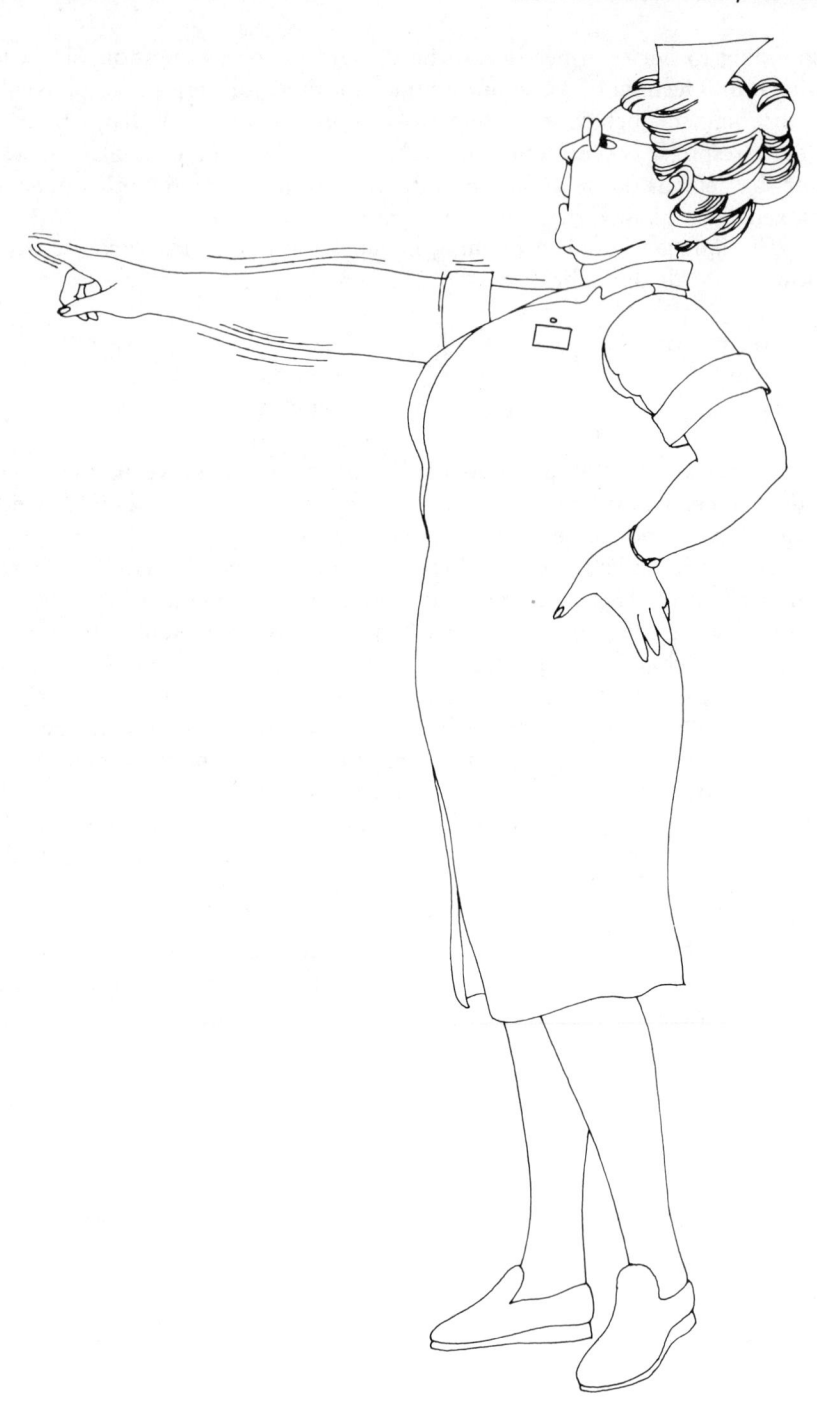

Exercise 1 in Blaming

1. Pair up. One partner will be *A*, the other *B*.
2. *A* puts the following statements into blaming terms by tone of voice, gestures, or changing the words. *B* listens and gives feedback, telling *A* if *A* is a "successful" blamer. You are allowed to be dramatic as you do this.

   Statements
   a. "I disagree with you."
   b. "Do you like me?"
   c. "What is your problem?"
   d. "Did you sleep well?"
   e. "What time is it?"
3. Then, *B* will practice blaming *A* by changing the following statements into blaming statements. *A* listens. Again, *B* can be dramatic.
   a. "You need to take your medicine."
   b. "How are you today?"
   c. "Can you try harder?"
   d. "You will be well in a week."
   e. "You have a lot of visitors."

Exercise 2 in Blaming

1. Pair up. One partner will be *A*, the other *B*.
2. *A* will say the following statements two ways; first in a caring way and then in as blaming a manner as possible *without* changing the words. *B* listens and asks *A* to do it again if *A* does not blame well.
   a. "You do not look well."
   b. "What's the matter with you?"
   c. "Please sit up."
   d. "Put out your tongue."
   e. "Show me the medicine you have."
3. Switch roles. *B* will then say the following statements two ways; first in a caring manner, then in a blaming manner. (*A* listens and makes *B* do it again if *B* does not blame well.)
   a. "Your gown is on backwards."
   b. "Do you have a problem?"
   c. "I'm very busy now."
   d. "Is your daughter home?"
   e. "Did Mr. Jones die?"
4. Discuss the subtle ways in which blame can be added to statements.

Placating

The second response Kim gave in the situation described earlier was: "You're right. I was wrong. It was my fault. I'm so sorry I do my job badly." In this instance, Kim is respecting John's view but is not respecting herself as a person. She "puts herself down," assumes total responsiblity for everything, and is overly apologetic. (It *is* possible to apologize without placating.) Figure 3–3 presents a diagram of the placator's communication. Similar to the blamer's ignoring the feelings of the other and yet putting responsibility on oneself, the placater ignores his or her own feelings yet takes responsibility for everyone else. ("It's my fault, I made you do it.") What a way to communicate! Yet, again, the placater is trying (unsuccessfully) to say, "I count, I'm OK."

The language of the placater is agreement. A placater will make peace at any cost, appease others, agree to conflicting opinions. In other words, a placater tries to be nice no matter what.

When we placate we are acting as if the only way to be "OK" is to agree. How many times have we agreed to things we did not want to do just to be nice? How many clients nod their heads yes in agreement as if they understand instructions but really do not? In the same manner that the blamer disagrees, the placater automatically agrees with everyone.

Phrases and words commonly used to placate include:

Yes	You are right
I made you do it	I don't deserve you
I'm so sorry	I apologize
It's my fault	I'm wrong
I'm to blame	I should do better

These words can, of course, be used without placating; but with the proper intonation, physical gestures, and body language, they can give a strong placating impression.

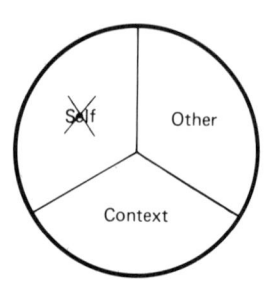

FIGURE 3–3. Representation of the placater's denial of the aspect of "self."

Communication Styles   69

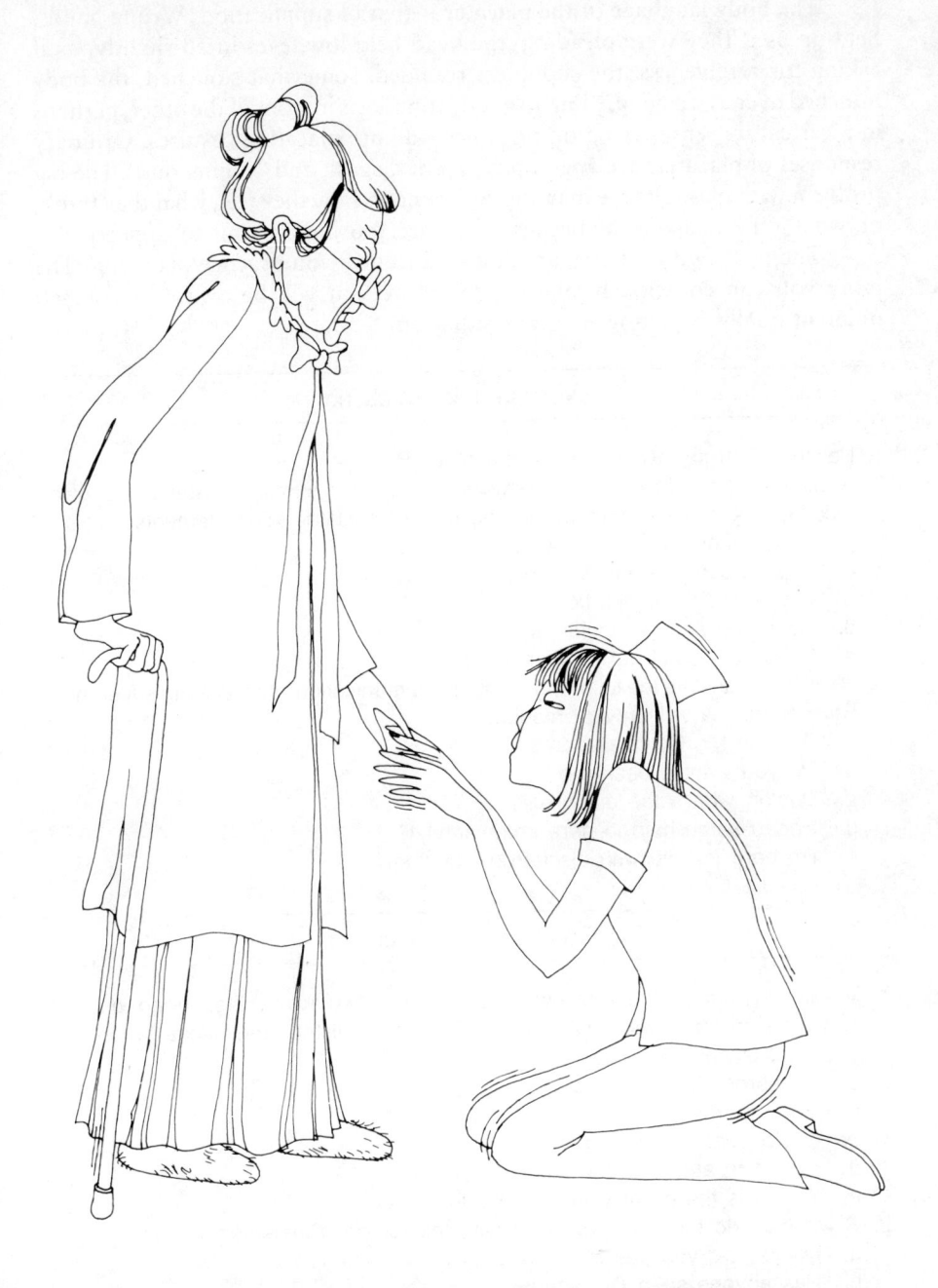

The body language of the placater is that of supplication. Wrung hands, held up as if they were pleading, the head held low, eyes lifted slightly, as if asking for forgiveness, the shoulders rounded, somewhat slouched, the body hunched over as if saying, "I'm no good," one leg is in front of the other, perhaps in a caricature sense, being on one knee—all are placating gestures. Ordinary responses of placaters are anger, pity, slight disgust, and "tuning out." The big problem with placaters are that one never knows how they feel, what they think, or what they really want because they are too busy trying to appease.

The next two exercises are designed to give you practice placating. The more you can consciously placate, the more you will be aware of yourself unintentionally placating in other situations.

Exercise 1 in Placating

1. Pair up. One partner will be *A*, the other *B*.
2. *A* will put the following statements into placating terms. *B* listens and gives feedback. *A* can be dramatic as she or he translates the statements.
   a. "I need more help with my clients."
   b. "Doctor, can you see Mr. Jones?"
   c. "Where is the client's chart?"
   d. "Have you seen a doctor recently?"
   e. "Does your child eat a balanced diet?"
3. *B* will then translate the following nursing communication into placating statements. Be dramatic. *A* will provide feedback.
   a. "What is Mr. Smith's address?"
   b. "Do you want a back rub?"
   c. "Doctor, what's the diagnosis?"
   d. "I need some help in here immediately!"
   e. "I'm here to help with discharge planning."

Exercise 2 in Placating

1. *A* will say each of the following statements two ways, first in an ordinary conversational tone, then placating. Be dramatic. (*B* listens and makes *A* repeat if *A* does not placate well.)
   a. "I'm sorry I had to wake you."
   b. "Good morning, I'm the V.N.A. nurse."
   c. "Doctor, can I help you?"
   d. "I need to ambulate the client."
   e. "Where is the client who is going to surgery?"
2. *B* will then do the same exercise with the following statements:
   a. "Doctor, did you see Mrs. Bova?"
   b. "Has anyone seen Dr. Cartone?"

c. "I didn't mean to disturb you."
d. "I was wrong to call you in for this."
e. "I'll be through with you in a minute."

Being Superreasonable

The third response Kim made was to be superreasonable: "Studies have shown that in 75 percent of cases similar to these, a different nurse has more success. Thus, I decided to use research data in coming to the problem solution." When people are being superreasonable, they appear to be quite intelligent but are, in fact, using their minds to avoid their feelings. What comes out sounds rational but is not truly creative thought. No attention is paid to the feelings of self or other. Thus, a diagram of the three aspects for a superreasonable communication would be represented by Figure 3–4. All that matters is the content. Feelings are to be avoided at all cost.

There are times when it is quite appropriate to communicate only content. Giving data about a client at report is one example. The difference between useful factualness and superreasonableness lies in how the brain is being used. Does what is being said involve ignoring relevant feelings or beliefs? If so, the communicator is being superreasonable.

The language of superreasonable is impersonal. Facts are substituted for "I believe" or "I feel." There is a frequent use of categorical statements such as "It is clear that" or "It is true that." Other phrases commonly used when people are being superreasonable include:

Let the facts speak for themselves
It said in the paper (book, article)
There is no logical reason
There is every logical reason
Let's be rational about this

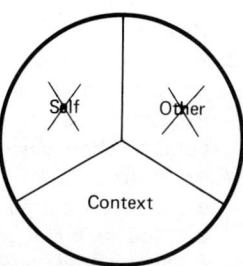

FIGURE 3–4. Representation of the denial of the aspects of both "self" and "other" in being superreasonable.

The body language of the superreasonable person is rigid and upright. There is no eye contact, since a superreasonable person is interested only in the facts. The caricatured superreasonable person is standing ramrod straight, arms at the side, looking off into the distance. The tone of voice is a monotone, and his or her words are spoken as if they came from a computer printout.

It is very difficult to respond with compassion to a person who is being superreasonable. Some common responses people have to superreasonableness include feeling they don't exist, feeling hurt, frustration, or even becoming superreasonable in return. The following exercises will give you practice in experiencing and identifying superreasonableness.

Exercise 1 in Superreasonableness

1. Pair up. One partner will be A, the other B.
2. A will "translate" the following set of statements into superreasonable communication. For example, a superreasonable "translation" of "Do not upset the client" is "Are you aware of the fact that the way you are communicating has been shown to elevate clients' blood pressures?" B listens and has A do it again if A is not superreasonable.
   a. Do not upset the client.
   b. It's time for the report.
   c. This client needs a bath.
   d. That temperature is very high.
   e. You really seem depressed.
3. Now switch roles. B translates the following statements into superreasonable communication:
   a. I am not sure the medication is correct.
   b. There must be an explanation for this.
   c. Have you been following your regimen?
   d. Your father is in room 29.
   e. Is everything OK?

Exercise 2 in Superreasonableness

1. Pair up. One partner will be A, the other B.
2. A will repeat each of the following sentences in two ways: first in a conversational and caring manner, then in a superreasonable manner. B will listen and have A do it again if A is not superreasonable enough. (Hint to A: be sure to make no eye contact when you are being superreasonable. Staring above B's head is an excellent tactic.)
   a. "Did you eat all of your meal?"
   b. "You look like you are in pain."
   c. "Is the tourniquet too tight?"

Communication Styles

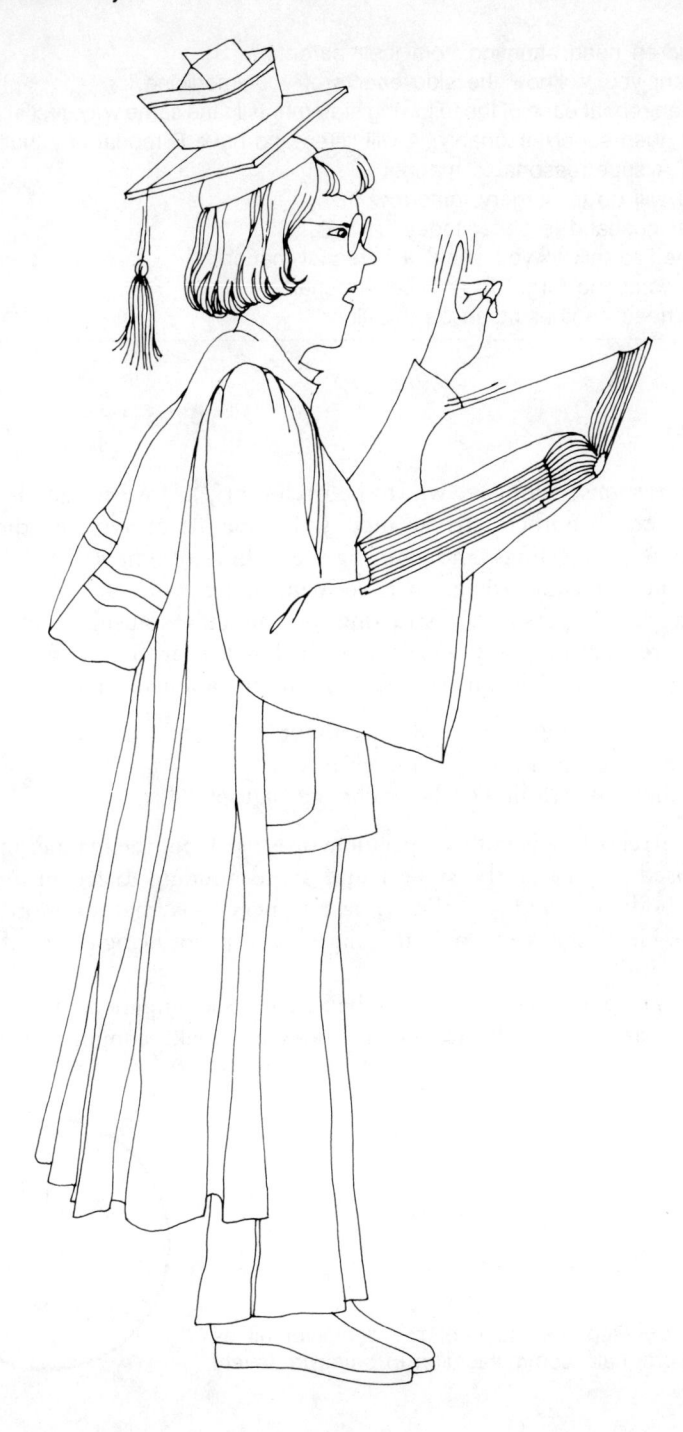

d. "Children need attention from their parents."
e. "I want you to know the side effects of your medicine."
3. *B* will then repeat each of the following statements in the same way, first in a caring manner, then superreasonably. *A* will listen and have *B* repeat any that are not done in a superreasonable manner.
   a. "You will go to surgery tomorrow."
   b. "Your husband is better today."
   c. "I need to talk to you about a personal matter."
   d. "Did someone forget to replace the chart?"
   e. "We need another nurse on this floor."

Irrelevance

The fourth response Kim gave was to be irrelevant: "He wasn't good-looking enough for me to bother." Irrelevancy is the fine art of avoiding the issue, ignoring your own feelings, and ignoring the feelings of others. The irrelevant response communication diagram is seen in Figure 3–5.

An irrelevant person is distracting, occasionally amusing, and hard to follow. There may be many words spoken, but few are to the point. Some common phrases used in an irrelevant communication include:

"Wait a minute, let me tell you about..."
"That reminds me of the one about..."
"By the way" (followed by a change of topic)

The key to irrelevancy is not the specific words used, but the manner in which they are used to change the subject and avoid alluding to feelings.

The body language of the irrelevant person is that of motion and distraction. He or she is "all over the place" (except for being centered on the matter at hand).

Others respond to irrelevance by being confused, impatient, anxious, and occasionally angry. Clearly, irrelevance does not make communication any better.

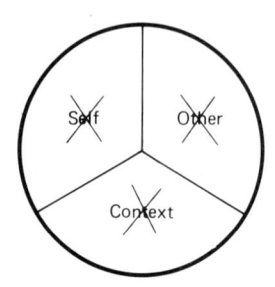

FIGURE 3–5. Representation of the denial of all aspects of appropriate communication in being irrelevant.

Communication Styles

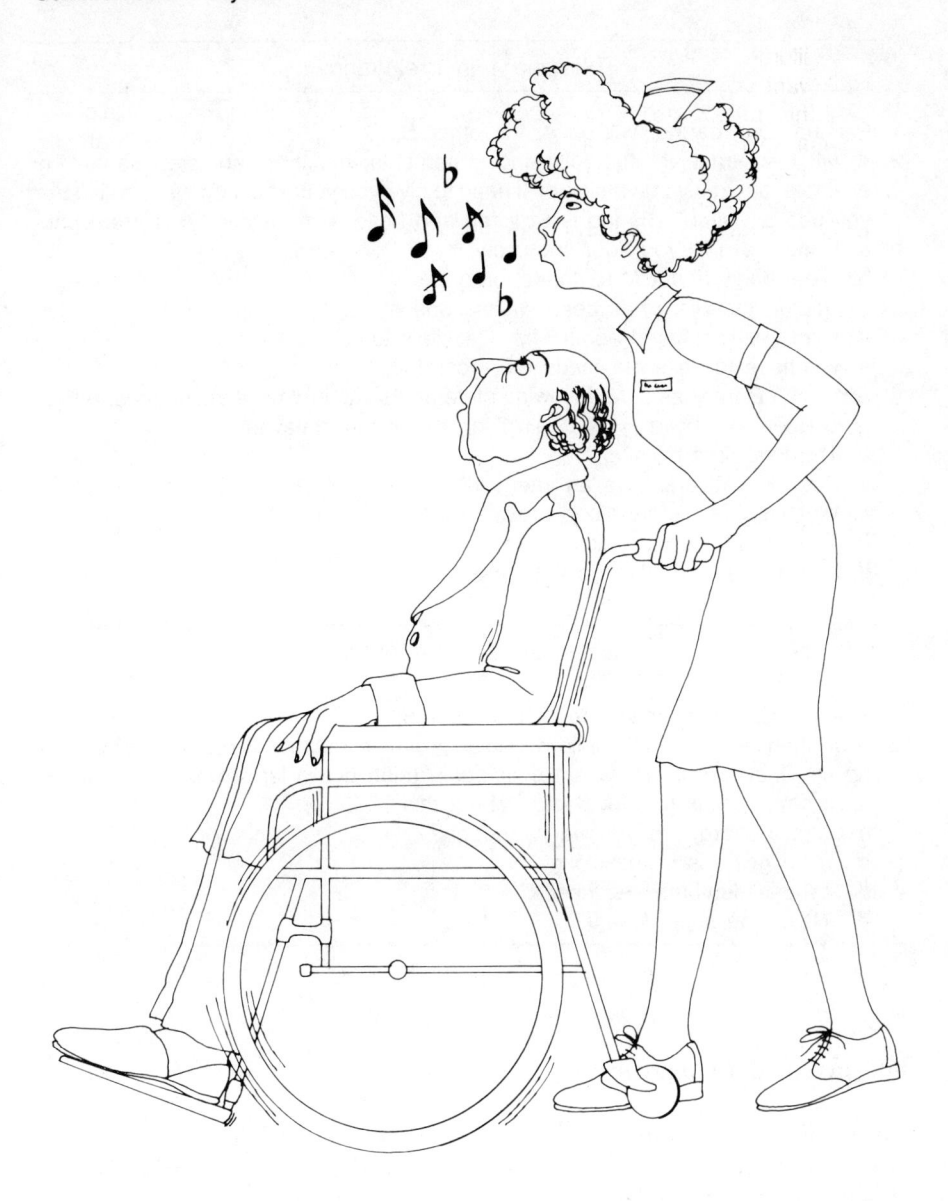

At the same time, levity, humor, and perspective can be beneficial in a work setting. Irrelevancy can be distinguished from these attributes in that self, other, and context are ignored, and the irrelevancy is inappropriate for the situation.

The following exercise will help you practice being irrelevant.

Exercise 1 in Irrelevancy

1. Pair up. One partner will be A, the other B.
2. A will then translate the following statements into irrelevant statements. For example, an irrelevant version of "I need to give you your shot now" is "I notice that you had a visitor." B's job is to listen and have A make sure A is irrelevant.
   a. I need to give you your shot now.
   b. I feel badly about Mrs. Jones' progress.
   c. Doctor, the client has been waiting one hour.
   d. I am very confused about Mrs. Castillo's tumor.
   e. We have to pass out meds more carefully.
3. Switch so B translates the following statements into irrelevant statements. A's job is to listen and have B try again if he/she is not irrelevant.
   a. The kardex is missing.
   b. Does Mr. Rivera have an internist?
   c. What is this client's blood pressure?
   d. This child's cast is cracked.
   e. How many cigarettes do you smoke a day?

Exercise 2 in Irrelevancy

1. Pair up. One partner will be A, the other B.
2. A will then say each of the following in an irrelevant manner. B listens and makes A do any that are not irrelevant over again (hint: use a lot of body distraction).
   a. "I have to talk to you, doctor, about this."
   b. "Mrs. Buffard, are you warm enough?"
   c. "Your gown is in the closet."
   d. "Whose dentures are these?"
   e. "Have you seen Joseph?"

Interpersonal Incongruency

Earlier in this text, the possibility of two people, each using one of the incongruent communication styles was mentioned. It is not uncommon to find blaming, placating, irrelevancy, and superreasonableness all going on at the same time. Many people will use more than one of the incongruent types of responses when they are in stress. What we would like to demonstrate in the next exercise, however, is how two or more incongruencies inhibit effective communication.

Communication Styles

Exercise in "Small-Group Incongruity"

1. Form groups of four. One person will be *A*, another *B*, another *C*, and the last *D*.
2. Take the following roles for the entire exercise.
   a. Doctor
   b. Nurse
   c. Middle-aged client who had recent surgery
   d. Social worker
3. For three minutes, pretend you are all at a meeting to discuss *C*'s postoperative plans; how long will *C* be in the hospital? In a convalescent center? On a special diet? Have exercise restrictions? See next step.
4. As you do step 3, take the following roles:
   a. Blame
   b. Placate
   c. Superreasonable
   d. Irrelevant
5. Repeat step 3, only this time, take the following roles:
   a. Irrelevant
   b. Blame
   c. Placate
   d. Superreasonable
6. Repeat step 3, only this time, take the following roles:
   a. Superreasonable
   b. Irrelevant
   c. Blame
   d. Placate
7. Repeat step 3, only this time, take the following roles:
   a. Placate
   b. Superreasonable
   c. Irrelevant
   d. Blame

How many were able to reach a sensible decision? How many felt *good* about their "case conferences?"

Congruence

There is a fifth choice in responding to stress. This choice is to be congruent; that is, the words and actions in a communication fit the inner experience of self and are appropriate to the context. A congruent response takes the other person's feelings into account and does not allow feelings of "low" self-worth to influence the communication process. A congruent response is healthy, as opposed to the other four responses—which are not. By healthy, it is meant that tension is decreased and self-worth is at a high level.

Being congruent does not mean sharing everything that is thought or felt all the time. However, the congruent person can comment about the situation or feelings, as well as respond to questions or other situational needs.

There are no magical congruent phrases (phrases that are *always* congruent) or magical congruent postures; no one stance of a person is necessarily congruent in all situations. However, certain phrases and statements from the four noncongruent categories can be restated in a more congruent manner. That is, they can be restated differently, taking away implied blame, placation, superreasonableness, and irrelevance. Generally, the "translation" includes using the word "I" for ownership of feelings or beliefs ("I think that...," "It is my feeling that...") or a lessening of categorical phrases ("always," "should," "never") to a more accurate statement of reality ("for now," "at this moment").

BLAME: Mr. Jones, why are you being so stupid? You should never leave the bed by yourself!!!

CONGRUENT: Mr. Jones, you are not supposed to leave your bed without help according to the doctor. Please call me the next time you have to get up.

BLAME: I don't care if you're the head nurse, don't you ever talk to me like that!

CONGRUENT: I feel you are being hard on me.

PLACATE: I'm so sorry to bother you, Dr. Barker, but...it's my fault I know...Mrs. Bailey is complaining of pain. I'm sorry.

CONGRUENT: Dr. Barker, Mrs. Bailey is complaining of pain.

SUPERREASONABLE: Ninety-eight percent of all post-op patients have variable control over their locomotion and gait, Mr. Peterson.

CONGRUENT: It may take you some time to walk well after that operation.

IRRELEVANT: Hello, Jonesy, what's new? Did you have trouble parking? (Jonesy is 10 minutes late for her shift.)

CONGRUENT: You were 10 minutes late. I'd like you to be on time.

There is likely to be a time when we find ourselves placating, being superreasonable, or being irrelevant as a nurse communicator. One issue at this point is "What to do?" Some people have a tendency to "block off" the

Communication Styles

incongruent style, such as the nurse who might say, "I will never blame." An alternative is presented here, namely, to think about how to transform an incongruent style to a congruent and healthy response. The first step is to assume a position of high self-worth. This may not be easy to accomplish and may require substantial work to decrease anxiety and a sense of being threatened.

A second step is to include the missing aspect of a full communication, be it concern for self, concern for other, or concern for context. Thus, a tendency to blame, when transformed by adding high self-worth and respect for others, can become an assertive request. Placating, when transformed by adding high self-worth and self-respect, can become care for others. Superreasonableness, when transformed by adding high self-worth and respect for one's own and others' feelings, can become creative intelligence. Irrelevancy, when transformed by adding high self-worth and respect for self, respect for others as well as respect for context, becomes humor and a sense of perspective. These transformations are summarized in Chart 3–1.

Chart 3–1

Response	Missing Pieces	Congruent Transformation
Blame	+ Respect for other's feelings	= Assertion
Placating	+ Self-respect	= Care, concern
Superreasonableness	+ Respect for other's feelings + respect for own feelings	= Intelligence
Irrelevance	+ Respect for self + respect for others + respect for the context	= Humor, perspective, ability to make connections

Being congruent is not always easy. Most people know when they are not congruent, if only by a vague sense of unrest after the communication is over. In addition, there are common statements we have all heard that could be construed as condoning *incongruence*. We present them below with their *missing* pieces in parentheses.

BLAME: Stand up for your rights (and do not deny others theirs.)
PLACATE: Always be nice (and pay attention to your own needs).
SUPERREASONABLE: Let's look at the facts (and respect both our opinions and feelings as part of "the facts").

IRRELEVANT: Everyone loves a clown (if the clown fits the setting, respecting her or his own feelings and those of others).

CONCLUSION

All persons have unique and varying styles of communication. Six of these styles, as well as related exercises, have been presented in this chapter to enable nurses to assess their own communication styles and those of clients more accurately.

A knowledge of Satir's communication framework and its relation to the concepts of self-worth and stress provide a foundation for understanding defensive behavior. Defensive behavior occurs when one's self-worth is threatened or one feels under stress. Four patterns of defensive behavior —blaming, placating, superreasonableness, and irrelevancy—are usually unhealthy responses. A fifth pattern, congruence, is a healthy response. There are some nursing situations and role relationships in which nurses might find themselves using "non-congruent" or defensive behaviors, fully aware of their decision to do so. For example, if nurses needed help in a medical emergency, they might yell or "blame." What has been emphasized in this chapter is that nurse communicators can make choices, based on the situational needs, rather than responding from a position of low self-worth.

BIBLIOGRAPHY

Altrocchi, J. *Abnormal behavior*. New York: Harcourt Brace Janovich, 1980.
Bandler, R., Grinder, J. & Satir, V. *Changing with families*. Palo Alto, Cal.: Science and Behavior Books, 1976.
Blake, R.R. & Mouton, J.S. *Building a dynamic organization through grid organization development*. Reading, Mass.: Addison-Wesley, 1969.
Egan, G. *You & me*. Monterey, Cal.: Brooks/Cole, 1977.
Grinder, J. & Bandler, R. *The structure of magic II*. Palo Alto, Cal.: Science and Behavior Books, 1976.
Jourard, S.M. *The transparent self* (Rev. ed.). New York: Van Nostrand Reinhold, 1971.
Katz, D. & Kahn, R.L. *The social psychology of organization*. New York: John Wiley, 1966.
Rogers, C. *Client centered therapy*. Boston: Houghton Mifflin, 1951.
Satir, V. *Making Contact*. Millbrae, California: Celestial Arts, 1976.
Satir V. *Peoplemaking*. Palo Alto, California: Science and Behavior Books, 1972.
Smith, V. & Bass, T. *Communication for health professionals*. Philadelphia: J.B. Lippincott, 1979.

Chapter 4 Communication skills

BEHAVIORAL OBJECTIVES

By reading this chapter and participating in the exercises, students will be able to:

1. Identify two concepts which promote helping relationships: the development of trust and the nurse's therapeutic use of self
2. Define six basic therapeutic communication skills; attending to the client, the use of "I" statements, reflection, verbal reassurance, nonverbal reassurance, and the use of silence
3. Identify four techniques which promote in-depth nurse-client relationships; active listening, empathy, sharing feelings, and the use of touch
4. Distinguish between procedural, caring, and therapeutic touch

Most nurses enjoy helping people; that is one of the major reasons they choose the field of nursing. Helping can be defined in several ways. We find ourselves helping others many times during the course of a day; responding to the requests of others or assisting in small tasks. These requests or tasks have a goal; they tend to solve a problem. They also foster a relationship between two people—a relationship that is essentially a partnership. Each partner gives and receives in the relationship in nearly equal proportions.

A helping relationship in a nurse-client interaction is different. Although the goal, that of problem solving, is the same, one person (the nurse) is giving more than the other (the client). It is an *unequal* partnership, that is, it focuses in one direction only—towards the client (Eriksen, 1979). The nurse is expected to bring to this relationship a special set of communication skills.

This chapter presents two concepts which foster helping relationships and promote intimate or in-depth communication. These two concepts, "the development of trust" and "the therapeutic use of self," contain both abstract and concrete elements. Thus, they are sophisticated techniques as well as concepts, and they require a high level of skill to implement. As nurses, we sometimes assume that clients will automatically trust us or that we have the natural ability to act in a therapeutic mode. The truth is that both these concepts require a high level of awareness and knowledge, both of which are developed over extended periods of time. These concepts are characterized by low visibility; their presence is difficult to assess. For example, how does one measure the level of trust between client and nurse?

Not all nurse-client interactions demand that the nurses establish a level of trust or use themselves therapeutically. Many interactions and relationships begin at a superficial level and progress over a period of time to an intimate level. Superficiality in a relationship is characterized by limited self-disclosure, and the communication content is on general or nonpersonal topics. The intimacy level implies an intimate sharing of feelings, with nurses responding in an accepting, nonevaluative way and using themselves therapeutically; an atmosphere of trust is present (Coad-Denton, 1979).

THE DEVELOPMENT OF TRUST

Trust is central to a therapeutic nurse-client relationship. Without a sense of trust, the interaction is superficial, with little personal involvement of either the client or the nurse.

What exactly is trust? Trust is relying on someone without question (Lewis, 1973). Trust implies confidence, dependability, and credibility in a relationship. One essential characteristic of trusting behavior is that it increases one's vulnerability to the other person (Rossiter and Pearce, 1975). The opposite of trust is suspicion. Trust is developed through communication—communication that is forthright and honest.

Erikson identified trust as the first stage of psychosocial development in the human life cycle (Erikson, 1963). According to his view, trust represents the degree to which the infant has confidence in self as well as the people who surround her or him. Trust then becomes reliance and faith in others.

It usually takes an extended period of time for persons to develop a sense of trust with each other. In nursing interactions, one hears the term "levels of trust"; that is, the development of trust progresses through a series of sequential phases. These phases are related to the three phases identified in the development of the nurse-client relationship itself; the orientation phase, the working phase, and the termination phase. Although the transition from one phase to another is gradual and each phase varies in length of time, there are characteristics which can be attributed to each, whether it be in the development of trust or in the development of the nurse-client relationship itself.

Phase I—Orientation Phase

This period is characterized by the superficial or beginning level of the relationship, and it can be marked by uncertainty and exploration. Both nurse and client are beginning to clarify their respective roles through the mutual provision of such information as name, how, when, how long and how often, and purpose of the interaction. There is a mutual "feeling out" of what is expected. In this initial phase, nursing goals and their related outcome are set. These goals can be either formal or informal, formal implying that a contract has been written. *The more visible these goals are, the better the nursing care outcomes* (Revell, 1978).

If trust is to be established, it begins in the orientation phase of the nurse-client relationship. Nurses who have had unhappy interpersonal experiences often find it difficult to undertake the risk of establishing a trusting relationship with a client. They must first test the trustworthiness of the other person.

Similarly, the demands of dependency and fears of the hospital setting can lead to situations in which the client tests the nurse's reliability by initial and concrete behaviors before a trust bond has been created. This is shown in the following example:

> Ann Smith, a 20-year-old college student, was receiving an I.V. because of dehydration. Her nurse told her, "I'll return to add the second I.V. bottle *before* the first bottle is completely empty."
>
> Ann, having some initial trust, waited until the very last minute, and when *all* the solution in the first bottle was gone, she rang for the nurse. As far as she was concerned, the nurse did not keep her word. The initial trust was then lost.

Trusting behavior on the part of nurses *sometimes* produces trust in clients, but distrusting behavior *almost always* produces distrust. (Rossiter and Pearce, 1975).

Phase II—Working Phase

In the second phase of trust development, the boundaries of the relationship are more flexible, as the stereotypic roles of "nurse" and "client" are shed. The nurse is no longer a symbol in a uniform, but a person; the client becomes a person with feelings. Both the nurse and client are willing to share feelings and discuss in greater detail those concerns touched upon in the orientation phase. They are now comfortable with an increasing awareness of self as well as their own goals and motivations, and they share this awareness with each other. The client has moved from an external to an internal frame of reference, and inner concerns central to the client (not the nurse) become the focus of the interaction. Confidentiality is established. The nurse may self-disclose, but only in the service of therapeutically attending to the client.

CLIENT: "Nobody cares what happens to me."
NURSE: "I feel the same way sometimes. It is not easy to face an operation."

Phase III—Termination

This phase occurs when encounters between the nurse and client are ending. It can begin on first contact when the nurse states the relationship will end (Brill and Kilts, 1980, p. 196). A sudden and unannounced departure, especially when there has been a strong personal investment, can leave the client in a state of mistrust and cause separation anxiety. This makes it all the more difficult to develop a sense of trust in future relationships.

Student nurses, by virtue of their short contact with clients, often fall prey to a sense of mistrust on the part of the client because they fail to inform clients when they will terminate the relationship. Clients, as much as they love students, often find it difficult to share feelings because of the temporary nature of the nurse–client interaction. A direct acknowledgement by the nurse of both the shortness of the contact and feelings about it are beneficial in preventing a sense of loss and in developing a sense of trust in these circumstances.

In developing trust with clients, nurses have an advantage. They know more about the client than the client knows about them. They have read the client's chart, heard reports about the client, know the client's age and diagnosis, and so forth.

THERAPEUTIC USE OF SELF

There is a difference when you are talking to your friend and when you are talking to a client. In both interactions, you bring the totality of your experiences—your values, feelings, and attitudes into the communication;

however, the basic objectives of these two interactions differ. You usually talk to your friend to socialize, to get to know each other better, to obtain or share information. While you may talk to clients for these same reasons, you also talk to them to establish trusting relationships, to allow for expression of feelings, or to help them to realize personal goals which will help them to regain their independence.

The nurse's role in such helping relationships is a therapeutic role, that is, the nurse interacts with the client for the express purpose of benefiting the client. The use of self in a therapeutic way in which the client's needs are the central focus characterizes communication interactions. The nurse *guides, directs, and structures* the communication interactions in such a way that the client is able to verbalize feelings. Rogers (1961) defines a helping relationship as one that "intentionally promotes growth and development, improved functioning and improved coping with life of the other."

Therapeutic use of self *does not* have to be done dramatically. Many normal nursing functions can be performed in a therapeutic manner. For example, many clients recovering from a stroke or a long bed rest have difficulty walking in part due to low confidence in their physical powers. When the nurse takes such a patient's arm and walks with him or her, the nurse is able to act as a prosthesis or extension of the person. But there is something more. There is kinesthetic communication. It is as if the confidence and stability of one person (the nurse) passes to the other (the client), and the client is able to walk with confidence and can assume a more normal gait. Although this is an example of the nurse extending herself or himself therapeutically to fulfill a client's physical need, psychological needs are fulfilled in much the same manner.

The following two exercises are designed to help you begin to conceptualize how to use yourself therapeutically in nursing activities. Keep in mind that the therapeutic use of self is a complicated skill that can require months or even years of training.

Exercise 1 in Therapeutic Use of Self

In the large group, discuss each of the following procedures in *two* ways; first, in terms of *how* to perform the nursing procedure; second, how to utilize "therapeutic use of self" while performing the procedure.

1. Taking a blood pressure
2. Bathing a client
3. Administering medication
4. Discussing medication compliance with a client
5. Home safety assessment.

Exercise 2 in Therapeutic Use of Self

1. Pair up. One partner will be A, the other B.
   A is to think of a situation or problem that is of real concern and one that A would like to change.
3. A shares the problem with B. Be brief and specific, but at the same time, share some of the reasons for your concern.
   B's task is to guide the interaction in such a way that A is able to focus on the concern. B should resist the temptation to talk about him- or herself.
5. Switch roles and repeat steps 2–4.
6. Discuss the interactions, asking yourself if you were able to demonstrate the "therapeutic use of self."

THERAPEUTIC COMMUNICATION SKILLS

There are many specialized communication skills and techniques that can facilitate the development of trust or the use of self in nurse-client relationships. These skills are presented in this chapter in two groupings. In the first group, the skills are more basic; they help to encourage the transformation of a relationship from a superficial to an intimate one. Their use emphasizes the client as a feeling human being with health problems. These skills are attending to the client, the use of "I" statements, reflection, verbal reassurance, nonverbal reassurance, and the use of silence.

Attending to the Client

Effective attending to the client means that the nurses should make sure both the physical arrangement of the space and the nurse's own attention maximize good communication with the client. One would not, for example, want to communicate for a long period of time about personal matters to a client in a wheelchair in the middle of a busy hall while standing up. At the same time, a brief and fairly non-emotion-laden message (e.g., "it's time for lunch") could be adequately communicated in the hall.

There are a few simple points to remember in attending to the client:

1. Find a place that is private. This may mean asking a roommate who is not bedridden to leave the room.
2. Make sure the client is physically comfortable (in the chair, on the bed, etc.).
3. Maximize your ability to hear the client and the client's ability to hear you. Generally, sitting three feet apart is recommended.

Communication Skills

4. Reduce external distractions (close doors, turn off TVs—though be sure to ask first).
5. Avoid extensive use of records, charts, questions written on paper, or any other prop that will distract you from the client. Some helpers spend too much time on their notes and no time attending to the client (Brammer, 1973). The client then may feel not listened to.

The second aspect of attending to the client is focusing one's own attention to the communication at hand. This means putting aside the experiences immediately preceding one particular interaction or not letting the negative encounter with one client put one in a "negative set" for the next interaction or not being so concerned with a meeting that will take place in an hour that one ignores virtually everything the client says.

Arranging the physical space and your own internal focus of attention are important prerequisites to good communication with the client.

"I" Statements

Counselors have written about the use of the word "I" as a way of helping clients own their own feelings (e.g., Gordon, 1970). The general view behind this is that as an individual says "I feel" or "I believe" (as opposed to "you make me feel" or "the truth is"), he or she will make a more accurate statement and come across in a less dogmatic or pedantic fashion.

The first issue is when to use "I." Obviously, there are times when "I" is inappropriate. For example, if it's time for a client's bath, you would say something like "It's time for your bath, Mr. Jones" or possibly "I see it's time for your bath." The common use of the word "we" to mean "you" is *not* recommended. In the example above, saying "It's time for our bath" is incorrect. Only one person is being bathed, and that is the client. The inappropriate use of the word "we" is at best confusing and at worst condescending.

So the question still remains as to when do you, the nurse, use "I"? The following contexts serve as a partial list. Can you think of any others?

1. Requesting information (I would like you to...)
2. Asking the client to comply (I would like you to...)
3. Giving your opinion (I think that...)
4. Discussing feelings (I hear you saying...)
5. Giving suggestions (I think you could...)

As is the case with any technique, "I" statements can also be misused. For example, it is possible to communicate defensively with an "I" statement, such as "I feel so sorry, it's all my fault, doctor" (placating) or "I hate you, I won't do it!!!" (blaming). It is also possible to dominate a conversation or overdo "I" statements. If every sentence a nurse says begins with "I think," others will start to tune out the nurse's communication.

Exercise 1 in Use of "I" Statements

Convert each of the following statements on the left to an "I" statement or to an appropriate "you statement." Suggested answers are given on the right side. Cover them until you have made your guesses.

Nurse's Statement	Transformation
"Mr. Jones, you should go back to your room."	"Mr. Jones, I want you to go to your room."
(to colleague): "You're always late."	"It is my perception that you are always late."
"It's time for us to get out of bed."	"It's time for you to get out of bed."
"You are depressed today."	"I sense that you are depressed today."
"Don't we look nice today."	"I think you look really nice today."
"You don't make any sense."	"I do not understand you."

Exercise 2 in "I" Statements

1. Pair up.
2. Partners have a conversation about their nursing program or clinical situation using "I" statements and correcting each other if either partner slips up. (You may find yourselves changing sentences like "She's really mean" to "I feel she's really mean.") Pay attention to the differences both as communication sender and receiver to "I" statements.
3. Discuss your reactions in the large group.

Reflection

Reflection is a particularly useful skill in helping a client experience feelings. In reflecting, the nurse verbally gives back the feeling parts of the client's communication. Thus, if a client said:

CLIENT: "It's been quite a long day today. They gave me tests and didn't give me results; the doctor hasn't come—it's scary."

An appropriate reflection response is:

NURSE: "It's scary for you."

There are two important aspects of this interaction. The first is that the nurse reflects the affective (feeling) words as opposed to answering the implied complaints in the rest of the client's communication. Reflection is a tool to be used to obtain feeling responses, not to exchange information. It will serve to help the client focus and explore his or her own feelings, with the nurse serving as a guide or ally.

By using reflection, the nurse stays with the feeling and ignores extraneous avenues of approach. For example, if the nurse had taken another tack, such as saying, "Why do you feel scared?" (an ineffective technique in itself, as is explained in the following chapter), and the client then proceeded to analyze his or her motives, the result would be quite different from the client continuing to explore the feeling of being scared. Similarly, if the nurse chooses to be reassuring, the feeling level will lighten instead of deepen for the client. Reflection focuses on feelings and tends to result in a deepening of the feeling state as the client responds to the nurse's verbalization and restatement of the client's feelings.

A second major point about reflection is that it can carry with it "unconditional positive regard" for the client (Rogers, 1961). That is, the voice tone, gestures, body posture, and facial expressions of the nurse should be congruent with the message, "You are OK." This empathic response imparts to the client an important covert message of positive self-worth, which can be stronger than a direct verbal message of the same sort. The appropriate message sent by the nurse, then, is not blaming, placating, superreasonable, or irrelevant! It is consistent and focused on the client's self-worth and feeling state at that moment in time.

Some beginning nurses will become too parrotlike in reflecting feelings. They will repeat any and all feeling words a client says. Obviously, this is misuse of the skill of reflecting feelings. Reflecting calls for some judgment about when to reflect, how to phrase the reflection, and what should be reflected. What we choose to say will be determined to a large degree by how well we listen, observe, feel, and perceive what is going on with the client. In fact, all of the therapeutic skills are based on our having accurate perceptions of the client. There will be moments when we figure out what is going on and let it pass or other moments when we carefully choose different but related words to reflect the feelings. (Consider the choice of expression, the channel language, what is known about the client's culture, age, sex, race, and so on.)

The following exercises give you an opportunity to practice reflection as a therapeutic tool.

Exercise 1 in Reflection

For each of the following statements, think of how you could reflect the feeling words or "tone" of the client's communication. Some possible reflections are included on the right side of the page. (Keep them covered until you think of your answers.)

Client's Statement	Nurse's Reflection
Nurse, what time is it? My sister was supposed to be here an hour ago.	You seem anxious. You're concerned.
I don't feel like doing anything today...go away. I'm too upset to talk.	You're too upset to talk?
(upset) Why are you bothering me? I'm just going to die.	You seem upset. You feel you're going to die?
Why do you want to talk to me?	You sound uncertain.
(Says nothing, just sits and looks out the window—no eye contact.)	You seem distant.
(sadly) Nobody cares about me. No one knows I'm here.	You seem down.
I don't know if I'll ever get better (sobbing).	You feel as if you have no hope?
I'm so worthless.	You feel worthless?

By reflecting feelings in several of these cases, the nurse not only focuses on feelings, but also enables the communication to continue. The focus of the communication is on the client's feelings, not on others—including the nurse. Many times the client will respond directly to the reflection and stop blaming others for his or her feelings. By focusing on the client's feelings, the nurse is keeping the communication in the "here and now," where there is implied hope for change, development of self-worth, or awareness that at least one other person (the nurse) has unconditional positive regard for the client.

Exercise 2 in Reflection

Discuss the following questions in the large group:

1. How do you reflect feelings with a relatively uncommunicative client?
2. When is reflection of feeling useful in dealing with other staff, aides, physicians, or other health professionals?
3. When is it awkward *for you* to reflect feelings?
4. Which feelings does it seem hardest to reflect?

Communication Skills ────────────────────────────── **91**

5. In which kinds of nursing situations is it easier to use a lot of reflection? In which types is it hardest?
6. How can reflection be misused to keep the nurse from having to answer a difficult question?

Verbal Reassurance

Along with reflection, a commonly used communication skill is to give verbal reassurance to clients that they are being listened to, that we understand what they say, that good care is being given. By giving reassurance, we play a very important role as a care giver, that of validating the client's self-worth and creating a sense of hope. What one also has to do is to be sure that the reassurance is real and truthful. Otherwise we are giving "false reassurance."

What kinds of things, then, can be reassured? A list would include:

1. That there is hope.
2. That one is listening.
3. That care is available.
4. That certain disconcerting changes are expected (such as slow recovery from a stroke).
5. That the client is being treated like a person.
6. That the problem is understood.

The basic ways in which verbal reassurance can be given include acknowledging any and all of the six points above.

Exercise 1 in Verbal Reassurance

For each of the following situations, think of what you could say to justifiably reassure the client. Some suggested responses are given on the right side of the page. Cover them until you have thought of your own.

Client's Statement	*Nurse's Response*
My stroke was four months ago, and I don't think I'll ever get better.	I know you are concerned, but four months is not a long period of time for recovery.
I don't think anyone here cares what happens to me.	I am here, I care.
I read in the paper that the clinic doesn't have enough money to oper-	In any procedures we do in the clinic we use good equipment. While there

ate. Can they take care of me?

What difference does it all make? You're just a number here anyway.

are some questions about funds, the only way we will stay open is if we can give high quality care.

I consider you to be a person, Mrs. _____ (be sure you know her name!).

Exercise 2 in Reassurance

1. Pair up. One partner will be A, the other B.
2. B thinks of a situation in which she as a client might need reassurance.
3. B then tells A about the situation.
4. A and B "play out" the communication three times, with A as nurse and B as client. A will reassure B each time. A will also try different verbal approaches to reassuring B.
5. Switch and repeat steps 2–4.
6. Discuss the methods you developed with the rest of the class.

Nonverbal Reassurance

Along with verbally expressing reassurance, there are several nonverbal ways the nurse can use to show that the client is cared for and listened to. Nonverbal reassurance refers to everything excluding words that the nurse can do to reassure the client. The use of nonverbal reassurance becomes very important as a subliminal message during the communication sequence, and it should be practiced until it is an active and easily accessible part of the nurse's communication skills.

There are visual, auditory, and kinesthetic ways in which the nurse can reassure the client. Visual ways include the following:

Visual

Smiling (at the right time)
Leaning forward
Nodding head in an affirmative fashion
Looking concerned (eyebrows down, mouth closed)
Certain gestures (arms open)
Maintaining eye contact
"Open" body stance (arms, legs not crossed)

All of the behaviors in the list indicate "I am receptive to what you have to say" and should serve to reassure clients. It is expected that we will not necessarily do all of these at once, but will practice and learn how to include these symbolic actions as part of our communication repertoire.

Auditory forms of nonverbal reassurance include the following:

Auditory
Use of "um-humm"
"Soft" tone of voice
Relaxed speed of speech
Allowing the other to finish speaking

The major kinesthetic form of reassurance is, obviously, touch. As mentioned in Chapter 2, there are many ways to touch another. A gentle, reassuring touch can be used to convey nonverbal reassurance in the following ways:

Kinesthetic
Shaking hands to say hello
Touching the lower or upper arm
Touching the shoulder
Holding the client's hand while communicating
Hugging from the side (arm around shoulder)
Frontal hug (pick the *appropriate* time and place)

At this point, a word of caution is offered. Some clients dislike being touched. Nurses must approach touching as a form of nonverbal reassurance carefully. This is discussed in greater detail later in this chapter under the use of touch. If nurses are not comfortable touching others, they transmit incongruent messages. Furthermore, because of the possible sexual overtones to touching in our culture, you may get some surprising responses to touch from clients of the opposite sex. This does not, however, mean you should never give reassurance through touch. Rather, it means you should practice it so that you can communicate quite clearly whatever message *you* want to send.

The following exercises should help you develop and refine your nonverbal reassurance skills.

Exercise in Nonverbal Reassurance

---

1. Pair up. One partner (*A*) will pretend to be a client with one of the following problems—health problems like diabetes, acne, psoriasis. *A* will describe how the problem affects *A*. The other partner (*B*) will listen to the problem and *visually* show nonverbal reassurance. (*B* can also give verbal reassurance.)
2. Switch roles.

3. *A* will again be the client. This time *B* will add auditory and kinesthetic components of nonverbal reassurance. Experiment with varying degrees of each until you find a good mix that seems to fit you, your partner, and the context of the problem.
4. Switch roles.

Use of Silence

The use of silence is one of the most effective and difficult skills for professional helpers. Often, the nurse has a series of questions to ask. In addition, many interviewers are uncomfortable with even as little as five seconds of silence. Somehow they feel nothing is being accomplished if either they or the client is not communicating something at every moment.

Yet silence has many therapeutic uses. It allows the client to dialogue internally and to process information. It also allows time to search for words to describe feelings or situations. Whereas the act of finding "the right words" in and of itself can be therapeutic, allowing the client time to find the words is obviously a useful therapeutic skill.

In most two-way communication, a pattern of responding emerges in which one person talks for a set time, then the other, then the first person, and so on. In terms of therapeutic communication, a silent response, coupled with a nonverbal gesture of reassurance, such as a head nod may *allow* the client to continue the train of thought. All that is required is the ability to keep quiet for 5 to 10 seconds. The client will usually pick up his turn.

Obviously, silence can be overused; it can become an excuse for having nothing to say or be the result of tuning out the client. When used judiciously, however, silence is a useful and powerful tool in therapeutic communication. Practice the following exercises until you feel comfortable with silence.

Exercise 1 in Use of Silence

1. Pair up.
2. Sit without talking until you *think* a minute has passed. Check to see how long it has actually been.

Exercise 2 in Use of Silence

1. Pair up.
2. Partner *A* will talk to *B* about an *imaginary* circumstance that makes *A* upset (health, school, family, etc.)
3. *B* will respond, be empathic (as usual), and consciously use silence at three points in the conversation. Take two to five minutes.

Communication Skills

4. Switch roles.
5. Discuss how it felt to use silence and what thoughts you had as *both* client and interviewer during the silence. What kinds of thoughts emerged? How helpful was the silence?

The communication skills that have been presented are not necessarily effective in all nurse-client interactions. Differences in the use of these skills are reflected through subtle gestures, tone of voice, or expressions. In addition, clients respond in different ways to the same communication skills for a variety of reasons, including channel awareness, "where they are at," and the context in which communication takes place. Effective use of these skills helps to establish an initial rapport between the nurse and the client. However, because each client and each nurse are unique, it is impossible to give a single specified formula that will indicate what skills should be used in order to create rapport. Some clients may not like attending behavior or reflection statements, while others may prefer nonverbal reassurance and silence. Rapport building can start with a series of "tests" of various skills by nurses to find out which skills work most effectively with a client. Nurses can then become better "guessers" of what will work with a given type of client based on appearance, sounds, and reports from the nursing staff.

Exercise in Establishing Beginning Rapport

1. Form into groups of three. One member will be *A*, one *B*, and one *C*.
2. *A* will role play a client with an emotional reaction to a health problem (for example, diabetes or hypertension). *B* will be a nurse making a home visit. *B*'s goal is to establish beginning rapport with *A* through the utilization of the six therapeutic skills presented.
3. Play the scene for three minutes. *C* will be an observer and note which skill *B* utilizes, as well as which channel language (visual, auditory, or kinesthetic).
4. At the end of three minutes, *C* will review his or her observations; how did the use of skills help (or not help) the development of beginning rapport?

TECHNIQUES RELATED TO TRUST AND THERAPEUTIC USE OF SELF

There are four communication techniques that nurses can incorporate within the broader concepts of trust and therapeutic use of self. The use of these techniques promotes more personal, in-depth interactions. These four techniques are active listening, the use of empathy, sharing feelings, and the use of touch. They require the use of channel language; for example, active listening is primarily auditory, while the use of touch is kinesthetic. Their use, either in combination or alone, allows nurses maximum flexibility in developing trust and extending themselves therapeutically when caring for clients.

Active Listening

One of the most effective means of assessing the status of clients is to listen to what they tell us. While information on physical and psychological status can be obtained through the different communication channels, what clients state about themselves is most important. Listening then becomes a primary source of communication for nurses.

The levels of hearing and listening were discussed in Chapter 2. Nurses hear a multiple of messages in the course of their work. This does not mean they have listened to those messages. The average person, after listening to another person talk, remembers only one-half of what is heard no matter how much the person was concentrating. In order to listen, nurses must be "actively" engaged in the receiving and decoding or retranslating of the client's message.

Active listening therefore implies that the nurse attends to the content of the message, *how* the client stated the message, and what feelings the client had when the message was stated (Gordon, 1970).

Benjamin (1974), describes a simple test nurses can use to determine if they are beginning to listen with understanding. If during the interaction, nurses can (1) state in their own words what clients have said and (2) convey in their own words the feelings clients have expressed, and clients can acknowledge what nurses have stated in (1) and (2) is what clients really feel, then nurses probably have listened to clients (Benjamin, 1974).

Nurses who actively listen are able to paraphrase what the client has stated to his or her satisfaction. They are also able to tune into the client's message through observation of body language, eye contact, and nonverbal behavior. In other words, they incorporate all sensory information, including visual, auditory, kinesthetic, and olfactory cues. In addition to receiving communication from all channels, the nurse is actively integrating the information to form a complete picture of the client's emotional state, and this facilitates therapeutic communication. Thus, the nurse is working at all three levels of integration (Level I, sensory; Level II, single channel integration; and Level III, full channel perception).

Active listening is a cognitive process that is developed over a period of time. It is hard work. One of the most effective ways to develop active listening skills is to begin to listen to ourselves. How do we transmit messages? How do we decode a client's message and then verbalize or feed back the decoded message? How effective is our ability to put into our own words what the client has said, as well as letting this client know he or she has been heard? Asking ourselves these questions will enable us to begin to develop the high-level technique of active listening.

Empathy

The use of empathy promotes an effective communication interaction, especially with clients who are under stress. Empathy is the ability to enter into the life of another person and accurately perceive his or her current feelings (Kalish, 1973). A nurse who is able to empathize is able to look with the client's eyes, listen with the client's ears, and feel the feelings of the client. The nurse is able to do this and still maintain his or her own identity.

Empathy differs from sympathy. A sympathetic nurse loses his or her identity and actually assumes the identity of the client. The client and the nurse become one person emotionally. The sympathetic nurse is subjective as opposed to the empathetic nurse, who maintains a sense of objectivity. The sympathetic nurse offers condolence and pity, whereas the empathetic nurse offers support and understanding. A skilled nurse communicator empathizes rather than sympathizes. The difference between empathy and sympathy is shown in the following example:

> A nurse's assignment included Jimmy, an eight-year-old boy who had been hospitalized with leukemia for several months. Jimmy's mother was often present when the nurse gave care. The mother had adapted to Jimmy's illness and wanted to have as much contact as possible with her son.
>
> However, the nurse was responding to the situation with sympathy. She felt very sorry for Jimmy and was often on the verge of tears while working with him. She also found herself close to tears when the mother was present. The nurse felt that neither mother nor child would understand her tears, so she would frequently leave the room. The nurse did not include the mother in bathing her son or in other appropriate procedures.

By feeling sorry for the client, the nurse in the above situation ended up being an obstacle to caring communication rather than a facilitator of good care. With an empathic approach, the nurse could have included the mother in the care, and the nurse could have shared tears with the family. Note that crying is not necessarily unprofessional, as long as it fits the context and the relationship between the nurse and others. The idea of "sharing tears with" (an empathic approach) is quite different from "shedding tears for" (a sympathetic approach).

The difference between sympathy and empathy is summarized in Chart 4–1.

**CHART 4-1
Empathy Versus Sympathy**

Area	Empathy	Sympathy
Relationship to client's feelings	"Borrows" client's feelings	"Takes on" client's feelings
Sense of identity	Maintains self-identity	Loses self-identity
Objectivity	Objective	Subjective
Perception of others' feelings	Accurate perception of true feelings	Inaccurate perception of true feelings
Nurse's emotional resource	Understanding and support	Condolence, pity

Kalish (1973) points out the importance of the relative here and now in the use of empathy. The empathetic nurse responds to the client's *current* feelings at the moment of confrontation. This must be utilized at the moment of impact; it is not something the nurse can think over and return to at a later point in time when the client's feelings might have changed.

If, in your role as a nurse, you stop to think about it, empathy is easier to come by if you can relate the client's experience to ones you have experienced. If you have been in the client's shoes, you can use that experience to empathize about the particular situation. Similarly, clients who know that the nurse (or person) has had a similar experience will appreciate his or her ability to tune into their feelings. The Reach for Recovery program sponsored by the American Cancer Society trains volunteers who have had a mastectomy to teach and listen to clients who have just undergone a similar operation during their immediate postoperative course. These volunteers are able to communicate effectively with the client because of an identical experience.

Not all nurses have to have had similar experiences to the client's in order to empathize. Empathy can be developed. A beginning step is to ask yourself questions such as:

"How would I feel if I were in her shoes?"
"What would I need in this situation?"

Empathy means responding in the client's language and terms. It can mean using the same feeling tone of voice as the client; sad if the client is sad or fearful if the client is fearful. It takes some people longer than others to develop empathy. Research has demonstrated that nurses usually do not perceive themselves as having high empathetic ability. On the other hand, most clients perceive nurses as "highly empathetic" (Forsyth, 1979).

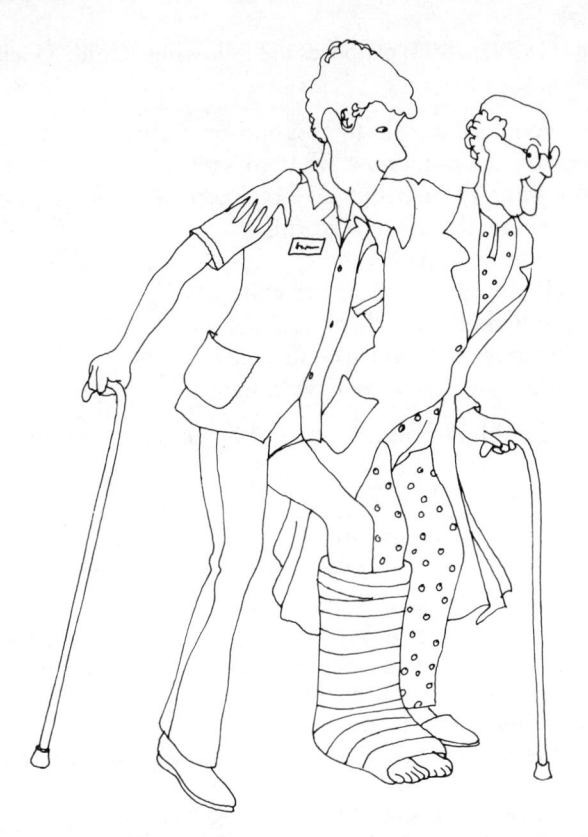

Ehmann (1971), has developed a model for the empathetic process based on four phases of understanding:

1. *Identification.* The first phase in which one loses consciousness of self and becomes engrossed in the personality and situation of the client.
2. *Incorporation.* The second phase includes the act of taking the experience of the client into one's own; it incorporates the feelings of the other person into one's self. This phase is difficult to separate from the first phase of identification.
3. *Reverberation.* While the first two phases describe what the client is feeling, there is now an interplay between two sets of experience; between the actual "me" and the "me" that has identified with the client, or put another way, one's own experience and the feelings of the client. This phase allows one's own responses to aid in uncovering the client's often unconsciously delivered message.
4. *Detachment.* The last phase involves a withdrawal from our subjective involvement and a resumption of our own identity.

LaMonica (1979, p. 494) proposes the following "Golden Helping Rule" for nurses:

> Whenever you feel unable to respond to a client;
> Whenever you do not know what to say;
> When you want to help but do not know what would be helpful;
> Place yourself in the client's world;
> Be in that time and space;
> Ask yourself the questions asked you;
> Feel what you think the client feels...
> Then say what you would like to hear;
> Do what you would like to have done.

Empathy is the ability to place yourself "in the client's world" and to "be in that time and space."

Exercise in the Use of Empathy

1. Pair up. One partner will be *A*, the other *B*.
2. *A* introduces him- or herself to *B* (who is a "new" client) trying to be as empathic as possible. *A:* Think of two or three sentences that will get your *empathic* message across to this new client and say them. For example: "Hello Mr. _____, I'm your nurse. Please let me know if I can help you."
3. *A* then introduces him- or herself to *B* being as *non*empathic as possible.
4. Switch roles.
5. Discuss the experience in light of the following questions:
    a. How did it feel to receive both the "empathic" and "nonempathic" greeting?
    b. What did you or your partner do that was *different* to create or destroy empathy?
    c. What are some good ways to create empathy?

Sharing Feelings

Clients in institutional settings are often not allowed to act out feelings in ways that are beneficial to them. Hospitals are relatively inflexible and demand conformity on the part of the client. In addition, the ill client is apt to be immobile. Expressing feelings through verbalization therefore assumes great importance in the institutional setting.

Nurses, to allow for the expression of feelings on the part of clients, must be able to share their own feelings. Along with this goes the ability to observe clients, to decode their behaviors, and to share feelings congruent with the observed behavior while at the same time insuring that the feelings are consistent with the nurse's own behavior. This progression can be summarized with the following hypothetical sequence.

Action: The client is worried about impending operation.
Observed behavior of client: Client clenches jaw, looks anxious, says nothing.
Nurse's perception of client's feelings: Client is fearful about operation.
Nurse's communication of own perception and feelings: "You seem anxious, Mrs. Smith. I feel you are really worried about the operation."
Nurse's behavior: Stands by bed, places hand on client's shoulder.

Although no substantive research has been done in the area, nurses with many years experience find that when helpers correctly "tune in" to the behavior of clients and then share their feelings, clients will then directly express feelings (crying, verbalizing, or in other ways) almost all of the time. The sharing of positive feelings almost always enhances the relationship with the client. The sharing of negative feelings may be the beginning of greater understanding of what can be done to solve the problem and thus improve the nurse-client relationship. Nurses are cautioned not to use the sharing of feelings in an effort to *force* a change in the client, however.

Nurses who cannot cope with their own feelings about the client may end up "labeling"; that is, instead of eliciting the client's feelings and understanding the client's frame of reference, nurses may make inaccurate assumptions about the client. Consider the following situation:

> Mrs. Gifford, a nursing home resident, was found to be hoarding soap. When the nurse looked in her bedside stand, she found 20 bars of soap. The nurse reported to the headnurse: "Mrs. Gifford is selfish!"

The nurse could have elicited Mrs. Gifford's feelings and an explanation of her behavior through a sharing of feelings in this situation. In this instance, it is also important to know that some institutional residents may hoard food or soap as an attempt to be independent, or even to have something to call "one's own."

One important consideration in handling clients' feelings is that nurses first understand their own feelings. Nurses cannot help clients to express their feelings without knowing how they themselves react to their own feelings. Do their feelings match their behavior? Are they congruent?

Your own feelings and behavior do not necessarily match those of your clients.

Exercise

1. Think how you *act* in the following situations:
   When I feel happy I usually _____
   When I feel depressed I usually _____
   When I feel overworked I usually _____

When I feel fearful I usually _____
When I feel anxious I usually _____
When I feel confident I usually _____
2. Write your responses on paper.
3. Think how you react in each situation. Does your feeling match your action in every situation? Can you detect any incongruent responses in yourself?
4. Now write how clients *act* in the following situations:
When clients feel anxious they might _____
When clients feel depressed they might _____
When clients feel pain they might _____
When clients feel ignored they might _____
5. Discuss with a partner or share your results with the whole group.

The Use of Touch

The use of touch is a form of nonverbal communication that can be therapeutic because it encourages expression of feelings. Touch is used in many nursing procedures, as well as with hospitalized or seriously ill patients (Barrett, 1972; Beaumont, 1974). There are several ways in which touch can be used. Two common distinctions are between procedural and caring touch. In addition, nurses are beginning to explore new areas of health care based on the use of touch.

Procedural Touch. Procedural touch is an essential aspect of nursing. It would be difficult to perform such nursing procedures as a bed bath or an injection without touching clients. Nursing procedures that involve touching the client invade the client's personal space, that is, the "bubble" that surrounds our bodies and defines the limits of space that are strictly "ours." One of the things that happens in the nurse-client relationship is that certain uses of procedural touch are expected and accepted within territorial limits of the client that might not be tolerated in other circumstances. The assumption of the client role allows for the invasion of his or her space by the nurse without question. While all health professionals tend not to question the ill client's right to maintain his or her personal space when performing routine procedures (doctors probe and palpate, nurses lift arms and legs and rub backs), it is questionable how much is actually communicated through the use of procedural touch.

Caring Touch. Caring touch concerns the use of touch in client situations that do not involve physical care. Caring touch can be more sensitive than procedural touch. A nurse who holds a client's hand or reassuringly pats the client's shoulder, communicates a message to the client. This message is

Communication Skills ──────────────────────────── **103**

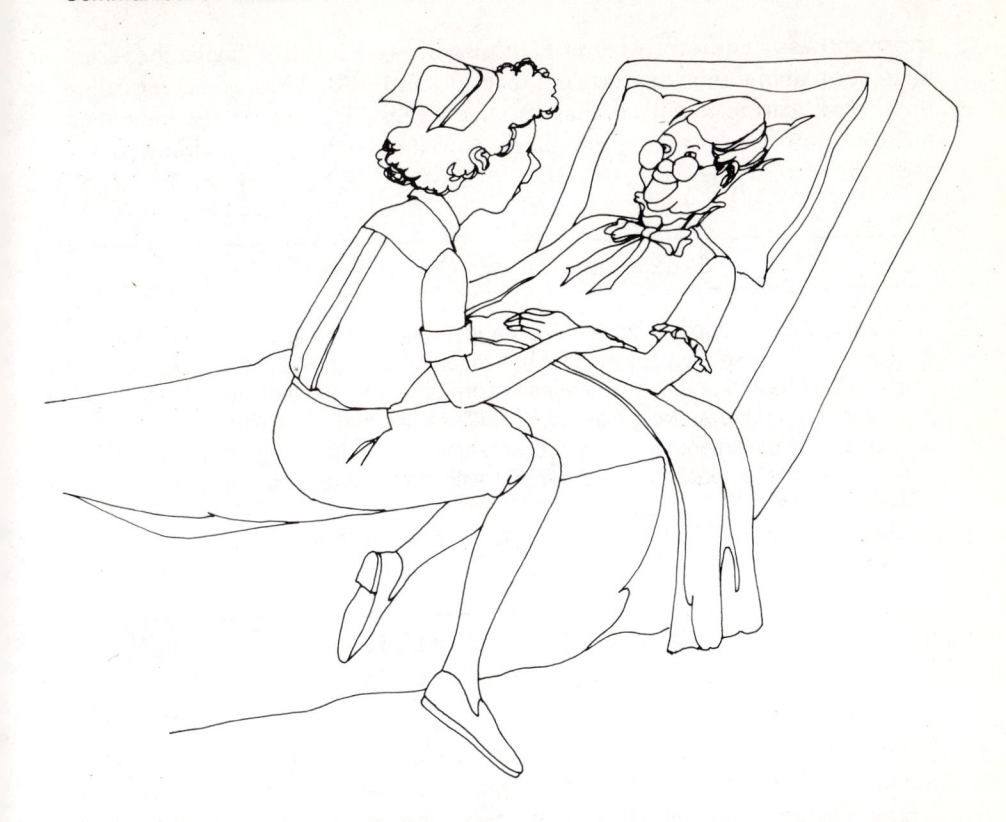

basically one of caring and concern for the client, who usually responds in some manner, be it positive or negative, to the nurse's action. In caring touch, the nurse conveys kinesthetic messages of concern and empathy. Research indicates that caring touch is normally perceived by clients as a therapeutic gesture. Not only does it establish and maintain openness of communication and development of rapport, it often transcends oral communication and promotes contact with reality (Farrah, 1979).

The use of "caring touch" by nurses involves a certain element of risk taking. It can be easily misconstrued by clients. Some nurses have difficulty using caring touch, especially those nurses who have not been accustomed to this sense of touch within their own families. However, the use of caring is a skill that can be developed with experience. Nurses who work in extended-care facilities with elderly clients for long periods of time have ample opportunity to develop the use of "caring touch." This caring touch encourages a closeness, a sense of trust, and reassurance.

The therapeutic effectiveness of "caring touch" has been the subject of nursing research. One study revealed that in seriously ill patients, the response to treatment was significantly better in those who were touched during the verbal interaction than those who were not (McCorkle, 1974). A basic tenet regarding the use of "caring touch" is that its effectiveness depends on the individual nurse's comfort in initiating the touch, as well as each client's comfort as the recipient of touch (Farrah, 1979).

Exercise on Use of "Caring Touch"
---

1. Break up into groups of three. One partner will be *A*, one *B*, and the other *C*.
2. *A* and *B* converse on a subject that has meaning and feeling to them. An example might be the observation of insensitive treatment of a client by another health professional. Use statements with "I feel" rather that "I think."
3. *C* observes this interaction. When *C* agrees with a statement from *A* and *B*, *C* will communicate empathy and agreement with both words and a touch.
4. Switch roles.
5. Discuss. How did *A* or *B* feel when *C* used touch to signify approval.

NEW AREAS OF HEALTH CARE BASED ON TOUCH

"Therapeutic Touch" (TT) is beginning to gain wide acceptance as a nursing modality. TT is related to the ancient practice of "laying on of hands" (Kreiger, 1979). Theoretically, the transfer of energy through the use of touch from a healthy body (the healer) to an ill body (the healee) helps the client to "repattern his energy level to a state that is comparable to the healer," and the resultant physiological changes have healing effects. The toucher-healer "listens" with her hands as they are placed over the areas of accumulated tension in the client's body and redirects these energies. TT is effective in two distinct areas: relaxation and pain (Kreiger, 1979, p. 17).

Kreiger (1979, p. 35) lists four phases to TT.

1. Centering oneself physically and psychologically, that is, finding within oneself an inner reference of stability.
2. Exercising the natural sensitivity of the hand to assess the "energy field" of the healee for cues to differences in the quality of energy flow.
3. Mobilizing areas in the healee's energy field that the healer may perceive as being nonflowing, that is, sluggish, congested, or static.
4. The conscious direction by the healer of his or her excess body energies to assist the healee to repattern his or her own energies.

Dr. Kreiger recounts in her book, *The Therapeutic Touch. How to Use Your*

Hands to Help or Heal, of her personal experiences with many clients in implementing these four phases. Therapeutic touch is in its infancy and provides an interesting area for further exploration.

An additional use of touch is found in the "Touch for Health," which uses acupressure and acupuncture meridians as the basis for strengthening muscle groups and relief of physical tension (Thie, 1979). One of the most interesting aspects of Touch for Health is that physical and mental tension are considered as related, a key tenet of the current holistic health movement. In addition, the authors stress the importance of touch to help another person, not just to perform a procedure.

The basic concepts in Touch for Health are based on work developed by Goodheart and others in the chiropractic profession. However, they can be adopted by other helping professionals. Touch for Health training is credited for nursing continuing education units and is licensed in California.

All of these uses of touch suggest that touch is a powerful tool in empathic communication.

THERAPEUTIC COMMUNICATION SKILLS AND A PLAN OF CARE

An example of how several of the communication skills presented in this chapter can be incorporated into a specific care plan follows. The care plan presented covers only one facet of the total care plan—relating to the client's psychosocial needs and the utilization of several communication skills.

> Mrs. Smith, a 47-year-old white married woman was admitted to the orthopedic unit with a medical diagnosis of a pelvic fracture which she sustained in an auto accident. Her husband, with whom she was traveling, was killed instantly. She was placed in a pelvic sling with traction for three weeks. After this period, she began to ambulate with a walker in the physical therapy department. Because the nurse recognized that Mrs. Smith was not able to finalize her husband's death, *one* nursing diagnosis was "delayed grieving." This diagnosis was based on the following signs: "Overconcern with self and bodily functions. Cries when she leaves the room and tolerates leaving for short periods only. Minimal reference to late husband or accident. Always joking or happy appearance. States, "I hate to leave the room—when I do, I realize that I have to face the world again. In my room, I feel safe. I expect to see him walk in the door any minute!"
>
> The nurse set the following goals:

Short-term goal: To encourage client's participation in the grieving process
Long-term goal: To support client's participation in ADL and social activities directed toward independent functioning in the community.

Nursing interventions to accomplish these goals were:

1. Demonstrate a caring for the client by building a *trusting therapeutic relationship* and fulfilling a fundamental need for love. This could be accomplished over a period of time and through a *therapeutic use of self* by the nurse.
2. Encourage the client to verbalize through helping her to *share her feelings*. Increase her self-worth by letting her know her feelings are normal and OK.
3. *Actively listen* to the client through the use of *empathy* and encourage her to grieve by crying.
4. Let the client know she is not alone, especially when she leaves the room. *Use touch* in a caring way to let her know you support her.
5. Develop a sensitivity to the client and her feelings by *observing her body language* (gestures, facial expression, posture). Discuss plans for discharge only when she is ready in order to establish positive aspects and existing life-support systems.

The therapeutic use of self and the utilization of knowledge, skills, and understanding were achieved by the nurse working with Mrs. Smith in such a way that it enhanced the client's self-worth, as well as the nurse's own self-worth as a caring individual.

CONCLUSION

The development of specific skills such as the use of "I" statements, reflection, and verbal reassurance enable nurses to use their communication in a therapeutic manner. Knowledge in the use of techniques such as active listening, empathy, allowing clients to share feelings, and the use of touch facilitates the nurse's therapeutic use of self and helps to create a sense of trust in the relationship.

Therapeutic communication is a concept that can be utilized in almost any nursing interaction. Although usually considered crucial in terms of client communication, the opportunity for therapeutic communication with peers or other co-workers may arise. Being therapeutic does not mean the nurse is becoming a junior psychiatrist or psychotherapist. The nurse who is able to respond to others' feelings in a caring manner along with performing other nursing duties is essentially performing at the highest level of the profession.

Yet, therapeutic communication is not the only skill needed by nurses. Nurses need to be able to obtain information, get facts, take histories, and communicate at a content level with clients. The skills nurses use to go about gaining information from clients are the topic of the next chapter on information gathering.

BIBLIOGRAPHY

Barrett, K. A survey of the current utilization of touch by health team personnel with hospitalized patients. *International Journal of Nursing Studies,* November 9, 1972, 195–209.

Beaumont, E. (Ed.) Touch helps nurses relate to seriously ill patients. *Innovations in Nursing, Nursing* 1974, 4, August, 28.

Benjamin, A. *The helping interview* (2nd ed.). Boston: Houghton Mifflin, 1974.

Brammer, L. *The helping relationship: process and skills.* Englewood Cliffs, N.J.: Prentice-Hall, 1973.

Brill, E. & Kilts, D. *Foundations for nursing.* New York: Appleton-Century-Crofts, 1980.

Brill, N. *Working with people* (2nd ed.). Philadelphia: J.B. Lippincott, 1978.

Coad-Denton, A. Therapeutic superficiality and intimacy. In Longo, D.C. & Williams, R.G. (Eds.), *Clinical practice in psychosocial nursing: assessment and intervention.* New York: Appleton-Century-Crofts, 1978.

Ehmann, V. Empathy: its origin, characteristics, and process. *Perspectives in psychiatric care,* 1971, 9(2), 72–79.

Erikson, E. *Childhood and society.* New York: Norton, 1963.

Eriksen, K. *Communication skills for the human services.* Reston, Virginia: Reston Publishing, 1979.

Farrah, S. The nurses reported use of touch. Master's Thesis (unpublished), University of Illinois, 1979.

Forsyth, G. Exploration of empathy in nurse-client interaction. *Advances in Nursing Science,* 1979, 1(2), 53–61.

Gordon, T. *P.E.T., parent effectiveness training: the tested new way to raise responsible children.* New York: P.H. Wyden, 1970.

Kalish, B. What is empathy? *American Journal of Nursing,* 1973, 73(9), 1548–1552.

Kreiger, D. *The therapeutic touch. How to use your hands to help or to heal.* Englewood Cliffs, N.J.: Prentice-Hall, 1979.

Kreiger, D., et al. Therapeutic touch. Searching for evidence of physiological change. *American Journal of Nursing,* 1979, 79, 660.

LaMonica, E. *The nursing process: a humanistic approach.* Reading, Mass.: Addison-Wesley, 1979.

Lewis, G. *Nurse-patient communication.* (2nd ed.). Dubuque: W.C. Brown, 1973.

McCorkle, R. Effects of touch on seriously ill patients. *Nursing Research,* 1974, 23 (March-April), 125–132.

Revell, C.J. The effect of public health nurse-patient contracts in developing self-care ability. Masters Thesis (Unpublished). Case Western Reserve University, 1978.

Rogers, C.R. *On becoming a person.* Boston: Houghton Mifflin, 1961, pp. 39–40.

Rossiter, C. & Pearce, W.B. *Communicating personally.* New York: Bobbs-Merrill, 1975.

Thie, J. *Touch for health.* Marina Del Rey, Cal.: DeVorrs, 1979.

Chapter 5
Information gathering techniques

BEHAVIORAL OBJECTIVES

By reading this chapter and participating in the exercises, students will be able to:

1. Define specific effective information-gathering skills (open-ended questions, appropriate use of focused questions, use of probes, exploring "personal" habits, testing discrepancies, clarification, paraphrasing, summarization, closing)
2. Demonstrate the effective use of these skills in an interview
3. Define common pitfalls in interviews (advice giving, blaming the client, inappropriately changing the topic, defensiveness, false reassurance, judging the client, leading statements, moralizing, multiple questions, overuse of closed-ended questions, parroting, patronizing, placating, rationalizing, stumped silence, "why" questions)
4. Distinguish between effective and ineffective interviewing skills
5. Demonstrate how to transform pitfalls into effective interview skills.

THE INTERVIEW: AN ASSESSMENT TOOL

The first phase of the nursing process, the assessment phase, begins with the nursing history. The purpose of this assessment phase is to elicit as much information as possible about the client in order to identify nursing goals related to wellness and illness (Yura and Walsh, 1978). This information is collected through a specific tool, the nursing history. The communication mechanism is the interview.

This chapter presents some information-gathering techniques related to interviewing in order to enable nurses to process a large volume of information more accurately. A few examples of data to be elicited from clients during the course of an interview are: all past and present experiences with illness; how the client interprets the presenting illness; occupational and social roles, level of growth and development, and cultural patterns of daily living (Bower, 1977).

Both environmental (external) and personal (internal) factors influence the effectiveness of information-gathering techniques. External factors include the physical environment and the related sense of privacy the client feels. Distractions, interruptions, and noise affect the sense of privacy. Perhaps even more important is the attentiveness given the client by the nurse. The client should have the impression that she or he is the focus of the nurse's interest (Marriner, 1979).

Internal factors related to the nursing history include the unique personal attitudes of a particular nurse and client. The nurse displays a respect for the client not only by maintaining a high level of interest in the client, but also by acknowledging individual differences. Freedom in expression is encouraged by allowing the client to ask questions. Four concepts of an interview include accepting, observing, listening, and questioning.

The nursing history form varies depending on the specific hospital or setting (client's home, hospital, community mental health center, or outpatient clinic, for example). Each history form is designed to elicit essentially the same basic information. A type of checklist has been developed in some instances for the purpose of convenience and in the interest of time. However, in using checklists, nurses tend often to make them sound mechanical. Ideally clients should not be aware of this (Eggland, 1977). Time is a factor to consider with nursing histories, and a period that is long enough to obtain as much information as possible in an unhurried manner should be allowed. Often nurses develop a format of their own that will allow greater flexibility and adaptability for clients with a variety of problems (Yura and Walsh, 1978).

The purpose of the nursing history, to obtain information, may change during the interview. If the client expresses a need to talk or ventilate feelings,

Information Gathering Techniques ———————————————————— **111**

the nurse will shift the focus of the interview and utilize those techniques which encourage expression of feelings (see Chapter 4).

The techniques used to obtain information include:

>asking open-ended questions
>focusing
>probing
>paraphrasing
>clarifying
>testing discrepancies (confronting)
>exploring personal health-related habits (smoking, drinking, medication or drug use)
>summarizing
>closing

Asking Open-ended Questions

An open-ended question is one that gives the client a wide range of options as to how (and to what) to respond (Benjamin, 1974). Open-ended questions are quite useful at the beginning of an interview or at a point where a new topic is being introduced. They allow clients to describe an issue, a feeling, or a problem in their own words, giving as much or as little information as they wish. In some situations, such as in the emergency room or in a highly structured interview, open-ended questions may not be appropriate. However, in many other nursing situations, open-ended questions allow clients to describe their personal experience in their own words. Such questions may lead to unexpected yet pertinent information. Many nurses tend to focus too quickly on one problem or an aspect of the problem and miss other equally valuable information that the client has but does not share. An open-ended approach ameliorates the problem of focusing too quickly on one aspect of the client's functioning. On the other hand, a closed-ended question needs only a one word answer.

Examples of questions (or implied questions) that are open-ended include:

>"How are you today?"
>"How have you been?"
>"What brings you in today?"
>"How is everything going?"
>"Tell me about (your problem, your family, etc)"
>"What seems to be the problem?"

A client would have considerable leeway in how to respond to each of these questions.

Exercise 1 in Open-ended Questions

Judge each of the following questions. Is it open-ended or closed-ended? When would it be appropriate to ask?

"Is 4 o'clock a good time for us to meet?"	(closed)
"Tell me about your health history."	(open)
"Do you come here often?"	(closed)
"Is the pain in the arm or shoulder?"	(closed)
"Is your daughter well?"	(closed)
"What are you doing for the headache?"	(open)
"How have you been?"	(open)
"Doctor, do you think we should ambulate Mr. Jones?"	(closed)
"How has your daughter been?"	(open)
"Doctor, what should we do for Mr. Jones?"	(open)
"Do you take aspirin for it?"	(closed)
"When can we meet?"	(open)

Exercise 2 in Open-ended Questions

For each of the statements on the left side of the page, think of a more open-ended way to phrase the request. Some suggested alternatives are given on the right side of the page. Cover them until you have made your guess.

Nurse's Question	Open-Ended Alternative
"Where is the pain, when does it hurt, how bad is it?"	"Tell me about the pain."
"Have you been ill this week?"	"How have you been this week?"
"Do you have family, brothers, sisters?"	"Tell me about your family."
"You look blue—are you depressed?"	"You look blue—how are you feeling?"
"Did you have a good week?"	"How was your week?"

Focusing

A focused question is neither open-ended nor closed-ended but possesses characteristics of both. A focused question limits the area to which the client can

Information Gathering Techniques

respond but still encourages more than a yes or no type of answer. Open-ended questions presented earlier can be considered focused questions if used to pursue a point not covered in the preceding communication. Usually, requests for more information or history about a specific problem can be considered focused questions.

Examples of focused questions include:

> "You only mentioned your family briefly. Could you tell me more about them?"
> "Tell me about the pain in your arm?"
> "How has the foot been this week?"
> "You complained of anxiety the last time I saw you. How has it been since then?"

Exercise in Open-ended and Focused Questions

1. Form into groups of three. One person will be *A*, one *B*, and one *C*.
2. *A* will pretend to be a client at home. *B* will be a community health nurse. *C* will observe.
3. *B* will begin the dialogue with open-ended questions followed by a few focused questions.
4. At the end of a minute or two, *C* will tell *B* how *B* did.
5. Switch roles until each person has had a chance to take on the three roles.
6. Discuss how focused questions helped the nurse address the issues at hand.

Probing

A probe is any question or statement used to pursue further detail about an area. Thus, focused questions also constitute a beginning probe. Any other phrase, question, or remark the nurse makes to gain further information on the same topic is a probe. Probes can be open-ended, focused, or closed-ended. Some standard probes include:

> "Tell me more."
> "Can you tell me more?"
> "Is there anything you left out?"
> "How do you feel about that?"
> "And..."
> "Um-humm" (followed by silence)

Probes have to be handled carefully, so they do not seem to be an invasion of the client's sense of privacy. It takes a great deal of practice and sensitivity to be able to determine how far and how much to probe. If you see the client tensing up or hear defensiveness in the client's voice, it may be time to reflect or leave the probe until the client is more relaxed.

Exercise in Probes

1. Pair up. One partner will be *A*, the other *B*.
2. *A* will give *B* a few sentences about an imaginary health or psychosocial problem.
3. *B* then responds with a probe.
4. *A* then answers the probe. After the answer, *A* will tell *B* how the probe felt, how it could have been improved, etc.
5. Switch roles. This exercise is worth doing several times.
6. Discuss the reasons for and against pursuing (probing) issues that are discomforting for the client.

Paraphrasing

Another important skill in interviewing is the ability to paraphrase. Paraphrasing is giving back the client's meaning of a phrase or sentence in your own words (Beckell and Smith, 1975). Paraphrasing is similar to reflection in that it is focused on the client's inner process. The major difference is that while reflection attends to feelings, paraphrasing attempts to capture the meaning of what is communicated, be it cognitive or affective.

By using your own words, you are accomplishing two important tasks. First, you are translating the client's words into your own thoughts. Second, you are checking out the translation with the client. This gives the client the opportunity to verify your "translation" and to think further about the matter at hand.

One question that continually arises about paraphrasing is, "How much do I change the words around?" Unfortunately, there is no hard and fast answer. A partial guideline lies in the answer to the following question: "How can I rephrase this so it is in *my* own words?" The answer to this question will vary depending on the nurse, the client, and the context, which are, after all, the three parts of any communication (Satir, 1972).

An example of paraphrasing occurs in the following interaction:

CLIENT: I've had the arthritis for a long time but it doesn't seem to get any worse.

NURSE: So, although you've had it quite a while, it's about the same?

Notice that the nurse rephrases "doesn't seem to get any worse" to "it's about the same," which is a reasonable choice. If the rephrasing had been "it's

Information Gathering Techniques — 115

probably better" or "it's hard to tell if it changes," it would not have been a good paraphrase, *even if the client agreed,* because the nurse expanded the client's meaning. Paraphrasing thus becomes a tool to be used carefully because it can be used to enhance or distort the client's meaning.

As is the case for other skills covered in this chapter, one becomes a good "paraphraser" by practicing paraphrasing. The following two exercises are good starting points.

Exercise 1 in Paraphrasing

For each of the following statements on the left side of the page, think of how you would paraphrase it. That is, how would you say it in your own words without changing the meaning? On the right side of the page are two possible ways of paraphrasing the statement—one acceptable, the other not. Cover them until you have thought of your own.

Client's Statement	*Nurse's Paraphrase*
"I'm originally from California, but I've lived in Florida most of my life."	*Acceptable:* "You're originally from the West and have lived in the South."
	Not acceptable: "You've moved around a great deal; is that unsettling?"
"The doctor told me to take one pill three times a day until the pills ran out, but I felt better the next day and stopped."	*Acceptable:* "Although the doctor told you to take all the medication, you stopped when you felt better."
	Not acceptable: "You did not understand the doctor."
"My child has a 100-degree temperature and has been coughing. What should I do?"	*Acceptable:* "You need some help on what to do about your child's fever and coughing."
	Not acceptable: "That sounds like flu. Don't worry about it."
"I haven't been sleeping well. I get up every morning at 3 A.M. and stay awake looking at the ceiling."	*Acceptable:* "You've been having trouble sleeping, especially in the morning."
	Not acceptable: "Sounds like you're depressed."
"I don't believe all this garbage about smoking. I've smoked a pack a day for 35 years with no problems."	*Acceptable:* "You're not convinced about the dangers of smoking because they haven't affected you."
	Not acceptable: "You won't believe that smoking is dangerous until you have a heart attack!"

"I'd like to lose weight, but you know, the holidays are coming up."

Acceptable: "You think this is a tough time of year for you to lose the weight you want to."
Not acceptable: "You don't have the will power, that's all."

"Nobody in this place gives a damn about you unless you're a private patient."

Acceptable: "Sounds like you feel you're not being treated like a person here."
Not acceptable: "So you think that getting state aid is accepting charity?"

Notice that many of the possible responses by the nurse begin with the word "you." This might seem to be a paradox in light of the discussion in Chapter 4 about the use of "I" statements. A more linguistically correct way to phrase them would be "I think that you...." If this method works for you, use it. Many professionals will use the "you" beginning, assuming that by careful paraphrasing, gestures, facial expression, and voice tone, they will convey the covert message that they are staying with the client's meaning as opposed to judging or interpreting the behavior or words.

Exercise 2 in Paraphrasing
---

1. Pair up. One partner will be *A*, the other *B*.
2. Have a discussion about the "highlights of your last week" for five minutes using the following rules:
    a. *A* makes a statement (one or two sentences).
    b. *B* has to *paraphrase A*'s statement before responding to it.
    c. *A* has to *paraphrase B*'s response before giving *A*'s next response.
3. Discuss the exercise in a large group using the following questions as guides:
    a. How much "work" is it to paraphrase?
    b. When is paraphrasing *appropriate* in nursing communication?
    c. When is paraphrasing *inappropriate* in nursing communication?
    d. Did anyone get so absorbed in the paraphrasing that they forgot what they were going to say next?

Clarifying

Often, a client will say or do something in the course of an interview that the nurse does not understand. When this occurs, there is an immediate question of judgment that has to be answered: "Do I need to understand this now?" If

Information Gathering Techniques

the answer is that you do, then a request for clarification is appropriate. Other choices can include requesting clarification later on (especially if the client is quite upset and not listening too well) or in a subsequent interview.

If the request for clarification is presented with warmth and empathy, it is likely to be perceived by the client as a sign of interest and an honest attempt to create understanding. It also "models" asking for clarification, and hopefully the client can use the same skill with the interviewer.

There are many ways to request clarification. Some examples include:

"I'm not sure I understood that completely. Could you repeat it?"
"I missed the last few words you said."
"I don't follow you. Can you say it another way?"

Exercise in Clarification

1. Pair up. One partner will be *A*, the other *B*.
2. *B* will be the client, *A* the nurse. *B* will think of a confusing sentence to say to *A*, such as:
   "Things are so nice here, I feel so terrible."
   "So you're the nurse who doesn't like me."
   The idea is to confuse *A*.
3. *A* will respond by asking for clarification.
4. Repeat this two times and then switch roles. If you are having trouble thinking of confusing statements, think about all the confusing things that have been said to you in the last week. You should have no problem finding one that fits the nurse-client setting.
5. In the large group, share your experiences from the pairs, including the "most confusing statements" and listing all the ways members of your group seek clarification.

Testing Discrepancies

In many interviews, there will be information, feelings, explanations, and even body language expressed by the client that are not consistent. For example, a male client with tears in his eyes may deny his feelings by saying, "I feel fine." Or, an older client in a nursing home might at one point tell you that the family visits every day and then later complain of feeling lonely. Neither of these instances is congruent; that is, the messages do not make sense when put together. The question then is, "What do I, the nurse, do about this?"

Discrepancies such as the ones given above can be categorized into two groups: "Incongruity of message" and "conflict of information." Incongruity of message refers to an inconsistency between the words, tone, gestures, and body language of the client in a single message. Conflict of information means that the data presented by the client at one moment in time differs from that presented at another.

When the nurse notes a discrepancy, a decision has to be made about what to do. There are basically three choices: ignore it, explore it, or note it for further probing at a later time. Assuming that the choice has been made to explore the discrepancy, a suggested guideline is to empathically present the client with a verbal summary of the discrepancy and ask the client to "put it together." This allows the nurse to be nonjudgmental, to obtain the client's understanding of his or her own discrepancies, and to gain insight into the client's thinking processes. The following exercise should help you begin to develop strategies for exploring discrepancies in your client's behavior.

Exercise in Testing Discrepancies

For each of the situations on the left side of the page, think of a way you could verbally explore the discrepancy with the client. Suggested answers are on the right side of the page. Cover them until you have thought of your answers.

Client's Discrepancy	*Nurse's Response*
A client sits in a health clinic, eyes wandering and generally distracted. When asked how he feels, he says, "Just fine."	"You say you're just fine, but your eyes and body seem tense. I'm confused about how you really feel." (use of "I" statement)
An older person gives you two different numbers on the same street as his address.	"You just gave me another number a few minutes ago. Can you remember which is the right one?"
A mother complains about her child's behavior with a slight grin on her face.	"I'm sure you're upset, and I notice you smiling at the same time. How does that fit?"
A hospitalized client says how the family always visits. Later the client admits to feeling lonely "all of the time."	"You say you're lonely all of the time. Before you told me that the family visits. How do you make sense out of that?"
A client claims to never get drunk, yet complains of blackouts, poor attendance at work, and bad headaches in the morning.	"To what do you attribute the blackouts and the problems at work?"

These situations are not easy ones. Yet, they are common. After you have finished the exercise, discuss the following related questions in a large group.

Information Gathering Techniques ——————————————————— **119**

1. How can you approach an older person about a memory problem with respect and a professional attitude?
2. How much can you challenge an alcoholic or a mother who gives conflicting messages to children *without losing the client* (important for community health work).
3. If you explore the discrepancy and the client cannot "explain" it, what can you do? Do you have to do anything?

Exploring Personal Health-Related Habits

One area of interviewing that gives many new nurses difficulty is asking questions about "personal" information. Personal information includes areas which the culture considers private, taboo, or not to be discussed openly. In health settings, "loaded" topics that need to be discussed include alcohol consumption, smoking, drug usage, and sexual functioning.

The aspect of these topics that distinguishes them from other areas that might create anxiety for a client is that the nurse may feel that even broaching the area is an invasion of privacy, given the cultural taboos. The nurse may therefore gloss over these areas, not probe effectively, or fail to reflect feelings, even though the topic may be one in which the client needs the most help. The nurse needs to be as comfortable as possible in discussing these areas, being able to put aside personal feelings so as to be capable of responding empathically to the client while at the same time obtaining the needed information. It is helpful for some nurses to realize that these areas are being discussed in a professional, confidential setting for the benefit of the client. To ignore or obtain inadequate information in these areas could have detrimental effects for the client and thus be a disservice rather than a sign of respect for the client's privacy.

Keeping these thoughts in mind, an initial criterion for approaching these areas during an interview is that a sense of trust and respect should have been developed between the nurse and client using the information given in the previous chapter. It would be most awkward, for example, to start an interview by immediately getting into serious health concerns without any "warm-up" or relationship building, even if the relationship aspects last only a few moments.

Assuming an atmosphere of trust has been established, how does one raise the issue of drinking, smoking, sex, and drug use? As noted, these can be sensitive areas. The manner in which the issue is raised is as important as the way in which the questions or requests are phrased. Several of the authors referred to in this book (e.g., Rogers, Satir) imply that the nurse convey (by manner, posture, voice tone, breathing rate, facial expression, and rate of speech) that anything the client says or does in response to these questions is

OK. A sense of unconditional acceptance for the client will yield much more useful information in these areas than a stern, judgmental, anxious, or moralizing manner.

In a sense, once an atmosphere of trust and acceptance has been established, asking questions about sex, smoking, drinking, and drug use is like talking about any other topic. Open-ended or focused questions can be used to begin, followed by probes, requests for clarification, and summation. A healthy dose of verbal and nonverbal reassurance is quite useful, since many clients will be struggling to find the words to describe private and occasionally frightening experiences.

In addition, the following focused/closed-ended questions can be useful as lead-in statements to personal areas of functioning:

Drinking: "Do you ever take a drink?"
Smoking: "Do you smoke?"
Drugs: "Have you ever used drugs?"
   "What medication do you take?"
Sex (for adolescents): "Do you have a boy/girl friend? How do you spend your time together?"
(for adults): "How do you and your (partner, wife, husband, etc.) spend your time together? What's the nature of your sexual relationship?"

After any of the lead-ins, watching and listening carefully to the client's response allow the nurse to quickly evaluate the direction in which the interview should proceed: more information (probes, focused questions), empathy (reflection, verbal/nonverbal reassurance), or temporarily leaving the topic. In choosing the latter case, a comment by the nurse about the situation (meta-comment) is reassuring, such as "I see that this is uncomfortable for you. Should we come back to this later?"

Exercise 1 in Interviewing about Personal Issues

Below is part of a hypothetical dialogue between a nurse and client. Assume they have been talking for 10 minutes at a high school health clinic. The client is a 16-year-old girl. After each statement by the client, think about what you would say or do. Then read the nurse's response and the type of skill/questioning procedure used. Are there any options that are better than the ones suggested?

CLIENT: So that's why I came in. I'm having trouble sleeping and wondered if you could get me anything for it?
NURSE: Um-hmm, could you tell me about your social life? (Lead-in)
CLIENT (looks down, fidgets, blushes): Well, I haven't gone out too much with guys, if that's what you mean.
NURSE: And? (Tone of voice reassures; "and" serves as a *gentle* probe.)

Information Gathering Techniques — **121**

CLIENT: Well, there's this one guy I met at a basketball game a few months ago from another school.
NURSE: Sounds like you liked him. (Reflects)
CLIENT: I did, but we went out a few times without my parents' knowing about it; then they found out and wouldn't let me see him again. They said he's the "wrong type for me."
NURSE: How did you spend your time together? (Focuses, leads in)
CLIENT: We went to a few parties, drank a little. You know.
NURSE: Do you remember how much you drank at the parties? (Probe)
CLIENT: Oh—you mean did I get drunk? (Giggles) Well, once I drank two beers and felt, you know, light-headed, but that was it.
NURSE: Have you been drinking since then? (Probe)
CLIENT: No, I really didn't like it.
NURSE: Were there any drugs at the parties? (Said in empathetic, understanding, professional tone. Lead-in)
CLIENT: Are you gonna tell?
NURSE: I'm concerned primarily with you right now (Reassures). What I do with the information depends on what it is.
CLIENT: Well, one night a couple of kids were passing a cigarette around—like I'm not sure, but it *could* have been a joint.
NURSE: Did you try it? (Probe)
CLIENT (agitated): Just don't tell my folks any of this. They'd kill me.
NURSE: You seem scared of your parents. (Reflects and changes focus)
CLIENT: It's terrible. Whenever I come home, I get the third-degree. "Where'd you go, what did you do, with whom, be careful"—it's awful.
NURSE: Are you doing anything with your boyfriend that they would be concerned about? (Lead-in)
CLIENT: Like what?
NURSE: Are you sexually involved? (Probe)
CLIENT: Oh, that. No, I mean we kissed and all that, and they would be concerned about that, believe you me.
NURSE: Although I'm not sure about your own use of drugs, I know you've drunk a little, you're not sexually involved with your boyfriend, but you're having some hassles with your parents. (Summarizes) Is that right?
CLIENT: That's it, but I don't use drugs, I don't even smoke. Just please don't tell my folks I've been at a party where there were drugs. They'd *kill* me.

After you have read and thought through the scenario, discuss the following questions:
1. How much probing was appropriate?
2. Could you, as a nurse, do this sort of interview keeping your personal values separate from your professional role?
3. How could you have given reassurance without "taking sides" on the issues?
4. Of all these issues (sex, drugs, alcohol), which are easiest for you to discuss? Can you think of ways to begin to make the difficult areas easier for you to handle with clients?

Exercise 2 in Interviewing about Personal Issues

1. Form into groups of three. One person will be *A*, one *B*, and one *C*.
2. *A* will be a client at a health screening clinic. *B* will be the interviewer. Pretend you have been talking a few minutes, have developed rapport, etc. *B* will then do a lead-in (focused or open-ended question) and probe for each of the following topics:
   a. Smoking
   b. Drinking
   c. Medication
   d. Drugs
   e. Sexual activity
3. At the end of these questions, *C* (who should have observed the communication) will comment on how *B* did, that is, how the questions sounded, did *B* seem relaxed, what gestures were used, and what was the body language? *A* will also comment on how it felt to be asked the questions by *B*.
4. Switch roles so each person gets to be the client, the interviewer, and the observer.

Summarizing

At the end of an interview or at a logical breaking point in an interview, many effective nurse communicators find it useful to summarize what the client has said. Summarizing means verbally capturing the essence of what the client presented, including pertinent facts, feelings, discrepancies and untouched areas (Brammer, 1973). Consider the following example:

> A nurse has been talking with a 46-year-old male who is getting ready for hospital discharge following a heart attack. The discussion has included a review of his recovery plan, including exercise and diet, as well as his perceptions of the family's response to his illness. He has also voiced concerns about his sexual functioning to the nurse, but not to his wife and has openly wondered about what the effect of all of this will be on his work as a vice-president of an advertising agency.
>
> One way of briefly summarizing all of this is as follows:
>
> "Let me see if I have everything we talked about. We have reviewed your recovery plans and your family's reaction to the heart attack. You still have some concerns about its effects on your work at the advertising agency and on your sexual relationship with your wife, although you have not yet discussed this with her. Is there anything else?"

The purpose of summarization is threefold. First, it forces you, the nurse, to pull pieces of the interview together for future recording. Second, the client has a sense that the nurse has understood what has been said, which is a good rapport-building experience. Third, the client has a chance to review the information and add any missing pieces. Many clients wait until the last

Information Gathering Techniques

minute to give nurses the most important information (e.g. "By the way, I've been having slight chest pain," in the type of case presented above). Summarization makes a logical place for this information to emerge.

The following exercise is one way to begin thinking about summarization.

Exercise in Summarizing

For each of the "case notes" on the left side of the page, figure out how you could summarize the "interview" in one or two sentences. A suggested summary is given on the right side of the page. Cover it until you have figured out your own.

Cases	Summary
1. A female client came to a health clinic upset over migraine headaches. She had gone to three doctors over the last two years who "do nothing." The client had just been fired from a job she needed to support two children. At the time, she smoked two packs of cigarettes a day.	As I understand it, you have had migraine headaches for a while, but the physicians you have seen have not helped. You also have to support your two children and currently have no job.
2. An elderly man's blood pressure was found to be elevated at a health screening clinic. He said he had medicine but did not take it because he felt OK. He hadn't been to a doctor in a year.	Your blood pressure is high. You've had it before but don't take the medicine because you feel all right. You haven't recently checked with your physician.
3. A postoperative phlebitis client feels tired but hopeful of fast recovery. Her husband has not been in to see her, and she expresses worry over where he is.	From what you've said, you're still feeling the aftereffects of the operation. You would like to get on your feet soon and are concerned that your husband has not been in to visit you in the hospital.

Closing

Along with summarizing at the end of the interview, the nurse should give the client a sense that the time has come for the interview to end. This is important when the interview is time-bound; for example, when there are usually other clients waiting, closure should be done smoothly so the client feels finished as opposed to cut off.

One way of doing this includes acknowledging the end of the interview and the time spent with the client, as in, "Well, I see our time is nearly up. It's been really nice talking with you today." Other statements that could be made are:

> "I have to finish in a minute."
> "We need to wrap up now."
> "That's about all the time I have—would you like another appointment?"

PITFALLS OF INTERVIEWING: COMMON WAYS OF HINDERING COMMUNICATION

Up to this point, the focus of this chapter has been on effective strategies, tools, and techniques with which the nurse can perform a successful interview. "Effective" suggests that the way in which the communication is given is respectful of the client and nurse's self-worth, that the content message is clear, that the communication promotes trust and that the client has a maximum opportunity to express his or her own feelings or views without being overly influenced by the nurse.

The aspects of effective interviewing mentioned earlier in this chapter meet all of these requirements. The "Pitfalls" enumerated below do not.

Pitfalls in communication are strategies, styles, or techniques that are nontherapeutic; they create distrust and restrict the response of the client. Nontherapeutic communication leads to decreased self-worth of either the client or nurse.

We all use nontherapeutic techniques at various times when we communicate with others. An awareness of our use of these pitfalls is the first step toward more effective communication interaction with clients. Sixteen pitfalls are presented in alphabetical order in this section; and although there is overlap between some pitfalls, each will be discussed separately [many of these are also discussed in Brammer (1973) and Benjamin (1974)]:

1. Advice giving
2. Blaming the client
3. Changing the topic inappropriately
4. Defensiveness
5. False reassurance
6. Judging the client
7. Leading statements
8. Moralizing
9. Multiple questions
10. Overuse of closed-ended questions

Information Gathering Techniques

11. Parroting (instead of reflection)
12. Patronizing the client
13. Placating the client
14. Rationalizing feelings
15. Stumped Silence
16. "Why" questions

Pitfall 1—Giving Advice

Giving advice on advice giving is relatively simple: *don't!* There are several reasons for limiting advice giving in a clinical setting. The first is that the advice generally will not be taken. The second is that if the client "takes it to heart," the nurse who gave the advice may be blamed if anything goes wrong. And the third reason is that clients are likely to misinterpret the advice and not follow it carefully.

What exactly is advice? The dictionary defines it as an opinion. When clients ask nurses for an opinion or advice about what to do, the nurse may well (inadvertently) set him- or herself up to take inappropriate responsibility for clients' decisions. If it is a question of an "informal nursing opinion," nurses can use the tactic of giving clients information and exploring options as opposed to giving advice. The client is viewed as an active participant in the health process; for this reason the giving of advice is not advocated.

The following statements on the left side of the page represent advice. Some nonadvice ways of rephrasing the statements are on the right.

Advice	Preferred
"If you want my opinion, I think you should..." (in situation where client has two choices).	"What are the pros and cons of each choice for you?"
"You've just got to try harder, that's all."	"What is holding you back?"
"Anyone can see that the way to discipline is...."	"What are some ways you could try to discipline the child?"
"Generic drugs are better than brand names."	"Do you know the difference between generic and brand name drugs?"
"My advice is—go on a diet."	"How can you lose the weight you need to?"

There is also occasionally a context in which it is appropriate for nurses to make suggestions. When this happens, ideally the suggestion should be presented as another option clients can consider along with any others. It can sometimes be difficult for nurses to allow clients maximum responsibility for their own choices because nurses' power as authorities in the clinical context may influence those choices.

Pitfall 2—Blaming the Client

Blaming was presented in Chapter 3 as an ineffective communication style. Blame carries with it decreased self-regard for the client who is directly or indirectly being told "It's your fault." However, there is a subtle but important distinction between blame and responsibility.

Clients can be responsible for many aspects of their own health and well-being. They can be educated as to how certain aspects of their lives led up to their current state of health (eating, exercise, life style, job pressure, smoking, drinking, etc.). When the educational aspect turns into a put-down and an implied message of accusation, then the client will feel blamed and guilty and experience lowered self-worth. Along with these nontherapeutic aspects of blaming, most psychological research has demonstrated that simple punishment—for example, blaming—is not an effective way to change behavior. What often happens is that only certain patterns of behavior change; the client will stop coming to the clinic or making appointments, for example. In this way the client avoids blame and punishment.

Blame can also come under the guise of advice. There are an infinite number of ways to blame the client. Some are obvious, some not. Many are unintended. Some examples of blame are:

> "Well, you should have called earlier to make an appointment."
> "Don't you know that smoking is bad?"
> "You're supposed to eat everything on your plate."
> "Look, we told you to take your medication three times a day. What's the matter with you?"

One way to work on blaming behavior is first identifying it in ourselves and then transforming it into a message that indicates respect for ourselves as well as clients. The following exercise is a step in that direction.

Exercise in Blame Transformation

For each of the following blame statements on the left side of the page, first say it out loud and add appropriate voice and facial expression to make it blaming. Then change the statement (or the tone and expression) so it still conveys the correct content but also respects the self-worth of the client. Say this "transformation" out loud. If you cannot think of one, use the suggested transformation on the right side of the page.

Information Gathering Techniques

Blame Statement (remember to say these with appropriately blaming tone)	Transformation
"What are you doing out of bed?"	"You're supposed to be in bed. What's the problem?"
"Why haven't you been here for your last two appointments?"	"I see you missed two appointments. What happened?"
"What have you done to your child?"	"What happened to the child?"
"Why haven't you eaten your dinner?"	"You haven't eaten your dinner." (Change of voice tone is important.)
"You should have this checked immediately."	"This should be checked immediately."

Pitfall 3—Changing Topic Inappropriately

A third common pitfall in nursing communication is the inappropriate change of topic by the nurse. This is related to Satir's concept of "irrelevancy" discussed in Chapter 3. Generally, nurses change topics inappropriately more as a result of their own rising anxiety than for reasons specifically related to clients. Thus, the change of topic is inappropriate in that it is not a strategy that helps clients.

If nurses find themselves inappropriately changing topics while interviewing clients, an investigation of the following areas might help to suggest the source of their anxiety.

> The client is touching on a topic area about which the nurse feels uncomfortable (sex, emotional problems).
> The nurse is unsure of what to do and is uncomfortable just listening.
> The client is describing a problem that exists for the nurse.
> The nurse is embarrassed by what the client says.

Pitfall 4—Defensiveness

Defensiveness is a more general category than many of the other pitfalls reviewed in this chapter. As you may recall from Chapter 3, defensiveness is defined as "being hostile, aggressive, not listening, or responding as if one had been attacked." Nurses who have defensive approaches to clients usually indicate it in their words and nonverbal behavior. It is difficult, if not impossible to be empathetic, listen well, and give messages of reassurance when one is feeling defensive.

However, there are times when any nurse will feel defensive, be it triggered by something that happened at home, on the job, or during the interview. There are two schools of thought on what to do at these times. One is to finish the interview as if "nothing is the matter" and then work things through with a head nurse or supervisor.

The second school of thought is to comment on one's emotional state *briefly* to the client. This choice gives the client some understanding about how, you, the nurse, are acting, and it can model comments about feelings from the client, which can be therapeutic. Examples of how to acknowledge your own defensiveness briefly include:

"I feel somewhat uncomfortable about this topic but I am listening to you carefully."

"I want to let you know I'm upset by other things today. Please do not take my reactions as a statement about you."

There are reasons to share *and* not share one's own defensiveness with clients. The reasons for sharing include the following:

Models self-disclosure
Explains own behavior
Can build trust
Helps nurse to get over the defensiveness

The reasons for not sharing one's own defensiveness include the following:

Client could be overwhelmed
It could be taken as a sign of weakness or incompetence
The nurse could end up "being the client"
Clients can feel pressured into disclosing things they are not ready to disclose

Nurses will have to make choices as to which course of action is best in this matter, based on their own feelings, their perception of the client, and the context in which they work.

Pitfall 5—False Reassurance

One of the great temptations to any nurse is to "lighten the emotional load" of a distressed client. Ways in which an effective nurse communicator can give appropriate verbal and nonverbal reassurance have already been discussed in Chapter 4. However, there are times when, with good intentions, the nurse gives false reassurance. That is, in trying to reassure the client, the nurse promises something that may not happen, says something that is untrue, or provides comfort in an incongruent manner. Examples of the three forms of false reassurance are:

Case 1. Promising something that may not happen: "Don't worry. Everything will be all right."
Case 2. Saying something not true: "You have nothing to worry about."
Case 3. Giving incongruent comfort: "I feel for you" (when in actuality, the nurse is trying to figure out what to do next).

False reassurance may raise clients' anxiety. Rather than being reassured, the client will become suspicious and more concerned as the inconsistency in the message from the nurse is noted. By inconsistency, we mean that the nurse's message is inconsistent with the client's perception of the problem.

Exercise in Identifying and Transforming False Reassurance

For each of the following statements, decide if it is either "false" or "true" reassurance. If it is false, figure out a way to make it more congruent. Answers and suggested transformations are given on the right side of the page.

Nurse's Statement	Type of Reassurance
"I hear what you are saying. You seem to feel hopeless."	Reassurance
"Don't worry. Everything will work out for the best."	False reassurance. Transformation: "You seem worried. Is there anything I can do?"
"Look, it's not so bad. I've seen patients in worse shape than this who have gotten better."	False reassurance. Transformation: "I think you have every reason to hope for the best."
"It's OK to cry when you feel like it."	Reassurance
"There's no need to cry. It's not the end of the world, is it?"	False reassurance. Transformation: "It's OK to cry. I'll wait for you."
(Edgily) "Sure, tell me about it."	False reassurance. Transformation: "Other things are bothering me. Let me get collected. OK, what's the problem?"

Pitfall 6—Judging the Client

Judging the client incorporates any tendencies the nurse has to evaluate the client as being "good" or "bad." In general practice, more emphasis is put on negative evaluation of the client than positive evaluation. However, even positive evaluation (as opposed to *unconditional* positive regard) can have problems. For example, if nurses are in the habit of nodding their heads and saying "that's good" during an interview when they hear things they like, clients will quickly learn to tell only those things that get rewarded and they may leave out pertinent information concerning their health.

There is an important distinction that needs to be made between evaluating *behavior* and evaluating the *client*. For example, it is quite appropriate to tell a client that a self-administered procedure was done incorrectly. That is your job. However, there can be negative consequences if the message carries with it a negative judgment of the client as well. Most clients respond to "being judged" by becoming uncooperative.

A client can feel judged by seeing a raised eyebrow, a "stern" look, hearing a raised voice, or by being blamed. In all fairness, clients may feel judged even when no judgment is intended or made. However, because the client is likely to be extremely sensitive to judgment, it is important to take note of all the ways nurses can judge the client and work on developing nonjudgmental communication.

Exercise in Judging the Client

This exercise is designed to help you discover ways in which you and other nurses can come across as judgmental, as well as to give you ways to change your own judgmental communication.
1. Pair up. One partner will be *A*, one *B*.
2. *A* will read the following list of paired statements to *B*. Read the first statement in a judgmental tone, using judgmental gestures, facial expressions, etc. Be expressive and creative; then read the paired statement (which will either be reworded or remain the same) in a nonjudgmental manner.

Judgmental	Nonjudgmental
"You don't take good care of your child."	"Raising a child alone is difficult."
"I would never do that."	"What prompted you to do that?"
"You're stupid to eat sweets with your diabetes."	"I would like to talk with you about your diet."
"I see you're late for your appointment."	"I see you're late for your appointment."
"If you weren't so depressed people would like you."	"Have you ever thought that people may react to how you are feeling?"
"Your husband has no manners."	"How do you feel about your husband?"
"Hello, I'm your nurse."	"Hello, I'm your nurse."

Information Gathering Techniques

"How are you today?" "How are you today?"
3. Switch roles and do step 2 again.
4. Discuss how it felt to receive the judgmental and nonjudgmental statements.

Pitfall 7—Leading Statements

A common mistake of beginning interviewers is to "put words in the client's mouth" or make a leading statement. A leading statement is any one that indirectly makes the *interviewer's* interpretation or observation appear to be the client's. Several examples include:

"You're tired because you're depressed, right?"
"You probably forgot the appointment because you were worried about the holidays."
"It doesn't hurt too much, does it?"

The problem with a leading statement is that it does not give the client a full opportunity to decide if it is true or not, especially if the client is under stress.

Exercise in Leading Statements

Identify the effective interviewing strategies and leading statements by the nurse in the following interview. The type of statement is given on the right side of the page. Keep it covered until you have made your guesses.

CLIENT: Well, I just do not know how my husband will adjust to me recovering from this stroke. He spends time with me—but doesn't say much. I don't know what he's thinking.	
NURSE: You say you're not sure about your husand's reaction.	Paraphrase
You seem concerned.	Reflection
How long has he been upset?	Leading
CLIENT: Well, I had the stroke two months ago. He had to work and I was in no shape to talk, if you catch my drift. My arm still feels stiff. Anyway, he started to spend time with me one month ago.	

NURSE: I can understand how you and he don't know if you're ever going to get better.
What brought about the change in his behavior?

Leading ("Know if you're *ever* going to get better")

Probe

You will notice that the client does not necessarily respond directly to the leading statements. Also, the second leading statement, which was an attempt to reflect, could serve to plant or exaggerate an unsurfaced fear the client has. The way it is presented makes it difficult for the client to verbalize her own fears.

Pitfall 8—Moralizing

Moralizing is a specific form of judging the client. While there is no exercise on moralizing presented here, it is worthy of comment. Moralizing refers to any instance in which nurses judge clients based on their own personal values. Examples of moralizing statements include:

"How can you smoke at your age?"
"Why do you eat sugar when you are overweight?"
"Abortion is sinful"
"Abortion is OK for everyone."

A good question for discussion is: "How can I be an effective nurse with someone whose values differ significantly from mine on the issue at hand?"

Pitfall 9—Multiple Questions

A less emotionally charged pitfall is use of multiple questions. Multiple questions are really a series of questions that are asked as if they were one question. For example:

"Did you forget the appointment or did you have something else or did you call and the line was busy?"
"Where do you live—is it an apartment and what is your neighborhood like?"

Multiple questions are difficult to answer. Clients, especially when distressed, can easily get confused as to which question should be answered first. Many multiple questions get asked because the nurse is somewhat anxious and does not give the client adequate time to think of a response (Benjamin, 1974). The nurse assumes that the client is having a problem figuring out the question,

Information Gathering Techniques

and, without checking it out, asks another question (or two). The result can be confusing.

Any multiple question can be broken down into separate single questions that can then be posed to the client. In other words, nurses can ask one question at a time and wait for the client to respond before rephrasing or asking another question.

Exercise in Multiple-Question Transformation

Transform each of the multiple questions on the left side of the page into separate questions. Make the initial one open-ended. A suggested breakdown is given on the right side of the page. Keep it covered until you have made your choice as to how to separate the questions.

Multiple Question	Transformation
"Did you sleep well, enjoy breakfast, and have a good morning?"	"How was last night?" (Wait) "How was breakfast?" (Wait) "How has the morning been?" (Wait)
"Tell me about your family, your work, your hobbies so I can get to know you."	"Tell me about your family." (Wait) "Can you tell me about your work?" (Wait) "What kind of hobbies do you have?" (Wait)
"What caused the problem? Was it stress, diet, exercise or something you ate?" (This is also a leading question.)	"How did the problem come about?" (Note: Only one question is necessary here.)

Pitfall 10—Overuse of Closed-ended Questions

As mentioned earlier, closed-ended questions elicit one or two word responses. Obviously, there are certain closed-ended questions that are appropriate, such as requests for specific information (name, address, names of medication, etc.). However, these direct questions can be overused when the purpose of the communication is to open up a new area or probe further into a relatively unexplored one.

For example, a nurse who wants to explore an older person's drug use and "chooses" to use direct-closed-ended questions will come out with a series of questions such as the following:

Nurse	Client
"Do you take any medication?"	"Yes."
"Are any prescribed?"	"Yes."
"Do you have some for your heart?"	"Yes."
"For your blood pressure?"	"Yes."
"Do you take a laxative?"	"Sometimes."
"Does it work?"	"Sometimes."
"What is it?"	"Why are you asking me all these questions?"

By overusing closed-ended questions, the nurse becomes an interrogator, puts the client on the defensive, and has to do most of the talking. Except in the case where there is a checklist of items to be asked, open-ended questions, such as, "Tell me about your medication," followed by *appropriate* focused and occasional closed-end probes can be a more effective approach.

Exercise in Closed-ended Questions

Change each series of closed-ended questions on the left side of the page to a more general open-ended question. A suggested answer is on the right side of the page. Keep it covered until you have thought of your answer.

Closed Questions	*Open Question*
Series 1	
"Do you live in a house?"	Tell me about your living arrangements.
"By yourself?"	
"Do you have pets?"	
"What kind?"	
"How many rooms?"	
Series 2	
"Where is the pain?"	Tell me as much about the pain as you can.
"How much does it hurt?"	
"Does it hurt at night?"	
"By day?"	
"How did it start?"	
Series 3	
"Do you have brothers, sisters?"	I'd like to know about your family.
"Are you married, how long?"	
"Is your relationship with your spouse good?"	
"Do you have children?"	

Information Gathering Techniques 135

Series 4
"Do you eat a good breakfast?"
"How much coffee, tea do you drink?"
"Do you eat dessert? Which ones?"
"Do you eat a balanced diet?"

What kinds of food do you eat in a normal day?

Pitfall 11—Parroting

"Parroting" refers to the continual repetition of parts of the client's phrases as an attempt to reflect or paraphrase. While occasional repetition of portions of the phrases is effective in highlighting aspects the nurse would like the client to pursue, the overuse of this technique makes the nurse seem like a parrot, mechanically repeating whatever is said.

The following dialogue shows how parroting is used. Reflective statements are included in parentheses:

Client	Nurse
"I'm concerned about my son."	"You're concerned about your son." (Reflect: "You seem upset.")
"He seems to be losing weight."	"He's losing weight."
"He stays out all night."	"He stays out." (Reflect: "You're concerned.")
"He has tremors and I don't know what to do about him."	"You don't know what to do." (Reflect: "You feel unsure about what to do.")

Pitfall 12—Patronizing the Client

Often, nurses and other health professionals talk to elderly clients and children in an overly kind manner, as if the client needed to be "talked down to" or put on a lower level than the helper or nurse. It is not so much a matter of words but how the words are said that gives the impression that clients are being treated as if they were less than human. The words and voice tones are not hostile; they are, if anything, too sweet.

Patronizing the client refers to any and all ways the client is talked down to while being comforted. Several communication patterns that go along with patronizing the client include the nurse's keeping his or her eye level higher than that of the client (for example, standing while the client is sitting), talking in a sing-song voice, using "we" when either "you" or "I" is meant, and using (for lack of a better term) "baby talk" words, phrases, or voice tone.

The results of patronization are lowered self-worth and increased dependence (or anger) by the client. There is no valid reason to patronize a client. Even though many health professionals who do so are doing it unintentionally, all clients deserve to be treated as equals in the interaction.

Exercise in Patronization

This exercise is designed to help you learn how you could come across when you are patronizing.
1. Pair up. One partner will be A, the other B.
2. A will say each of the three statements below and be as patronizing as possible. After each statement B will then repeat it exactly as A did, with similar voice tone, gestures and facial expressions. A will closely attend to B to find out how A came across.
    a. "How are you today?"
    b. "It's time for us to get out of bed."
    c. "Oh, you didn't eat your lunch. Is something the matter?"
3. Switch roles and repeat.
4. Discuss the following questions in the large group.
    a. Have you ever seen anyone be patronizing in a nursing context?
    b. What was the effect of it?
    c. What would have been needed to help that person change? Who should have been involved (superior, client, peers, etc.)?

Pitfall 13—Placating the Client

A pitfall that is related to being patronizing is placating. Placating is one of Satir's communication categories referred to in Chapter 3. Placating the client means that the nurse agrees with everything, takes the blame for everything, and can't say no. Placating does not mean unconditional regard for the client.

The results of placating the client include decreased self-worth for the nurse, as well as either dependence or anger on the part of the client. However, the temptation to placate can exist when it is easier to say yes to a demanding client than to say no and have to defend oneself.

For an exercise on placating, refer to the other exercises in Chapter 3.

Information Gathering Techniques — 137

Pitfall 14—Rationalizing Feelings

Rationalizing feelings means finding an apparently reasonable excuse for having the feelings. In fact, the excuse is not reasonable, it is an attempt to explain away whatever is being felt. This form of pitfall is a result of being "superreasonable" at a moment in time. Superreasonable is another of Satir's defensive communication styles. It refers to using reasons to protect the self from uncomfortable feelings.

When rationalization is used, then, the nurse is probably feeling anxious. Some examples of rationalizing phrases are:

"Oh, well, that's probably because..."
"It's not important because..."
"Everyone feels a little..."
"I misunderstood you because I thought you were done."

The problem with rationalization is that feelings and behavior are subtly dismissed (e.g., "I only did that because..."). Rationalization also eliminates some of the unpleasant truths about the motivation for behavior in an interview. However, to rationalize the avoidance of a sensitive topic clouds the reasons for discontinuing, since it may be the nurse's problem not the client's.

The following exercise is designed to help nurses begin to recognize rationalization and transform it to a more accurate statement of reality.

Exercise in Rationalization Transformation

In each of the following communications, identify the nurse's rationalization. Then, change the nurse's rationalization to a more accurate statement of feelings or observation of what is going on with the client. Suggested answers are given on the right side of the page. Cover them until you have made your own.

STATEMENT 1

CLIENT: I've never talked about this problem. I'm not sure you can help me. It's private.

NURSE: I see. I'd like to help. You probably never talked about it because you were afraid. You do not have to worry.

Rationalization: Because you were afraid.
Transformation: It's been hard for you to talk about it. (Reflection)

STATEMENT 2

CLIENT: I've gained 25 pounds with this pregnancy. I read somewhere that you should only gain 15 to 20 pounds at my weight. What should I do?

NURSE: I wouldn't worry. It was probably an uninformed opinion. What have you been eating?

Rationalization: I wouldn't worry (because it was probably an uninformed opinion).
Transformation: You seem concerned. Would you like me to find out more on this for you?

STATEMENT 3

CLIENT: So I took grandfather home from the hospital and then, one night, he began to... (voice drags off).

NURSE: I didn't hear the end. I must not have been listening.

Rationalization: (Because) I must not have been listening.
Transformation: Your voice dropped. How are you feeling? (Focused question)

Pitfall 15—Stumped Silence

A stumped silence occurs when the client and the nurse are both stuck. There is an uncomfortable feeling that nothing is going on, that the nurse is confused.

A general guide in the instance of stumped silence is to meta-comment about the confusion. That is, the nurse can comment about being confused, which can then lead to the client's focusing on her or his own confusion.

Examples of appropriate comments to break a stumped silence are:

> "I'm having trouble figuring out what we do next. How are you feeling?"
> "At times it's hard to know exactly what to say. Let's see if we can continue in a few seconds."

Another option is to meta-comment and briefly summarize what took place:

> "I'm not sure where to go. Let's see, we were talking about ___, you said ___, and I said ___ just before we stopped. Do you have anything to add?"

Pitfall 16—"Why" Questions

One of the great temptations when a client says virtually anything is to respond "Why did you say that?" The problem with "why" questions is that they imply that clients should come up with the underlying motivation of their actions or

Information Gathering Techniques 139

feelings, which is not what the nurse usually wants. In addition, many clients will feel that the nurse knows why and is testing them. They then get into guessing what the nurse thinks rather than examining their own motivation. "Why" questions can also easily be asked or perceived as accusatory (Benjamin, 1974). For example:

"Why do you feel that way?"
"Why is the bandage off?"
"Why were you late?"

Almost any question can be rephrased as a less accusatory and more accurate statement. In the first of the examples given above, the nurse may really be asking for more information about the client's thoughts. A more accurate question would be, "What are some of the thoughts behind that feeling?" or more simply, "Tell me more about it." The second example could have been rephrased: "What happened to the bandage?" And the third could have been stated as, "You were late. What happened?" As a general guide, avoid "why" questions when interviewing clients.

Exercise in Transforming Why Questions

Change each of the following "why" questions on the left side of the page to another statement that gets to the same information. Suggested answers are given on the right right of the page. Cover them until you have made your guess.

Why Question	Transformation
"Why didn't you take your medication?"	"You didn't take your medication." "What happened?"
"Why do you feel anxious?"	"Tell me more about your anxiousness."
"Why are you depressed?"	"What's been going on?"
"Why do you think the clinic's bad?"	"What has happened to make you think the clinic's bad?"
"Why didn't you tell the doctor what you felt?"	"What prevented you from talking to the doctor?"
"Why aren't you happy about your new baby?"	"Tell me more about it."

INTEGRATING THE SKILLS WITH AVOIDANCE OF PITFALLS—AN EXERCISE

The following script of an interview has many examples of therapeutic and information-gathering skills, as well as a good number of pitfalls. As you read the script, identify each skill or strategy. When you find a pitfall, think about how it could be changed to promote increased self-regard and clearer communication.

A set of categorizations is provided with transformations of pitfalls on the right side of the page. Cover them until you have made your own choices. You may also want to use this method of interview analysis for analyzing role playing and taped interviews with clients. With practice, you will become adept at identifying your strengths and weaknesses as an interviewer and will, hopefully, attempt to correct ineffective techniques.

The Interview

The client, Mrs. C., is a home-bound senior citizen. She has arthritis, is recovering from a broken hip, and uses a walker. The purpose of the interview is a regularly scheduled check on her living situation and morale.

	Response Type
NURSE (Pulls chair over so the two are three feet apart and sitting):	Attends to seating
Hello Mrs. C., how have you been for the last week?	Open-ended question
MRS. C.: So-so. You know. (Sighs)	
NURSE: You sighed just then, but said "so-so." How are you feeling?	Shares discrepancy, focused question on feelings
MRS. C.: I don't know, I just don't have any energy.	
NURSE: You have no energy?	Probes
MRS. C.: I just seem tired today.	
NURSE: Don't worry. It's probably the time of day. What did you do last week?	False reassurance, inappropriate change of topic. Transformation: You look tired. What's going on?
MRS. C.: Well, I saw you on Tuesday. Wednesday I didn't do much at all, just watched TV.	
NURSE: Um-hmm.	Non-verbal reassurance
MRS. C.: Thursday that lady, the physical therapist, came. She made	

Information Gathering Techniques

me do all these exercises. (laughs) I thought I was in the gym.

NURSE: Does she work you too hard or have you do difficult things? — Multiple question. Transformation: What does she have you do?

MRS. C.: I don't know. I've never seen anyone do the things the way she does them.

NURSE (Waits silently) — Use of silence

MRS. C.: How long will she be coming to see me. Why does she even bother?

NURSE: How do you mean "why does she bother?" — Probe, request for clarification

MRS. C.: It's just that. (Sighs) I don't know, I just think I'm never going to (starts to cry, voice softens) get better. I'm so embarrassed.

NURSE: There, there, you'll feel better in a while. (Waits) — False reassurance. Transformation: It's OK to cry. Use of silence

MRS. C. (Continues to cry, stops. Neither speaks, both look uncomfortable) — Stumped silence

NURSE: Tell me, Mrs. Clark, what were you thinking just now? — Probe

MRS. C.: I was thinking about how I used to go to the community center before I fell. It was very nice there.

NURSE (Nods head) — Nonverbal reassurance

MRS. C.: I was just wondering what they were doing there this week.

NURSE: You'd like to be able to find out what's going on? — Paraphrases

MRS. C.: Um-hmm, I miss it. I have all of my friends there. There was even a special gentleman friend.

NURSE: What was your relationship like with him? — Lead-in to "personal" area

MRS. C.: We used to see each other a lot. He'd even come and visit me here on weekends.

NURSE: Did you have meals here together?

MRS. C.: Yes, occasionally.

NURSE: Did he visit every weekend?   Starts to use too many closed-ended questions. Transformation: Tell me about your relationship with the gentleman.

NURSE: Have you seen him since you were in the hospital?

MRS. C.: Only once.

NURSE: Why hasn't he come?   Why question. Transformation: What do you think his reasons are for not coming?

MRS. C.: I don't know.

NURSE: Well, I think you should call the center and find out.   Advice giving. Transformation: Have you considered calling to find out if he's OK?

MRS. C.: No, I couldn't do that.

NURSE: OK, it was just a suggestion.   Defensiveness. Transformation: Umhm.

MRS. C.: I just don't know what to do.

NURSE: About what?   Probe, Clarification

MRS. C.: Can you really help me?

NURSE: I'll try my best.   Reassurance

MRS. C.: Well, we were—we had been talking about living together like man and wife, but without getting married.

NURSE: You mean you'd do that without getting married?   Moralizing, judging Transformation: What would prompt that choice?

MRS. C.: We'd have to. Our social security checks would be cut if we were married. We can barely get by on the two checks as they are now.

NURSE: I see, you need both checks to get by.   Paraphrases

MRS. C.: Right, only I haven't heard from him and I'm very worried.	
NURSE: Is there anything I could do?	Focused question
MRS. C.: Could you call the center and see if he's OK? I just can't bring myself to do it.	
NURSE: Sure. I'll let you know in two days what I find out. Other than this, how is everything else?	
MRS. C.: Fine, I can't complain. I take my blood pressure pills. The arthritis bothers me a little bit, but no more than it usually does.	
NURSE: Good, I'm glad to hear it.	Reassurance
Let me be sure I have everything straight before I go. Everything is going along OK as far as your recovery goes. You're working with the physical therapist. You're taking your blood pressure pills. Your arthritis bothers you a little, but no more than usual. Your main concern is your gentleman friend.	
You haven't seen him and would like me to call the center to find out if he's OK. I'll get back to you in two days with the information.	Summarizes, closes
Did I leave anything out?	Gives the client a chance to add information
MRS. C.: No, but there is something important I should add.	
NURSE: What's that?	Probe
MRS. C.: His name. I don't want you to be bringing the wrong man around here to move in with me! (Both laugh)	

CONCLUSION

The first section of this book, Chapters 1 to 5, has presented content on communication models, communication channels, communication styles, therapeutic communication skills and information gathering skills and pitfalls. All these concepts and skills can be used in varying role relationships and in different nursing contexts. Role relationships between nurses and clients and between nurses and other health professionals are the focus of the next section of this book (Chapters 6 to 8).

BIBLIOGRAPHY

Bechnell, E.P. & Smith, D.M. *System of nursing practice: a clinical assessment tool,* Philadelphia: F.A. Davis, 1975.
Benjamin, A. *The helping interview* (2nd ed.). Boston: Houghton Mifflin, 1974.
Bower, F.L. *The process of planning nursing care: a model for practice* (2nd ed.). St. Louis: C.V. Mosby, 1977.
Brammer, L.M. *The helping relationship: process and skills.* Englewood Cliffs, N.J.: Prentice-Hall, 1973.
Craighead, W.E., Kazkin, A.E. & Mahoney, M.J. *Behavior modification, principles, issues and applications.* Boston: Houghton Mifflin, 1976.
Eggland, N. How to take a meaningful history. *Nursing 77,* 1977, 7(7), 24–30.
Marriner, A. *The nursing process: a scientific approach to nursing care* (2nd ed.). St. Louis: C.V. Mosby, 1979.
Okun, B.F. *Effective helping: interviewing and counselling techniques.* North Scituate, Massachusetts: Duxbury Press, 1976.
Rogers, C.R. *Client centered therapy.* Boston: Houghton Mifflin, 1951.
Satir, V. *Peoplemaking.* Palo Alto, California: Science and Behavior Books, 1972.
Yura, H. & Walsh, M.B. *The nursing process. Assessing, planning, implementing, evaluating* (3rd ed.). New York: Appleton-Century-Crofts, 1978.

SECTION II

COMMUNICATION AND ROLE RELATIONSHIPS

Nurses who work in hospital or community settings assume a variety of roles as they interact with clients. First, they assume the role of *care-giver*, that is, they administer care to clients in a systematic way. They also assume the role of *care-planner* (Manthey, 1974, p. 83). In this role, nurses assume teaching, collaborative, and client–advocate roles. In the dual role of care-giver and care-planner, nurses might choose one or more of the following alternatives for a client who is experiencing pain:

Alternative Nursing Action	*Type of Interaction*
Administer a medication for pain.	nurse–client (care-giver)
Question the client about the pain and/or instruct client about the pain medication.	nurse–client (care-giver)
Ask a nurse on the team to give a back rub to promote relaxation.	nurse–nurse (care-giver)

Ask the physician to reevaluate the order for pain medication because the client is complaining of pain before the three hour interval is up.	nurse–physician (care-giver)
Consult with the social worker about the client because the pain symptoms appear to indicate stress due to worries about finances and care of children.	nurse/co-worker

These examples of communication are dyadic. Dyadic communication is face-to-face interaction between two persons; in this case, the nurse and client or the nurse and a co-worker (nurse, physician, or social worker). A dyad is the basic unit of all communication interactions, with both persons in the dyad simultaneously interacting as senders and message receivers. As we have seen in the first section of this book, dyadic communication can vary, depending on the context, content, style, and channels used to convey messages.

A basic communication principle to be considered in the discussion of dyads and roles is: "All communication relationships are either symmetrical or complementary, depending on whether they are based on equality or inequality" (Watzlawick, et al., 1967, p. 70).

Symmetrical Relationships

Symmetrical relationships are based on equality; the partners tend to mirror each other's behavior (Watzlawick et al., 1967). That is, symmetrical relationships express or exchange the same basic communication behaviors; two friends talking about school, two clients sharing information about their surgery, or two staff nurses discussing their work in the hospital are examples of symmetrical relationships. In healthy symmetrical relationships, the partners can demonstrate a willingness to share feelings or give and accept constructive criticism.

Complementary Relationships

Complementary relationships are based on inequality; one partner assumes a superior or "one-up" position in the relationship (Watzlawick et al., 1967, p. 69). Examples of complementary relationships are parent-child, teacher-

Communication and Role Relationships — 147

student, or nurse-client. Complementary relationships are not necessarily unhealthy or "bad" relationships. There are situations in which this type of communication relationship is necessary—for example, in the case of an acutely ill client and a nurse who is caring for this client. The ill client is dependent on the nurse, who is the decision maker for the care that is to be administered to the client.

Similarly, symmetrical relationships are not always "good" or normal relationships. Unhealthy symmetrical relationships can be characterized by competitiveness and lead to escalating, unstable relationships in which the partners fight and quarrel (Watzlawick et al., 1967).

The key point here is that nurses can learn to communicate effectively with others (clients and co-workers) using both symmetrical and complementary communication patterns. Some interactions call for symmetrical relationships and others for the complementary relationship, depending on the social or cultural context. Complementary and symmetrical communication patterns can even exist within the same relationship.

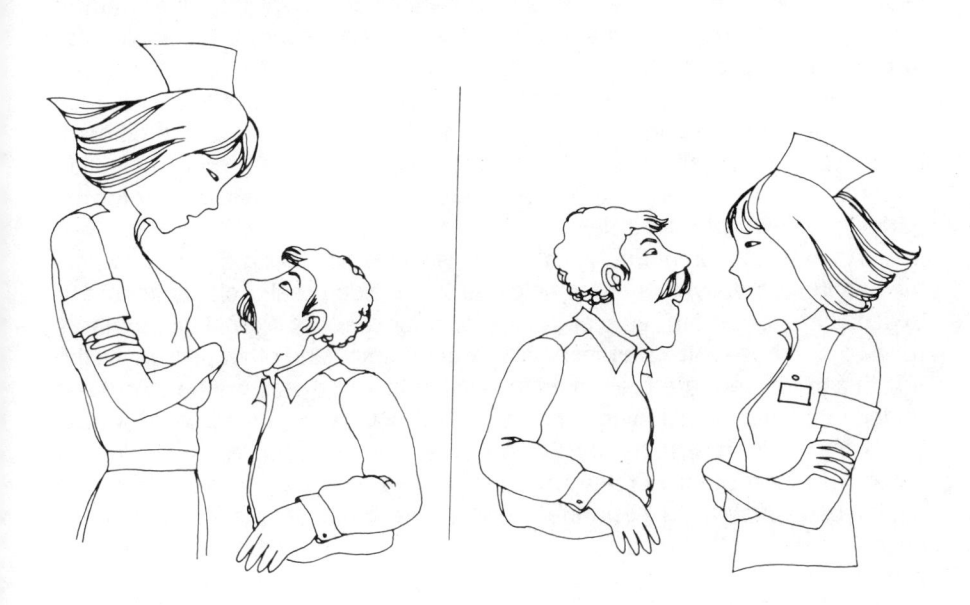

For example, two nurses (A and B) work in a geriatric extended-care facility. Nurse A asks Nurse B to help her with one of A's assigned clients (complementary). Nurse A is instructing Nurse B how to help her in this situation. Later at lunch, Nurse A and Nurse B exchange information about the client (symmetrical). In the afternoon, the head nurse shares some information about the client with Nurse B. Nurse B relays this information with Nurse A (complementary with Nurse B one-up). Relationships that alternate between symmetrical and complementary patterns such as in the example of the two nurses just presented tend to be healthy relationships; this is to say that each pattern of behavior has a tendency to stabilize the other when there is unhealthy competition (symmetrical) or rigidity (complementary). These changes from one pattern to the other (complementary to symmetrical or symmetrical to complementary) can be thought of as "homeostatic" (Watzlawick et al., 1967, p. 110). In other words, nurses relate to others in symmetrical and complementary relationships depending on many different factors and influences.

Communication conflicts arise when patterns of symmetry and complementarity are used in unhealthy ways. For example, professionals who perceive themselves in relation to another as one-up (complementary) can use a defensive behavior such as blaming; other health professionals who perceive themselves as one-down (complementary) can use a defensive behavior such as placating. Another area where communication conflicts arise is when both partners do not agree as to who is subordinate, superior, or equal to whom. In other words, one partner acts as if the other partner were equal, while at the same time the other partner assumes a complementary relationship exists!

This issue of symmetry-complementarity is an important one for nurses as they communicate with clients and other health care workers in different health settings. Again, it should be emphasized that both communication patterns can be mutually supportive and can be used constructively for the partners involved in the relationship.

An examination of the types of role relationships that are present within the health care delivery system helps us to develop greater clarity about our expectations of others, as well as the confusing set of expectations others have of us. These role relationships between nurses and other persons in the health care system are presented in Section II. The dyads will be discussed under three major groupings: nurse–client in Chapter 6; nurse/co-worker (including physician), Chapter 7; and nurse–nurse, Chapter 8. While it is recognized that other nurses are, strictly speaking, also co-workers in the health care system, a separate chapter has been devoted to the nurse–nurse dyadic relationships because of the unique problems that exist among nurses.

BIBLIOGRAPHY

Watzlawick, P., Beavin, J. and Jackson, D. *Pragmatics of human communication: a study of interactional patterns, pathologies and paradoxes.* New York: Norton, 1967.

Chapter 6
Nurse/client dyads

BEHAVIORAL OBJECTIVES

By reading this chapter and participating in the exercises, students will be able to:

1. Describe the changing roles of the nurse and client and changing aspects of the illness role
2. Understand the concept of self-awareness and recognize its importance to the nurse-client relationship.
3. Describe the psychological aspects of illness and wellness states
4. Recognize labeling: "hostile patient," "good patient," and "good nurse."

Suppose for a moment that one of your friends sat down with you tonight and said, "OK, you're a nurse. You've seen some clients, you've learned some things. Now tell me, what's so special about what you do for the clients? Is there anything you do that couldn't be done by any other professional in the health care field?" How would you answer?

What the friend might be trying to do is get at the effects of the nurse's contact with the client. Obviously, the most positive results are realized when there is an effective relationship between nurse and client. The development of effective relationships is important for two reasons: first, exchange of information is more accurate when both persons are "open" to each other; and second, it can enhance the therapeutic qualities inherent in the client's return to a state of wellness.

Specific communication patterns in nurse-client dyads relate directly to roles. These roles are changing because of many influences. Patterns of change in three areas—the role of the nurse, the role of the client, and the illness role—are reviewed in this chapter, as are some of the influences that helped to create these changes.

THE CHANGING ROLE OF THE NURSE

Today, such terms as "expanded" or "collaborative" are often used to define the role of the nurse. The nursing role has been redefined to include nurses as care planners as well as care-givers. As a consequence, new nursing roles have evolved from the traditional role that characterized nursing.

The traditional role of the nurse focuses on the client's physical needs. The nurse-client dyad is primarily complementary; the nurse assumes a superior one-up relationship to the client. In this role, the nurse emphasizes the qualities of nurturing, assistance, and succoring, whereas the role of the client involves dependence and submissiveness.

Contrast this role with the collaborative role of the nurse, which includes specialized functions and activities related to wellness. One reason for this change is that the nature of health care has changed, with the client taking a more active role. Concepts such as health education, prevention, compliance, and health promotion are important parts of today's nurse's thinking and activities.

This continuing state of change and expansion that typifies the role of the nurse causes such questions to be raised as, "How does one define nursing?" or "What constitutes the nurse-client relationship?" If one is able to define nursing, does that help to know what the nurse does or says in a particular nurse-client relationship? Nursing can be defined many ways, but for our purposes here, we focus on one facet of nursing that addresses the communication interaction in the nurse-client relationships, even if this results in a somewhat simplistic and broad definition:

> Nursing encompasses interactions between two people, one the client and the other the care giver. These interactions cannot occur without some form of communication.

The key word is interaction—interaction which occurs between the nurse and the client wherein the nurse's primary responsibility is to assist the client in the performance of activities the client is unable to carry out; in other words, the nurse's function is *to meet the client's needs,* which may be those of either high or low visibility (see Chapter 1). Any behavior which the nurse observes in the client constitutes communication about those needs. One way to categorize these interactions is to utilize the framework of the nursing process; each phase of the nursing process contains significant elements of communication.

The framework that has been chosen for the purposes of our discussion is the Szasz–Hollender Model (1956) as modified by Branch and Paxton (1976). This model presents three phases of the nurse-client relationship (Figure 6–1). Each phase is characterized by client's states of illness and wellness.

In Phase I, the client is acutely ill and is thus the passive recipient of nursing care. The nurse does something to the client, who is in a totally dependent state. The type of communication relationship is predominantly complementary, with the nurse one-up.

In Phase II, the client is ill but is able to cooperate with the nurse, who acts as teacher or enabler. The client is moving from a dependent to a more independent state. The communication is complementary but is moving towards a more symmetrical pattern.

In Phase III, the client and the nurse are involved in a partnership characterized by mutual participation. The communication relationship is more balanced, with both partners alternating in symmetrical and complementary patterns.

These phases of the model are not discrete, but rather are continuous in nature. The illness-wellness and complementry-symmetrical dimensions are continuous as well. One phase is not necessarily "better" than the others. Each phase is appropriate under certain circumstances. The phases are presented in the form of the model to highlight the face that as clients move along the continuum of illness-wellness, the nature of the complementary-symmetrical communication patterns change.

Some nurses have a tendency to judge themselves on their technical skills, rather than on the types of human relationships they foster. It is easier for these

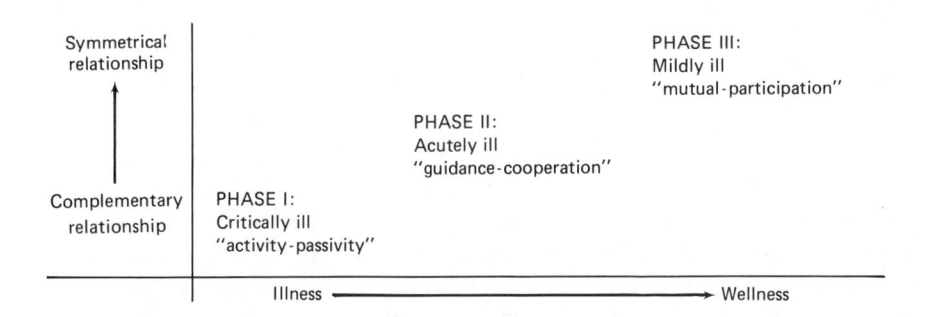

FIGURE 6–1. Three phases of the nurse–client relationship.

nurses to conceptualize complementary (as opposed to symmetrical) nurse-client dyads seen in Phase I, activity-passivity, of the model. If these complementary relationships become rigid and inflexible, the implication is that there will be more control over clients who want to please, to do the "right" thing. If the dyadic relationship is locked into one pattern, rather than alternating between complementary and symmetrical patterns, defensive behaviors can surface. For example, the nurse can blame, while the client placates. Healthy nurse-client dyads are dynamic and progress through phases (depending on the nature of the illness) in which both participants assume different roles. The goal of nursing care is to progress from doing everything *for* the client to assisting the client and finally, to planning *with* the client so that he or she can assume total responsibility for his or her health.

As the nurse-client dyad moves towards an equal or symmetrical pattern (or even a complementary relationship in which the client is one-up), greater demands are placed on nurses in terms of the complexity of the communication required. Communication often becomes an intricate process of sequencing patterns of behavior that are multidimensional in nature (Daubenmire et al., 1978) and take place over extended periods of time. How does one begin to understand these communication relationships? One of the best ways to begin is to attempt to understand ourselves clearly, to be self-aware.

Sense of Self-Awareness

If we ever stop to think about what we bring to the nurse-client dyad, the list would be long. Here are a few examples:

Feelings
Values
Fears
Motivations
Prejudices
Goals

Our unique make-up, our background, all the things that make us tick contribute to the nurse-client dyadic relationship. A knowledge of who we are, who we would like to be, how we think others see us, and what motivates our actions are all part of our own uniqueness. Such questions as "How well do you know yourself?" "How does this knowledge of yourself influence your perception of the client?" or "How does this knowledge influence the manner in which you decode and react to the client's message?" are often never answered. The relationships nurses have with clients are directly related to their perceptions of themselves. This is evident in two ways: (1) positive relationships and experiences with others usually result in a positive self-concept, and (2) a positive self-concept can translate into a positive regard for clients and others (Wilmot, 1975).

There are three ways in which self-concepts can be changed in interactions with others: *selective exposure* of self to others, *selective interpretation* of other's behavior, and *selectively choosing* goals to be achieved in a dyadic relationship (Wilmot, 1975). This ability to choose is not *always* open to the nurse in the nurse-client interaction. Nurses cannot selectively choose clients; they are usually assigned to them. They cannot selectively interpret; they must be objective at all times; and they cannot change goals—goals are mutually shared between both client and nurse. Contrast this limitation in selectivity to one's role outside nursing, in which one can choose friends, interpret one's own behavior in such a way that it becomes a positive experience, and can change goals if the initial ones set seem too difficult to achieve. The difference is that one role is personal, while the other is professional. In a professional relationship, the self-concept of the nurse becomes secondary and submerged in an interaction in which the central focus is on the client. The nurse is concentrating solely on the client.

Self-awareness is directly related not only to self-concept or how highly one values oneself, but also to the congruence between one's own feelings and the facts. Confusion between one's own feelings and the facts can lead to ineffective communication. The following situation serves as an example:

> Mr. Stone, who was 87 years old, was getting progressively more disoriented. His wife, a nurse, had been caring for him in their home. When Mrs. Dixon, the visiting nurse, made a home visit to see how things were, Mrs. Stone, who had previously been able to cope, burst into tears, and stated that the time had come to place Mr. Stone in a nursing home. "He keeps saying that he wants to go home. He doesn't know me and I can no longer communicate with him. Yesterday I had to call the police because he ran outside and down the street in his bathrobe, looking for his home. I'll just have to place him in the nursing home where I have reserved a bed for him."
>
> Mrs. Dixon then remembered when her grandfather was placed in a nursing home by his daughter (Mrs. Dixon's mother). The grandfather was not disoriented and actually became confused after his admission. He died soon thereafter. Mrs. Dixon's internal response was, "I'd never do that to my parents!" And she recommended to Mrs. Stone that Mr. Stone not be placed in a nursing home.

Mrs. Dixon's use of her own emotional feelings was not helpful to Mrs. Stone, who needed support for what was a difficult and possibly correct decision. However, this is not to say that the feelings should have been ignored.

The underlying concerns about when to institutionalize a loved one could have been used by the visiting nurse to empathize with Mrs. Stone. It should also be noted that the visiting nurse gave advice (an interviewing pitfall) rather than working with Mrs. Stone to make her own decision and feel good about it.

The whole issue about *how* to use one's inner reactions is complicated. The more self-awareness, the more one is likely to match relevant parts of experience to current reality. Most people work on developing an increased sense of self-awareness throughout their life. Increased knowledge comes through daily experiences interacting with all people, not just clients. Merely having the experience does not, however, mean that anyone, including nurses, automatically learns from what has transpired. Self-awareness is usually the result of active thinking about one's own interaction with others and consideration of both positive and negative feedback from others. It is through the process of experience and thinking and integrating it with knowledge that self-awareness emerges.

THE CHANGING ROLE OF THE CLIENT

Not only is the role of the nurse changing, but that of the client is also taking on new dimensions. Today's clients live in a society where they know more about disease and health care than the average physician did at the turn of the century (Norris, 1979). Health care today has become the right of all individuals rather than the privilege of a selected few (Bullough, 1976). And there is beginning to be an emphasis on health promotion and wellness within the health care system. Perhaps as a result of these factors, clients have become more assertive in their demands for quality health care. Two examples of this are the movements of self-care and peer practice.

Self-care has influenced the change in the role of the client through acknowledgment of the right of clients to take responsibility in developing their own health potential by defining health and their own priorities and options, as well as their own risk indices. Clients assume an assertive posture in the decision and planning for their care. Self-care participation demands a nurse who is open to change and willing to enter into a nurse-client relationship in which clients control the administration of their own health care through problem solving (Norris, 1979).

The second movement that has influenced the changing role of the client is that of nurse-client *peer practice*, which is characterized by the client acting as a peer or equal of the nurse in the setting of goals for his or her health. This movement developed out of clients' sense of dissatisfaction with the health care system, as well as with inconveniences encountered in illness (Bayer and Brandner, 1977). It is important that nurses encourage the right of clients to share in decision making. One way to do this is to help the clients learn how to solve problems by means of a problem-solving methodology.

Problem-solving is a task that confronts every person in daily life situations. From the moment we wake up in the morning, we are confronted with many decisions. However, we usually do not go through a series of steps to arrive at these decisions. In nurse-client encounters, problem solving is deliberate and objective. Clients need help in setting realistic and appropriate goals to bring about change. A problem-solving model, such as that in Figure 6–1, is systematic and can be used to help the client solve his or her own problems.

Problem-Solving Model
1. The problem is presented.
2. The problem is defined and/or refined.
3. Define specific criteria that ascertain if the problem is solved.
4. Solutions and/or options are listed.
5. Solutions and/or options are prioritized and/or decided.
6. One option is tried.
7. The option is evaluated (did it work?).
8. Recycle if necessary.

The model presented is a step-by-step process of inquiry which helps to facilitate the solution of the problem. The problem-solving methodology and nursing process are very similar in that each presents a systematic step-by-step methodology for arriving at the solution of the problem; the problem is presented (Assessment), the solutions are prioritized (Plan), one option is tried (Implementation), and the solution is evaluated (Evaluation). The problem-solving method presents a planned approach to help clients ventilate problems, and the orientation is client-centered.

Geach (1974) points out three hallmarks of the problem-solving approach in nurse-client interactions:

1. The nurse involves the client in the process;
2. The problem to which the client and nurse address themselves has immediate relevance to what is happening between them; and
3. There is some relatedness between the nurse and client so that the solution of problems is experienced from within a relationship, not in isolation.

When they begin to use a problem-solving model, nurses often say, "I don't know what bothers clients! I just can't get clients to say what is really bothering them." Problem definition is often the most difficult step in the problem-solving process. Once the problem is properly defined, which may require extensive discussion and examination of related issues, the subsequent phases of the problem-solving model are more easily handled.

While a set of guidelines has been presented, it should be stressed that no two problems are alike. Variations can occur with regard to the problem solution even with the same client, depending on the context, the nurse with whom the client is attempting to problem-solve, or even such seemingly unimportant things as the time of day.

THE CHANGING ASPECTS OF THE ILLNESS ROLE

Illness has always created some sense of dependency on the part of the client with respect to the nurse. This feeling has fostered a complementary role relationship with the nurse one-up. Ill clients perceive nurses as protective and physically supportive. All of us have felt this sense of dependency during an illness state at some point in our lives.

The illness role itself is changing with the advent of modern medical technology. A major factor influencing this change is the high degree of specialization in all areas of health care and which has resulted in sophisticated monitoring and life-support systems. Modern medical and surgical treatment is often more traumatic with regard to the physical needs of the clients and recovery.

In addition to the physical needs of clients, the psychological and sociological aspects of the illness role have come into focus. Thus, the nursing role has now become one of blending the physical, psychological, and sociological needs of clients to help them move towards a more symmetrical relationship with the nurse and develop a greater sense of independence.

Psychological Aspects of Illness

There are characteristic psychological aspects that are often associated with all illness states and transcend the specific illness symptomotology. They are summarized below*:

Illness	Wellness
Dependence	Independence
Passivity	Activeness
Heightened fear and anxiety	Lessened fear and anxiety
Self-rejection	Self-acceptance
Lowered feeling of self-worth	Strong feeling of self-worth
Identity loss and identity confusion	Sense of identity

*From Skipper and Leonard, 1965, p. 160; Purtilo, 1978, pp. 40–50.

In acute phases of illness, when clients are dependent and traditional health care (and cure) is given by others, there is heightened anxiety and concern. There is also a loss of roles and identity as a result both of removal from ordinary daily roles (worker, mother, father, friend, neighbor, child) and the anonymity of being a patient or client.

While a state of physical dependency is never a preferred state it is almost inevitable when a client is ill. However, the goal of the nurse–client relationship is for the client to gain independence of functioning as rapidly as possible. The psychological aspects of illness are related to how illness is viewed in our culture, to the nature of the illness itself, to the role of being ill, or to some interaction of all three. They may be caused by the onset of the illness. The point here is that they lead to several kinds of client response that unless picked up by the nurse, can become barriers and inhibit effective and therapeutic communication.

Sociological Aspects of Illness

Parsons (1966), in his description of the sociology of sick roles, states that sick persons are exempted from a certain type of responsibility for their own state. In other words, clients are not expected to be responsible for their illness or its recovery except in a peripheral sense (Spector, 1980). This is changing today. Often clients feel responsible for their illness and their participation in goal setting directly contributes to their recovery and well-being. Some clients will even blame themselves for their illness and therefore have a lowered sense of self-worth.

Barriers to Effective Nurse-Client Communication

Nurses, as well as others, often use role labels to categorize people. Placing people into categories can help us confront difficult situations more easily. This form of labeling utilizes defensive behaviors. We live in a world of labeling. Labeling limits effective communication. Labels are based on erroneous (or at least inappropriate) concepts about people and how they *ought* to behave. For example, nurses who assume either consciously or unconsciously that *all* older people (75 years and over) are disoriented will certainly be less effective in communicating with these clients than nurses who regard older individuals as "unique." Categorizing persons into groups with common patterns of behavior can block effective communication. Three labeling concepts are:

1. The "hostile client" label
2. The "good patient" label
3. The "good nurse" label.

The "Hostile Patient" Label. One kind of client response to illness is hostility, often directed at others. Some clients are hostile by nature, as well. In the hospital, hostile behavior can be shown by constant demands such as using the call light, asking for a bedpan, complaining about food, or anything to do with the hospital routine.

Hostile behavior presents a challenge for the nurse in terms of accurately understanding its meaning. Unfortunately, there is a tendency for nurses to stereotype these difficult clients with terms such as "complainer," "bad patient," or "pest." These labels are a form of blaming the client. The labeling of clients in this manner can also become a self-fulfilling prophecy: that is, nurses will reinforce the behavior of such clients by responding only to complaints or demands, which will then lead to further demands and complaints.

Once a client receives a negative label, the label can permeate the entire nursing staff of a unit, making it all the more difficult for the client to change. Many nurses who graduated within the last two decades remember the original version of a classic film *Mrs. Reynolds Needs a Nurse*. The film depicts an elderly woman who is acutely ill and has become a major problem on the unit, with her constant demands, numerous complaints, and overall hostile attitude towards nurses, doctors, and other health workers. The situation gradually worsens until a student nurse arrives on the scene. She actively "listens" to Mrs. Reynolds and begins to understand the reasons underlying her negative behavior. The film is a particularly moving one, as it hits at the heart of nursing. Although there was therapeutic nurse-client communication, the student had to *change the attitude* of an entire staff on the unit toward Mrs. Reynolds in order to change the client's behavior. Chapters 7 and 8 of this book are devoted to issues in role relations with other staff.

The "Good Patient" Label. A difficult problem to detect is the client who has, at some level, decided *not* to be a burden on the staff and suffers in silence. This client becomes the "good patient" who never complains, never uses the call light, never asks questions, and is "no problem" for the nursing regimen.

In terms of Satir's communication styles, these clients may placate by assuring the nurse they feel fine when, in actuality, they have pain. There may be a contradiction between verbal and body language messages, although an accomplished "good patient" can be quite successful in disguising inner feelings from the message that is communicated to the nurse.

Nurse/Client Dyads 159

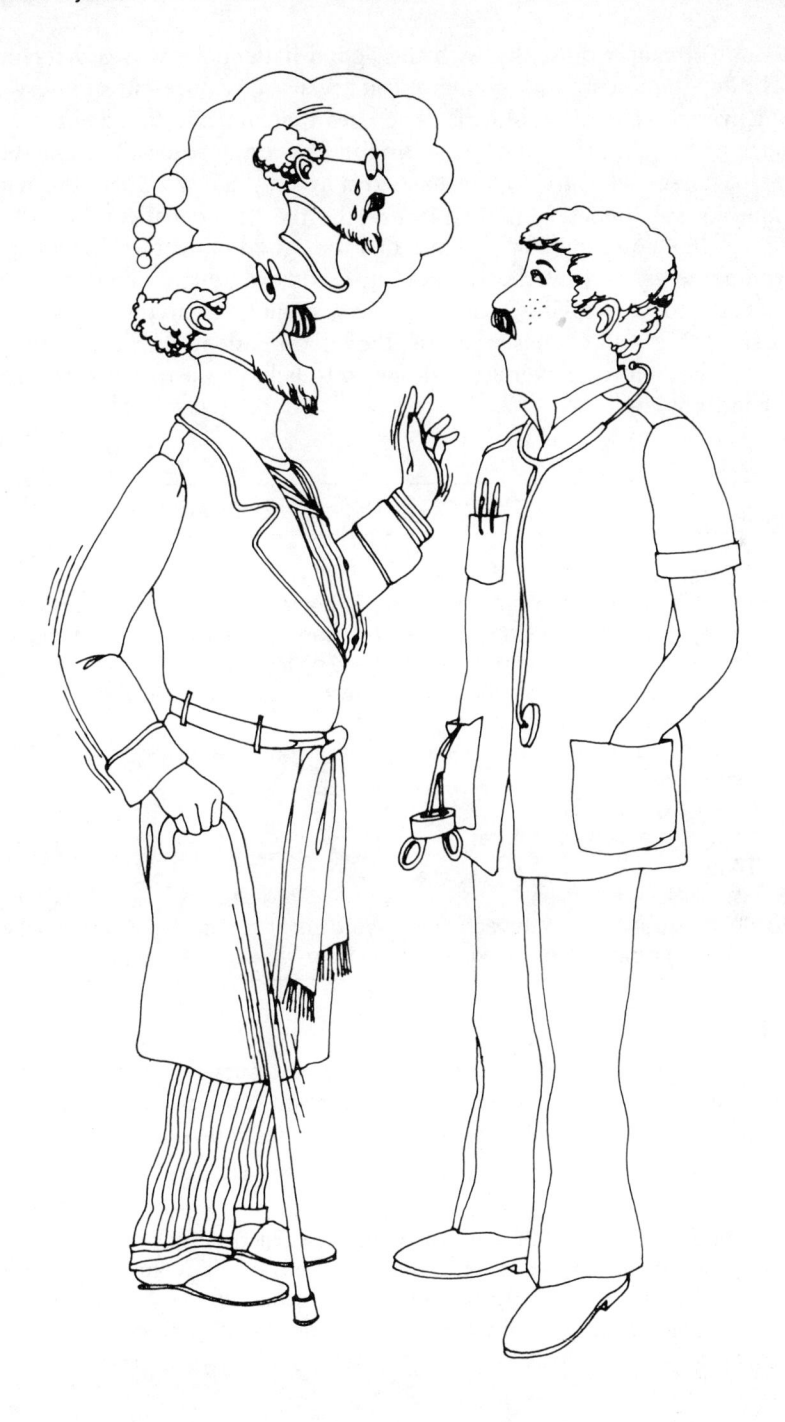

The major difficulty with the "good patients" involves detecting them. The "good patient" may go unnoticed because it requires direct intervention to uncover the client's problems. The cues that indicate the client is suffering, such as a slight grimace or hesitation in answering a question, may be subtle. Also, nurses who are feeling harried may only apply oil to "the wheel that squeaks the loudest"; this will never be the "good patient."

The "good patient" is rewarded for "good patient" behavior by smiles, compliments, and overheard messages. For example, a client may overhear, "That's Mrs. Williams, she is always smiling, even though she just had surgery." For all of these reasons, the "good patient" is difficult to uncover.

The following exercise is designed to help you learn how to discover the "good patient."

The "Good Patient" Exercise

1. Pair up. One partner will be *A*, the other *B*.
2. *A* pretends to be a client recovering at home from an illness (stroke or a heart attack). *B* will be checking up on *A*'s recovery. *A* will act *as if* everything is all right, but in one aspect pretend to be the "good patient." That is, *A* will "cover up" some problem, but will give subtle clues that things are not all right.
3. *B* interviews *A* as if doing a checkup.
4. *B* listens to *A*, watching for the following nonverbal cues:
   Eye contact
   Facial expression
   Body movements (posture)
   Tone of voice.
5. *A* and *B* switch roles.
6. Share experiences with each other. Were either of you able to figure out when the other was being the "good patient?" If so, what were the cues?

The "Good Nurse" Label. The "good nurse" is task-oriented rather than one who is person-oriented. This nurse gives top priority to high-visibility tasks, at times, to the detriment of client care, as shown in the following story.

A nursing instructor we know was hospitalized for a cataract operation. She was told that she had a p.r.n. post-op pain medication ordered. The first evening after the operation she was experiencing considerable pain. She saw the medication nurse passing out meds in the room across the hallway and asked if she might have her p.r.n. medication as she was in some pain. The nurse said that she had to finish one side of the hallway and then work up the other side and after that, then she would bring her the medication, a task that might take anywhere from 30 minutes to more than an hour.

This situation, as ridiculous as it sounds, is not uncommon. The nurse was totally consumed with carrying out the task to the exclusion of caring for the client. The "good nurse" is always busy, always carrying out the doctors' orders, and usually feels overworked. The "good nurse" rarely stops to listen, *really* listen to clients. There is a tendency to be superreasonable or a bit blaming. The overall orientation of the "good nurse" to nursing is similar to a computerized exercise in which the nurse collects, analyzes, and produces data. The "humanistic" approach to the client is nonexistent.

Jourard attributes the stereotyped role of "good nurse" behavior to nurses' attempt to obliterate or deny individuality in clients (Jourard, 1971). "Good nurses" hide behind the armor of a stereotype not only to avoid their own self-disclosure, but to prevent clients from sharing their feelings and experiences in stressful situations.

Clients, on the other hand, consistently emphasize the caring aspect of nurses (rather than their technical ability) when recalling good care in stressful illness experiences. As one physician, who was himself a client, expressed it (Viner, 1975, p. 34):

> The most important thing I found was that the nurses were the most important people to me—more important in that narrowly circumscribed world than the doctors even, because they were with me all day. Some were absolute angels but others were just plain bitches. I don't know exactly what made the difference. I just know that the most important thing to a patient is that the nurse cares. Probably the least important thing to a patient is how technically capable she is. The single most frustrating thing that can happen to a patient is when a nurse doesn't listen to or believe him.

The intent here is not to negate the importance of physical high-visibility tasks, but rather to point out that from the clients' perspective it is equally important that nurses are able to use themselves therapeutically in total client care. An effective nurse should be able to handle both procedural and emotional aspects of nursing care.

Unfortunately, "good patients" reinforce "good nurses." Clients who do not wish to "take up a nurse's time," "cause trouble," "call a nurse if they can do something by themselves," (in spite of doctor's orders), or look on the nurse as busy and overworked (oftentimes true) help to foster the stereotyped role of the "good nurse."

CONCLUSION

Many forces and influences in the health care system have created greater demands on the ability of nurses to communicate effectively with clients. The nurse's rule is changing from the traditional bedside nurturing and caring of physically and psychologically dependent clients to that of mutual relationships. The client's role changes in a series of phases, from a passive to an active one in which he or she assumes the responsibility for the setting of goals by utilizing a problem-solving methodology. The illness role itself is changing, with increased emphasis on the psychological and sociological aspects of illness.

If nurses are to help others, an awareness of who they are is essential. Also, a knowledge of communication patterns—whether they are complementary or symmetrical—helps nurses to understand their own defensive behaviors better and to promote congruent responses. Examples of defensive behaviors utilized in labeling ("the hostile patient," "the good patient," and "the good nurse") help to futher clarify congruent communication responses.

BIBLIOGRAPHY

Bayer, M. & Brandner, P. Nurse/patient peer practice. *American Journal of Nursing,* 1977, 77 (1), 86–90.

Branch, M. & Paxton, P. *Providing safe nursing care for ethnic people of color.* New York: Appleton-Century-Crofts, 1976.

Bullough, B. Influences on role expansion. *American Journal of Nursing,* 1976, 76 (9), 1674–1681.

Daubenmire, J., Searles, S. & Ashton, C. A methodologic framework to study nurse-patient communication. *Nursing Research,* 1978, 27 (5), 303–310.

Geach, B. The problem-solving technique. *Perspectives in Psychiatric Care,* 1974, 12, 1.

Jourard, S. *The transparent self.* New York: Van Nostrand, 1971.

Manthey, M. Primary nursing is alive and well in the hospitals. *American Journal of Nursing,* 1979, 73 (1), 83–87.

Norris, C. Self-care. *American Journal of Nursing,* 1979, 79 (3), 486–489.

Parsons, T. Illness and the role of the physician: a sociological perspective. In W.R. Scott & E.H. Volkart (Eds.), *Medical care: Readings in the Sociology of Medical Institutions.* New York: John Wiley, 1966, p. 275.

Purtilo, R. *Health Professional Patient Interaction.* Philadelphia: W.B. Saunders, 1978.

Skipper, J. & Leonard, R. *Social interaction and patient care.* Philadelphia: J.B. Lippincott, 1965.

Spector, R. *Cultural diversity in health and illness.* New York: Appleton-Century-Crofts, 1979.
Szasz, T. & Hollander, M. A contribution to the philosophy of medicine. *Archives of Internal Medicine,* 1956, 97, 586.
Viner, E. Ordeal. *Nursing 75,* June 1975, pp. 31–34.
Wilmot, W. *Dyadic communication: a transactional perspective.* Reading, Massachusetts: Addison-Wesley, 1975.

Chapter 7
Nurse/co-worker dyads

BEHAVIORAL OBJECTIVES

By reading this chapter and participating in the exercises, students will be able to:
1. Describe the four major schools of thought about nursing roles
2. Identify four dimensions of reciprocal nurse/co-worker relationships
3. Describe the relationship among self-worth, the nurse's role, and communication in the nurse/co-worker relationship
4. Demonstrate an understanding of key aspects of the nurse-physician relationship (conditions for collegiality, differences in training and orientation, and emergence of the nurse clinician) that affect communication
5. Demonstrate an understanding of the three major factors that create barriers to effective communication in nurse-aide relationships
6. Explain how communication skills can be used to enhance nurse/co-worker relationships
7. Explain the concept of assertion in communication with co-workers

Suppose for a minute that the friend who sat down with you at the beginning of Chapter 6 approached you again. This time the friend stated, "OK, I understand how nurses communicate with clients. But what about physicians, social workers, other health professionals? Is communication any different with them than with clients?" What would your answer be?

Communication with other professions is becoming increasingly important for nursing. Both the way in which the nurse interacts with others and the relationships that develop affect interprofessional communication. This chapter is but a beginning of an exploration into relationships with other professions.

NURSE/CO-WORKER RELATIONSHIPS

The nurse rarely exists as a totally independent health care provider. Today's nurse interacts professionally as well as personally with a wide range of co-workers, including aides, clerks, pharmacists, physicians, psychologists, medical technicians, social workers, and health educators, as well as with other nurses.

This chapter includes the major co-worker relationships encountered in health settings (nurse-physician and nurse-aide), as well as raises general issues pertaining to communication between the nurse and other co-workers. Effective communication strategies with co-workers, including a section on the use of assertion in nursing, are also discussed.

History of Nurse/Co-worker Role Relationships

Nursing is currently in a state of transition in its relationships with the other health professions. A look at the history of nursing indicates that nursing's development has been characterized by a series of changes as the profession has coped with advances in social, professional, and health systems. A brief look at the four schools of thought influencing nursing (Abdellah, 1972) suggests that nursing is moving toward even more collaborative relationships with other health disciplines.

The service school of thought (1900–1943) supported the belief that nurses were prepared for service. Nurses were not only educated in hospital-based programs, but there was a great tendency for them to remain in hospitals after graduation. The major nurse/co-worker relationship was between nurse and physician, and it was characterized by submission on the part of the nurse to the physician and his orders. Nurses were reluctant to make decisions without clear-cut directives from the physician. There was teamwork in the hierarchical sense between these two professions because of a mutually agreed upon goal. The central goal of helping clients to regain their optimum level of health was accepted by both nurses and physicians.

The administrative school of thought (1944–1950) was an outgrowth of World War II and the beginning of dramatic developments in the advancement of medical science. This period was characterized by large government subsidies for the education of nurses in the field of administration, including supervisors, directors, and administrators. The movement of the most qualified nurses "away from the client" into areas of administration, as well as the introduction of auxiliary personnel into the health care system, was beginning. Although rapport between the nursing and medical professions was good, territorial boundaries—and their resultant defenses—were beginning to develop.

The academic school of thought (1951–1964) initiated the movement of nursing education onto the college campus. The lack of government financial support for nurses seeking advanced clinical training forced nurses into other areas, for example, academia. This period was characterized by the emergence of nursing as a bona fide profession. Territoriality developed between medicine and nursing largely because of the increasing use of technology and specialization in both these sciences. Lines of communication between the physician and nurse continued to be locked into traditional role relationships, as for example, in the "doctor-nurse" game, where the nurse made recommendations to the physician while at the same time appearing acquiescent and passive (Stein, 1967). The physician carried out the nurse's recommendations by writing orders in such a way that it appeared as though he or she had actually initiated the order. The center of focus in the physician-nurse relationship was often on the physician, even to the point where at times the nurse's desire to gain praise and approval from the physician superseded the need to be a competent professional in her or his own right (Kalish and Kalish, 1977). While "traditional" nurses accepted this role, many nurses saw a new model of health care emerging: that of a clinical nurse returning to the bedside in a caring, nurturing, teaching role with shared responsibility with the physician for decision making concerning client care.

The clinical school of thought (1965–present) grows out of a rebellion to the movement that had forced nurses into administrative and academic routes for recognition. New roles, such as the clinical nurse specialist and nurse practitioner, are developing, in part due to shortages in distribution of manpower in medicine. These roles carry greater responsibility for decision making, especially in client assessment. Nursing, having identified its professional boundaries, is now beginning to communicate with other disciplines. Mutual trust and reciprocity are beginning to replace the defenses that existed between the medical and nursing professions.

Four Dimensions of Reciprocal Nurse/Co-worker Relationships

Even with improved role relationships, if communication relationships between nurses and other co-workers are to be effective, they must be "reciprocal," that is, mutual or shared interactions (Phillips, 1979, p. 738). Such interactions imply openness, equality, and the opportunity to present one's information or point of view without being blamed. The state of reciprocity can be measured across four dimensions: task, authority, deference, and affect. These four dimensions, which provide a framework for examining nurse/co-worker relationships, were first conceptualized by Stevenson (1977) and adapted to nurse-physician relationships by Phillips (1979).

Task dimension. The task dimension relates to the division of tasks or activities delegated to the particular health care provider; what client-care tasks should be relegated to the nurse, the physician, or the social worker? History shows that many tasks have shifted among these professionals. For example, physical assessment of the heart, a task that was once exclusively carried out by the physician is now within the realm of the nurse.

Authority dimension. The authority dimension relates to how much power each health care provider has in relation to other health professionals, that is, which health care provider is at the top of the "pecking order" in the eyes of the other health care provider groups. The amount of power one has is usually determined by the amount of education or knowledge one possesses.

Deference dimension. The deference dimension is related to whose needs take precedence, the client's or the health care provider's. It is important that there be a reciprocal relationship between the health care providers if the client's needs are to be met. If everyone's opinions on what is best for the client are heard, then the decisions made are based on shared decisions. In this way a "therapeutic community" is created and the client benefits, especially if the client requires long-term care.

Affect dimension. The affect dimension is concerned with the feelings that health care providers have toward each other. Health providers are able to coordinate their efforts more effectively for the ultimate benefit of the client when they work in an environment of mutual respect for each other's role or profession.

Reciprocal relationships between the nurse and other health care providers begin with a respect for oneself. One needs a sense of self-worth not only to be emotionally supportive of clients, but to be able to work within health care environments with others.

In Chapter 3 of this book (Communication Styles), the term *self-worth* was introduced as an important concept in understanding defensive and

Nurse/Co-worker Dyads

congruent communication, and how blaming, placating, superreasonableness, and irrelevancy emerge as predominant behaviors when self-worth is threatened.

Self-worth can be affected differently by various role relationships. For example, a nurse may feel very good about clinical skills and nurse-client interactions and have a low self-image or feel threatened when presenting information to physicians or even when giving instructions to aides. The following exercises are designed to help you begin to raise your self-worth as a nurse and to understand how your self-worth might be involved in your dealings with other health professionals.

Exercise in Increasing Your Self-worth

1. Break up into groups of four.
2. Think of three traits, talents, or actions that you feel are positive or good about yourself in relation to your nursing role; for example, "I am well organized in my client care," "the other nurses like me because I am always willing to help out."
3. Write your three positive items on paper.
4. Share with the group.
5. Review and discuss. How difficult was this exercise? If it was difficult, was your own *low* self-worth getting in the way?

Now that you have listed your strengths, do you feel more positive about yourself? Do you see any advantage to continuing to do this periodically?

Exercise in Self-worth and Co-worker Relationships

1. How would you rate yourself on each of the following dimensions in terms of how you feel *when relating to a physician*? You can make an × in pencil on the appropriate line. (For example, if you felt a slight positive image, your mark might appear just to the right of the midline, but if you felt a strong negative self-image, your mark would appear at the extreme left near the words *Negative self-image*.)

Negative self-image		Positive self-image
Unimportant		Important
Undeserving		Deserving
Fear of other		No fear of other
Judged by other		Not judged by other

2. Now, rate yourself on the following dimensions as to how you feel about yourself when communicating with an aide or orderly.

Negative self-image					Positive self-image
Unimportant					Important
Undeserving					Deserving
Fear of other					No fear of other
Judged by other					Not judged by other

3. Now, rate yourself on the following dimensions as to how you feel about yourself when communicating with people from other health professions (social worker, psychologist, etc.)

Negative self-image					Positive self-image
Unimportant					Important
Undeserving					Deserving
Fear of other					No fear of other
Judged by other					Not judged by other

4. Compare your ratings in the three groupings. Which are different? Which are the same? What do you think made you rate yourself the way you did? If your responses were on the left side of the scales, what communication styles do you think you might use when you feel this way?
5. In the large group, discuss your answers to step 4 and answer the following questions:
   a. Is it necessary to feel superior or inferior in a hierarchical relationship?
   b. How is communication different when talking to a superior from talking to a subordinate?

While the focus of the rest of this chapter is on the interaction between the nurse and other co-workers, it is valuable to make frequent assessments of our own self-worth as we interact with others. When communication problems occur between professionals, figuring out "the" cause and "the" cure is difficult. By recognizing that our own self-worth is lowered in certain situations we can change our own behavior; this can result in doing things or communicating in such a way as to raise our level of self-worth and thus influence a solution to the problem.

The Nurse–Physician Relationship

One area in communication among health professionals that is undergoing change and resulting in role realignment is that of the nurse-physician relationship.

Consider the following situation:

> A doctor comes on to the unit where you are working and examines a chart. He notices the X-rays he ordered are not there. He turns to you and says, "Why aren't those X-rays on the chart? They were taken three days ago?"

How would you respond to this situation? You might say,

1. "I'm sorry, I'll call for them right now," or,
2. "I really don't know where they are; the X-ray department should be called."
3. Or you might pretend you don't hear the physician and not answer anything.

In the decades of the '60s and the '70s, many nurses might have responded with the first of these responses. But recent changes in the orientation of the nurse and physician roles evoke a different response. Today many nurses might utilize the second response. Can you discern the difference in the first two responses in the example given? What communication style was used by the nurse in the two responses? Does the third response (that of doing nothing) relate more closely to the first response or the second? Finally, how do you think the differences in these responses relate to the nurse-physician role relationship?

Significant role changes in the nursing profession have altered the physician-nurse relationship. The traditional relationship between nurse and physician was a complementary one—a relationship with roles mutually agreed upon by both parties. It was characterized by dominance-submission, order giving-order taking, and leading-following.

Today, there is more ambiguity in the nurse-physician role relationship, and there is often disagreement as to the rules governing the relationship. Many nurses are stating convincingly that they are colleagues in a *symmetrical* relationship. This is especially true with nurse practitioners or nurse clinicians, where nurses have specialized competence. At the same time, there can be obvious differences in skill, educational status, income, and responsibility between, for example, the head of surgery at a hospital and a newly graduated baccalaureate nurse. This raises one of the most fascinating role relation issues for health providers in the 1980s, namely, how can collegiality be achieved between medicine and nursing?

Conditions for Collegiality. Smoyak (1977) believes that nurses and physicians work best as colleagues when there is

1. Mutual agreement on a goal
2. Equality in status and personal interactions
3. A shared base of scientific and professional knowledge with complementary diversity in skills, expertise, and practices
4. Mutual trust for each other's competence.

The goal of quality health care for the client is at the heart of both the nursing and medical professions. But what of the status of equality in personal interactions? While nurses perceive the nurse–physician dyad as an alternating symmetrical-complementary relationship, many physicians still view the relationship as totally complementary with no feedback for correction or control. This has resulted in conflicting views of the two roles.

Studies have demonstrated that when doctors and nurses share a common view of their roles, communication is smooth; but when physicians perceive nurses as dependent and nurses perceive themselves as independent, communication blocks occur (Sutterly and Donnelly, 1973).

There are instances in which nurses as a professional group have a poor self-image and do not have reciprocal relationships with physicians, especially in the dimensions of deference and affect. Many nurses perceive the physician–nurse relationship as a totally "one-up" relationship in which the physician makes the decisions (as in the doctor–nurse game).

A study by Wesson (1972) demonstrated that while physicians initiated and directed 23 percent of their communication to nurses, nurses initiated and directed only 9 percent of their messages to the physician. The author concluded that persons of higher rank initiate interaction toward persons in lower rank more often than vice versa.

There are physicians who perceive the physician–nurse relationship as having symmetrical and complementary components. One study suggests that the opportunity for nurses to experience increased collegiality with physicians exists. When physicians were asked their opinion of nursing as a profession, they ranked nursing as the highest in prestige when compared with certain other professions (pharmacy, dietetics, physical therapy, occupational therapy, and hospital administration). It was also demonstrated in this same questionnaire that fewer nurses (50.8 percent) than physicians (58.8 percent) perceived themselves as equal partners with the physician in the care of patients (Wiley, 1979).

The purpose of this section is *not* to state how things should be but to alert nurses to the fact that the doctor-nurse relationship is changing and varies considerably from setting to setting. When the nurse desires a high degree of independence or collegiality, communication problems may arise from differences of opinion between the physician and the nurse, implied superior relationship (or double messages) from the physician, or from incongruent and mixed messages from the nurse. As was mentioned earlier, lowered self-worth only further confuses communication at these times.

Differences in Orientation. It is important to recognize that physicians and nurses have a shared base of scientific and professional knowledge. It is also important that each recognizes differences in behavior related to their professions. Physicians have traditionally been oriented to behavior targeted at "cure" (Linn, 1974). Behaviors which involve the expressive, emotionally supportive activities are oriented toward "care" and have been traditionally the domain of the nurse. Care involves client comfort and emotional support, as well as an understanding of health problems. Studies using attitudinal questionnaires have demonstrated this difference in orientation between physicians (cure), nursing students (care), medical students (cure), and nurse practitioners (care) (Linn, 1974).

This difference in orientation has been one source of conflict in the nurse–physician relationship. While some physicians feel that nurses have moved too far in the direction of care and have become guilty of ignoring physical needs, some nurses feel physicians have neglected the client as a person. When over 10,000 nurses responded in one study to a questionnaire with the question of how they would rate physicians on "psychological support given to patients," 77 percent rated them either "fair" or "poor" (Funkhauser, 1976).

There are several other traditional differences between nursing and medicine that indirectly affect professional communication. They are:

Educational level
Age
Specialization in one area
Income
Direct recipient of fees
Public attitude (status)
Sex distribution.

While all are important and changing, the latter (sex distribution), merits a few comments. Until the woman's movement, the majority of physicians were male, while nursing was predominately a female profession. Today the picture is changing. It is realistic to predict that these changes will continue and more women will enter medical schools, resulting in more female physicians (Hite, 1971). Conversely, as nursing roles continue to expand into highly specialized areas, the number of male students in nursing schools will also increase.

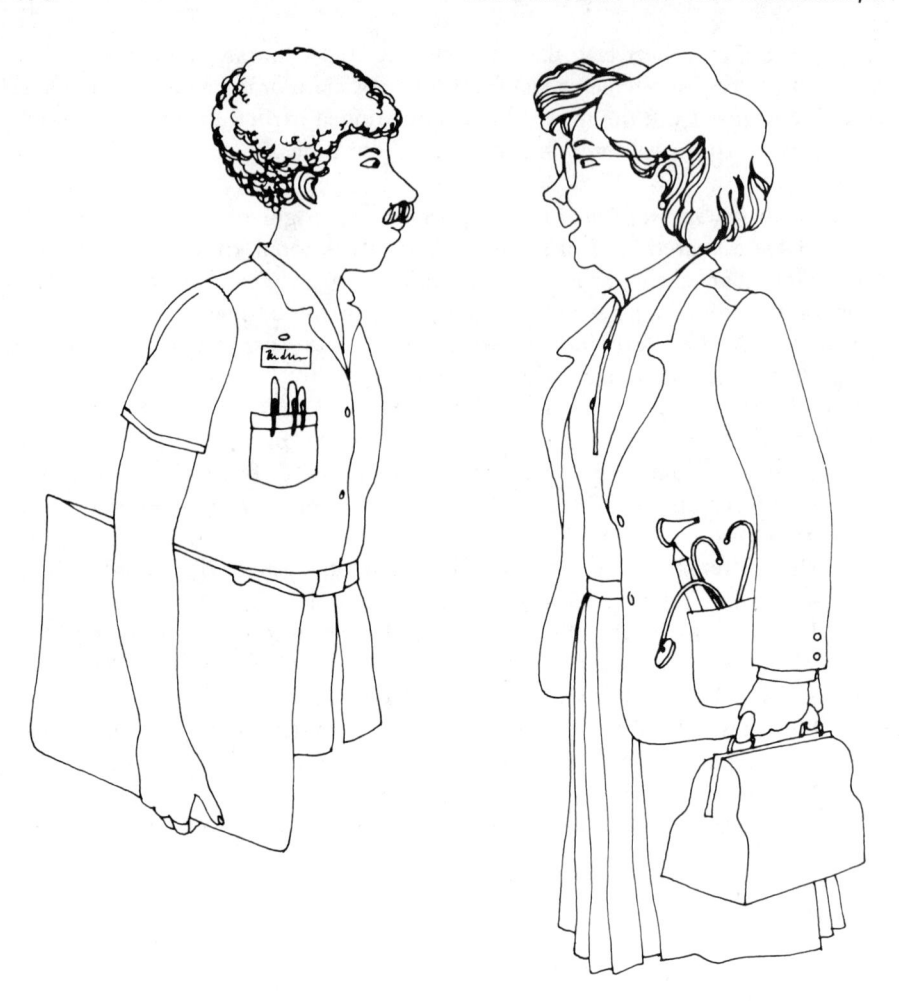

It is intriguing to speculate on how the change in sex distribution in these two professions will affect role relationships and communication patterns. One study measuring the acceptance of the nurse practitioner in the expanded role showed that female physicians accepted nurse practitioners more readily than their male colleagues in medicine (Reed and Roghmann, 1971). It may be inevitable that as the ranks of the two professions become more equal in terms of the numbers of men and women, communication patterns will be significantly improved.

Emergence of the Nurse Practitioner. A new facet in the nurse-physician relationship is the emergence of the nurse practitioner. A nurse practitioner is a licensed registered nurse who has taken specialized training in primary care. Nurse practitioner programs leading to a degree are, for the most part, graduate-level programs. They give the nurse experience in physical assessment, treatment, and related health aspects of a specific client group such as children, families, or the elderly. The emergence of this type of graduate-level education carries with it the impetus for nurses to expect more equality in their dealings with physicians.

There is no question that the emergence of the nurse practitioner has had an effect on the nurse–physician relationship. The nurse practitioner role has fostered positive communication relationships with the physician, since the practitioner has a higher level of education (master level), is usually older, and is specialized in one area. At the same time, some physicians are threatened by nurse practitioners, especially those physicians who are older and have been in practice for a longer period of time (Claiborn and Walton, 1979). Again reciprocity with reference to the four dimensions proposed by Phillips is emphasized; the physician and the nurse practitioner must know their specific tasks, who has the authority, that their mutual goal is to serve to client's needs, and that there is mutual respect for the other's health care role.

It was acknowledged earlier in this chapter that there are differences in the cure and care orientations of various health care professionals. Physicians are cure-oriented; nurses, care-oriented (Linn, 1974). One question that could be asked about the nurse practitioner is: Does the nurse practitioner change to a cure orientation after assuming a role which uses primarily the skills of assessment and data collection? The answer is no. The nurse practitioner is able both to integrate this extension of roles, one oriented towards cure into the traditional nursing role model, one oriented towards care, and to achieve a unique professional approach to health care (Linn, 1974, p. 644).

As the educational gap narrows between nurses and physicians, the collaborative role becomes more visible. "They (physicians and nurses) make better use of their own professional skills. They enjoy the opportunity to teach and learn from each other. They may feel a new kind of collegial relationship and find it helpful to share the burdens as well as the joys of clinical practice" (Bates, 1975, p. 705).

The Nurse-Aide Role Relationship

Aides usually have a clear-cut definition of tasks or activities. They are often experienced in these tasks, having worked in a particular health care setting longer than the nurse. Normally, aides do not question the nurse's authority; they know they are at the bottom of the "pecking order."

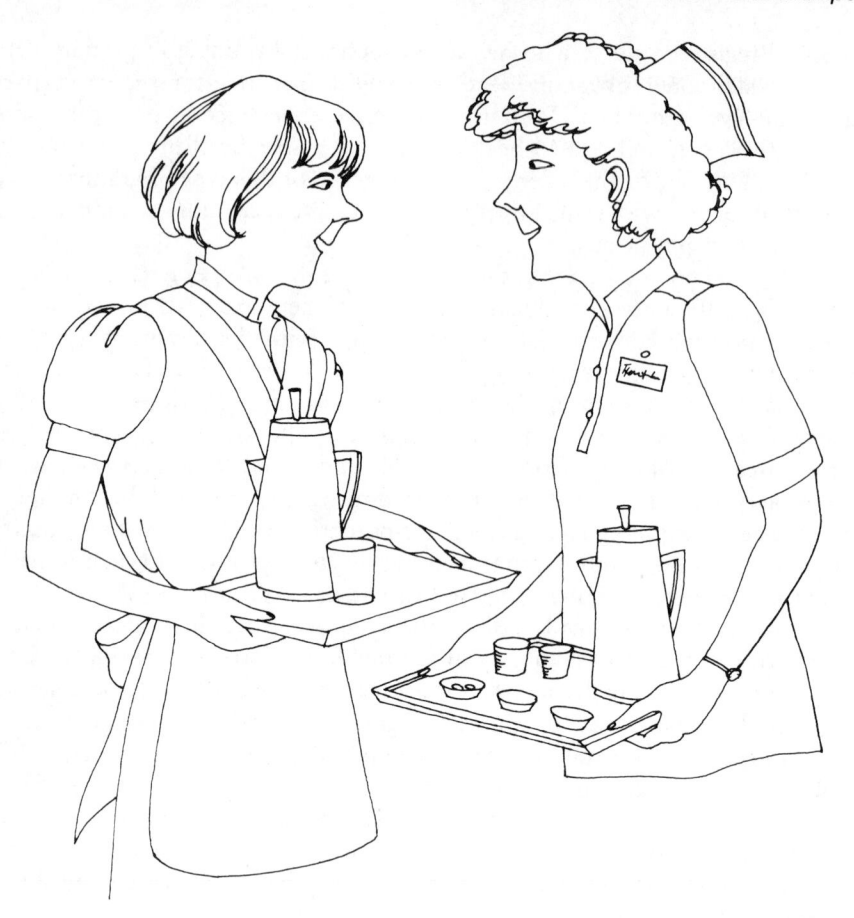

Wiley (1976, pp. 99–100) cites three major factors that create barriers to effective communication between the nurse (team leader or head nurse) and the aide; first, the aide does not always know what the nurse expects; second, the aide may feel that no credit is given for good judgment, and third, the aide may feel that nurse co-workers avoid giving help to aides.

In the first barrier, expectations in terms of tasks, the aide is stating that there is little opportunity to clarify expectations; that there is no reciprocity in the relationship. While the aide can be a constant in a health care setting, the leaders can change. Each nursing leader has different priorities. Thus, the aide plays a "guessing game" as to what the particular nurse in charge expects of him or her. In general, all nurse–aide communication should answer two questions: What does the aide *want* to know and what does the aide *need* to know (Kron, 1967, p. 43)? The nurse should attempt to give the aide as much information as possible. If these two questions are answered, the aide usually has enough information and facts concerning client care to be able to perform in a dependable way.

In nurse-aide interaction, the "what," "when," and "how" are sometimes given, but the 'why" omitted. The following two statements by the nurse to the aide demonstrate the difference between omitting and including the "why."

> Mrs. O'Brien, the aide, has the task of filling the water pitchers on the unit. The nurse in charge might say to her:

Statement A: "Do *not* fill the water pitcher of the client in Room 202."
Statement B: "Do not give Mr. O'Hara, the client in room 202 any liquids. He is on n.p.o. because he is on call for surgery."

In statement A, the nurse did not give a "why"; the aide concluded there must be a reason that the nurse did not want to tell her, and she attempted to fill in the answer herself (by thinking the nurse was angry with Mr. O'Hara). In statement B, the aide was given an explanation which would help her perform a simple task dependably because of the rationale given for the action.

The second barrier, the lack of credit for the aide's good judgment, demonstrates an absence of reciprocity in the nurse–aide relationship, particularly in the affect dimension. While the aide is expected to accept and respect the nurse, there is little sense of being respected in turn by the nurse. A word of thanks or praise by the nurse about the aide's performance is essential. Nurses themselves often are victims of the same syndrome, that is, lack of recognition or credit from *their* superiors.

The third barrier, no help from the nurse, demonstrates a lack of reciprocity across the deference dimension. The aide thinks that the nurse who does not help is placing a greater priority on serving a superior such as the head nurse or physician. The following is a common occurrence in the hospital setting:

> The aide is carrying out a procedure for a client (taking a temperature and pulse) and the call light flashes in the next room. The aide notes that the nurse at the nurses' station does not answer the light. When the aide answers the light, the aide sees the nurse sitting at the nurses' station desk charting. The aide assumes that the nurse *does not want* to answer the light, that his or her role in the eyes of the nurse if not important, and that he or she is not being recognized. Satisfaction with the role of the aide begins to diminish.

Up to this point, we have been talking about nurse-aide communication using the auditory channel, that is, verbal interactions. The aide often receives an assignment on a written assignment sheet, but other than that, all directives are verbal and often one-way. There is no provision for aides to respond even if they do not understand the orders. Effective nurse leaders take the time and opportunity to communicate face-to-face with aides, utilizing all channels (observing, listening, and feeling) in order to make accurate perceptions about what is happening. They also include aides in the planning of client care. A perceptive aide who has had contact with the client for long periods of time will often be able to come up with solutions to client-care problems that are creative and useful. In addition, if aides are included in the planning of care, they will feel that what they are doing is important and that they themselves are appreciated. If one stops to think about it, many problems in the communication interactions between the nurses and aides are the same problems that nurses have felt as students or "new" nurses with a leader. This communication can be termed "downward" communication (complementary) because the level of communication is directed by the leader to an individual who is at a lower level than he or she. This type of communication in relation to the organizational setting in which it occurs is discussed in more detail in Section III of this book.

COMMUNICATION WITH OTHER HEALTH PROFESSIONALS

The extent of communication interactions that nurses have with co-workers depends on the nursing role. Normally, nurses who administer client care do not consult with other co-workers—pharmacist, social worker, or occupational therapist—as much as head nurses or nurse clinicians do. When communication takes place between nurses and other health professionals, the major purpose of nurse/co-worker communication is to share and exchange information about the client and to make joint decisions.

Nurse/co-worker communication relationships are, theoretically, symmetrical. There is reciprocity in the relationship, with mutual agreement on a goal, that goal being to enable the client to function independently. The task dimension of each health care provider often overlaps with a nursing task; for example, the social worker and the nurse both interview the client and often seek the same information from the client. Often co-workers and nurses are not aware of expertise overlap or how much of a difference in perspective each has in their approach to client care.

In the ideal nurse/co-worker relationship, each partner excels in a particular area of expertise and works collaboratively in exercising the expertise to the benefit of the client. They both work to serve client needs (deference dimension); they also respect each other's opinion, as well as have mutual respect for the particular profession that the other represents (affect dimension). More discussion of nurse/co-worker relationships is to be found in Chaper 12 (Health Teams).

Communication Skills as They Relate to Nurse and Co-workers

One way of approaching communication between nurses and co-workers is to think about the kinds of communication skills that are useful in enhancing quality of care, understanding, and self-worth. When these three goals are borne in mind, it becomes obvious that open communication—that is, communication in which there is feedback, trust, and a willingness to comment—is preferable. Defensive communication, on the other hand, will work against the quality of care, understanding, and self-worth of both the nurse and co-worker.

Even with good will, there is likely to be misunderstanding between professions, if only because their language and ways of approaching clients and of organizing health care differ. The nurse may have to use several of the communication and information-gathering skills outlined in Chapter 5, such as summarizing, using focused questions, and asking for clarification to make meaning. The issue of using the other person's "channel," as discussed in Chapter 2, is also applicable.

There are always times when interprofessional communication becomes an emotionally charged issue, such as how to deal with the family of a terminally ill client. At these times, it is particularly important for the nurse to use active listening, self-disclosure, "I" statements, reflection, and paraphrasing. The purpose of using these skills at this time is *not* to make the nurse a therapist of a "one-up" relationship, but rather to help the nurse create symmetry in the relationship and model a willingness to share and be sensitive to the emotional needs of other professionals.

Unfortunately, there are plenty of situations in which all the active listening in the world does not seem to help matters. Like other people, health professionals (including nurses) are at times either not ready or are unwilling to share feelings. Some may be closed to an empathic approach. One has to be continually assessing what kind of style will meet ones goals with other professionals. In fact, one of the reasons some nurses give for maintaining the doctor-nurse game is that at least one goal is met, namely, the client gets the right care. Although this "manipulation" is disturbing at times, it accomplishes what nurses say it does.

The following exercise is presented to help you think about how to use the communication skills discussed in this and earlier chapters in your work with other health professionals.

Exercise in Communication with Other Health Professionals

For each of the following situations, think about how you could use each of the communication skills listed below it to insure the quality of client care, efficient information exchange, and heightened self-worth of both the nurse and the other. Use either Chapters 4 and 5 or the Glossary in the back of the book to refresh your memory of the skills if necessary. Some suggested uses of the skills are found on the right side of the page. Cover them until you have made your choice and then compare them. Remember, even as there are several skills that can be brought to each situation, there are many ways to use each skill. Our suggested use may be no better, or even worse, then the ones you develop.

Situation 1
   An aide comes up to you while you are busy with a client and asks you a question that could wait: "What time is Mr. Brown supposed to be ambulated?"

Skill	*Suggested Option*
Clarification	"Is something wrong with him now?"
"I" message	"I'm busy right now and will get to you when I can. (Said *without* blame.)
Reflection	You seem concerned about Mr. Brown."
Verbal/nonverbal reassurance	(touch shoulder) "Thank you for reminding me. I'll get to it in a minute."

Situation 2
   A physician comes over to you and asks a question about a new client you know little about. How do you handle it?

Skill	*Suggested Option*
"I" statement	"I'm a little short on information, the client is new."
Paraphrase	"You want to know ____. (Paraphrase the question.) I'll have to find out."

Situation 3
   The social worker comes over to you and starts discussing a client with a complicated illness. It becomes obvious that the social worker does not have full

information or understanding about the illness; she then asks: "Well, what is the prognosis—what should I tell the family?" How would you handle this?

Skill	Suggested Option
Focused question	"How much do you know about the illness?"
"I" message	"I feel we ought to talk about the illness first."
"Why" question (not recommended)	"Why do you want to know that?"

Each of these recommended skills represents a beginning to what could be useful communication. Can you also see what the negative consequences of blaming, placating, "why" questions, or patronization might be?

The Use of Assertion with Co-workers

In the previous exercise, you may have found yourself wanting to give a direct message to the other person about your needs or point of view. In the last 15 years, a whole "movement" called "assertion training" has grown around this type of communication.

Traditionally, nurses have been taught to be acquiescent, passive, and submissive in their relationships with other people in the course of their work. What is today thought of as nonassertive or passive was the mode of behavior normally expected of nurses, and women, in the past (Hutchings and Colburn, 1979). Passive, nonassertive nurses possessed those qualities most valued by others within the profession, as well as by those outside of it. Nonassertive behavior was associated with feminine traits; assertive behavior was considered masculine. It was logical that a female profession would emphasize those traits that were feminine.

Assertion training was initially introduced in the late 1960s as a therapeutic tool for psychiatric patients who were considered passive (Lazarus, 1973; Edinberg, 1975; Hutchings and Colburn, 1979). Others, mainly women's groups, were quick to adopt assertion as a way of helping individuals cope with feelings of inadequacy and inferiority. Virtually all nursing schools have introduced some sort of assertion component into their curriculum.

What exactly is assertive behavior? Assertive behavior is that type of interpersonal behavior that enables individuals to act in their own best interest, to stand up for themselves without anxiety, and to exercise their rights without denying those of others (Alberti and Emmons, 1974). Assertive behavior is a direct, honest, and appropriate expression of one's feelings, opinions, and beliefs (Jakubowski-Spector, 1973). Assertive behavior is also taking responsibility for the consequences of those actions.

Consider the following situation:

> A client is in acute distress and needs a blood replacement. You are required to stay with the client. The doctor comes by and orders the blood. He then asks you to go to the blood bank to pick it up.

As the nurse, you are aware that your job is not to pick up the blood at the blood bank; your first priority is to stay with the client. How would you respond?

Four assertive responses are:

1. "No, I cannot do what you requested; I'm not supposed to leave the client."
2. "Doctor, would you get the blood? I'm not supposed to leave."
3. "I feel that is not my responsibility, and it is unfair of you to ask me."
4. "Perhaps you and I should discuss this further with Mrs. Black, the head nurse."

However, some nurses would feel anxious with *any* of these answers, as they potentially provoke controversy and interpersonal conflict with the physician. One outcome could be the rationalization that the status of the client would not be jeopardized while the nurse took a quick run to the blood bank and picked up the blood. The nurse at that point might respond:

> "Yes, doctor, I'll pick up the blood immediately."

In this instance, the nurse is being passive. Passive behavior is interpersonal behavior that allows the individual's rights to be violated in one of two ways: (a) the person violates her or his own rights by ignoring them, or (b) the person permits others to infringe on his or her rights (Jakubowski-Spector, 1973). Passive behavior pays off by enabling the individual to avoid potentially unpleasant conflicts with others; however, various unpleasant internal consequences—hurt feelings and lower self-esteem—are then likely (Jakubowski-Spector, 1973). Another way of avoiding the whole situation in the above example is by ignoring the physician and walking out of the room on the pretext that something is needed for the client.

There is still a different way to respond to the situation. The nurse might say:

> "Doctor, you ordered it. I'm supposed to stay here, so you will have to pick it up!"

In other words, the nurse might try to control the situation; the goal is to "win" regardless of the client's or physician's feelings. In this instance, the nurse is using an aggressive response. Aggressive behavior is interpersonal behavior in which a person stands up for his or her rights in such a way that the rights of the other person are violated. Aggressive behavior dominates, humiliates, or "puts the other person down" as opposed simply to expressing one's honest emotions or thoughts (Jakubowski-Spector, 1973). Aggressive behavior is reactive, not planned. People who utilize aggressive behavior fail to take responsibility for their own action and beliefs.

Although the responses to the situation given in the example have been categorized into three major types of responses: assertive, passive, and aggressive, both the nonassertive and aggressive responses can be considered to be different ways of expressing the same behavior pattern, that of aggression. They are, in a manner of speaking, opposite sides of the same coin. Clarke (1978) notes the similarity of these two overlapping forms of behavior; they are reactive and reflect an underlying insecurity. Passive behavior or avoidance can be thought of as aggression toward oneself in which there is failure to take personal responsibility for one's own actions and feelings. Chart 7-1 summarizes the major attributes of each type of response.

CHART 7-1

Assertive	Aggressive–Passive (avoidance)
Speaking honestly, directly	Control another's behavior
Congruent behavior	Incongruent behavior
"I" statements	"You," "should," "ought" (blame) statements; also "my fault" (placate) statements
Symmetrical relationships	Complementary relationships
Goal-directed	Reactive
Self-regarding	Self-defeating

Types of assertion. Lazarus (1973) divides assertive behavior into four separate and specific response patterns:

1. The ability to say "no"
2. The ability to ask favors and to make requests
3. The ability to express positive and negative feelings
4. The ability to initiate, continue, and terminate general considerations.

Think a moment about yourself and how you would rate yourself on each of the above four abilities. You might think that you are deficient in one area (the ability to say "no," for example) but not the other three. Lazarus states that each ability requires specific training, since the degree of transfer from one area to another is slight. That is, if you think you lack the ability to say "no," this does not mean that you are unable to be assertive in the three other response patterns.

Situation specificity. Another aspect of assertion is that it is situation-specific (Edinberg, et al., 1976). That is, you might find yourself quite capable of being assertive in one situation but becoming passive or aggressive in another. One of the first steps to becoming assertive is to identify which situations give you the most trouble.

Appropriateness of assertion. There are certain situations in which the use of assertion is not appropriate. For example, if a client is in cardiac arrest, and the doctor yells at you in an aggressive manner, it is obviously inappropriate to confront the doctor at that time. In other words, the context in which the interaction occurs determines the appropriateness of the response. In most situations, however, the nurse's right to question the doctor's order or be assertive should not be denied.

Becoming more assertive. Several authors have developed strategies to help people become more assertive (Jakubowski-Spector, 1973; Alberti and Emmons, 1974). While this section of the book is not designed to provide extensive training in becoming assertive, some of the key steps include the following:

1. Identifying the situation
2. Deciding what an assertive response would be
3. Thinking how you would name such a response (covert rehearsal)
4. Watching someone else give the assertive response (modeling)
5. Practicing the response with others (rehearsal)
6. Finding out how you came across (feedback)
7. Actually giving the response in the situation
8. Evaluating how you did.

The following exercise is designed to help you differentiate between assertive, aggressive, and passive behavior.

Exercise in Identifying Assertive, Aggressive, and Passive Behavior

---

In each of the situations below, decide which of the responses is assertive, passive, or aggressive. We have put ratings done by nursing students on the right side of the page (Pa-passive; Ag-aggressive; and As-assertive). Cover them until you have guessed. Discuss your decision with the rest of the class. Which would be appropriate?

Situation 1:
You are ordinarily relieved by the night nurse at 11:15 P.M. However, she is continually

Nurse/Co-worker Dyads

tardy. Tonight is the third night in a row. She is 15 minutes late. Possible responses include:

Responses	Rating
1. "Excuse me, I'm sorry to bother you, but I hope you can get here a little earlier tomorrow."	Pa
2. "You are always late. I'm sick and tired of it."	Ag
3. "This is the third night you have been late. It annoys me that you are late. I would like you to be here on time."	As

Situation 2:
A doctor says, "Where is Mrs. Jones' chart?" You tell him it is in the chart rack. He responds, "It's not there, I can't find it and I need it now."

Responses	Rating
1. You stop what you are doing and go look for it.	Pa
2. "Doctor, can't you see I'm busy? You'll have to find it yourself."	Ag
3. "I'll be with you in a minute; if it's not in the rack, we'll look elsewhere."	As

Situation 3:
A doctor comes onto the floor on a busy day and asks why Mr. Bears hasn't been ambulated. (Mr. Bears has to be ambulated once a day.)

Responses	Rating
1. "If it is so important, why don't you ambulate him? We've been swamped today."	Ag
2. "I'm sorry. I'll do it right now."	Pa
3. "I'm sorry. I didn't know Mr. Bears hadn't been ambulated. I will get an aide to do it when there is time."	As

Situation 4:
You are having trouble with an aide who doesn't want to move a client. The aide yells at you saying, "You don't know what you are doing."

Responses	Rating
1. "Are you going to cooperate or am I going to call the supervisor?"	Ag
2. "OK, I'll get someone else to do it."	Pa
3. "I see you are upset. I would like you to move the client as soon as you calm down."	As

As a final step, act out the situations with a partner. Practice the assertive responses or make up ones of your own. These particular situations are ones that several nurses have designated for us as "assertion-appropriate" situations.

The four situations which have been presented can only serve as examples of what *might* happen to nurses in their work roles. It is impossible to predict exact situations in which one can tell nurses how to respond. This chapter has presented guidelines for understanding some of the communication interactions between nurse and co-worker. The best axiom for all interactions to use is: *never do anything that violates your common sense.*

CONCLUSION

Abdellah's four major schools of thought about nursing encapsulate a brief history of how nurses have related to other health professionals. Before meaningful professional relationships are established, it is necessary that they be reciprocal. This reciprocity is determined by examining four dimensions: task, authority, deference, and affect.

Communication interactions in one particular dyad, that of the nurse-physician, have shifted from what was primarily a complementary dyad to a more symmetrical one. The emergence of the nurse practitioner is one influence that has helped to create this change in emphasis.

Communication barriers can exist in the nurse-aide complementary dyad when the aides do not know what the nurse expects of them, when they feel no credit is given to them, or when nurses avoid helping them.

The use of assertion is one way to encourage congruent communication responses. All workers within the health care system have the right to be assertive and to utilize those communication behaviors that are honest, direct, and self-enhancing.

BIBLIOGRAPHY

Abdellah, F.G. Evolution of nursing as a profession. *International Nursing Review,* 1972, *19,* 319–327.

Alberti, R.E. and Emmons, M.L. *Your perfect right: a guide to assertive behavior* (2nd ed.). California: Impact Publishing Co., 1974.

Bates, B. "Physician and nurse practitioner: conflict and reward. *Annals of Internal Medicine,* 1975, *82,* 702–706.

Claiborn, S. & Walton, W. Pediatricians acceptance of PNPs. *American Journal of Nursing,* 1979, *79,* (2) 300.

Clark, C.C. *Assertive Skills for Nurses.* Wakefield, Massachusetts: Contemporary Publishing, 1978.

Edinberg, M.A. Behavioral assessment and assertion training of the elderly. Unpublished Ph.D. dissertation, University of Cincinnati, 1975.

Edinberg, M.A., Karoly, P., & Gleser, G.C. Assessing assertion in the elderly: an application of the behavioral analytic model of competence. *Journal of Clinical Psychology,* 1977, *33,* 869–874.

Funkhauser, G. R. Probe quality of care: Part I. *Nursing 76,* December 1976, 24–31.
Hite, R.W. New radicalism in nursing: prelude to an irrepressible conflict. *Supervisor Nurse,* March 1977, 14–16.
Hutchings, H. & Colburn, L. An assertiveness training program for nurses. *Nursing Outlook,* 1979, 27, 394–397.
Jakubowski-Spector, P. Facilitating the growth of women through assertive training, *Counsel Psychology,* 1973, 4, 75–86.
Kalish, B.J. & Kalish, P. An analysis of the sources of physician-nurse conflict. *Journal of Nursing Administration,* January 1977, 7, 50–57.
Kron, T. *Communication in Nursing.* Philadelphia: W.B. Saunders 1967.
Lazarus A. On assertive behavior: a brief note. *Behavior Therapy,* 1973, 4, 697–699.
Linn, L.S. Care vs cure: how the nurse practitioner views the patient. *Nursing Outlook,* 1974, 22, 641–644.
Phillips, J.R. Health care provider relationships: a matter of reciprocity. *Nursing Outlook,* 1979, 27, 738–741.
Reed, D. & Roghmann, K.J. Acceptability of an expanded nurse role to nurses and physicians. *Medical Care,* 1971, 9 (4), 372–377.
Smoyak, Problems in interprofessional relations. *Bulletin of the New York Academy of Medicine,* 1977, 53, 51–59.
Stein, L.I. The doctor–nurse game. *Archives of General Psychiatry,* 1967, 16, 699–703.
Stevenson, J.S. *Issues and Crises During Middlescence.* New York:Appleton-Century Crofts, 1977.
Sutterly, D. & Donnelly, G. *Perspectives in human development nursing throughout the life cycle.* Philadelphia, J.B. Lippincott, 1973.
Wesson, A.F. Hospital ideology and communication between ward personnel. In Gartley, J.E. (ed.), *Patients, physicians and illness* (2nd ed.). New York: Free Press, 1972.
Wiley, L. Communications: understanding the gravity of the situation. *Nursing 76,* April 1976, 97–101.
Wiley, L. What doctors really think of nursing—and nurses. *Nursing 79,* August 1979, 73–77.

Chapter 8
Nurse–nurse dyads

BEHAVIORAL OBJECTIVES

By reading this chapter and participating in the exercises, students will be able to:

1. Differentiate between personal and professional nursing identity
2. Describe the purpose and nature of nursing relationships (student-student, student-nurse, nurse-nurse)
3. Identify the internal and external factors that influence student-nurse communication
4. Recognize how nurses confront conflict when it occurs in nurse-nurse communication.

Suppose for a moment that your friend who asked you about nurse-client relationships in Chapter 6 and co-worker relationships in Chapter 7 was quite curious and pursued the conversation one step further. The friend might now ask, "How about your work with other nurses? How do you communicate with them? Is it the same or different from communication with clients or other professionals?" How would one answer this question?

Even though there are many roles, functions, and degrees that are associated with the nursing profession, nurses are often stereotyped, that is, seen as all being identical. The purpose of this chapter is to address the issues in role relationships and communication between nurses.

In addition to time spent with clients and other professionals, nurses spend a portion of their time communicating with other nurses. Who are these "other nurses?" They include supervisors, students, charge nurses, nurse clinicians, RNs, BSNs, ADNs, and LPNs. In this chapter, nurses have been divided into two groups for the purpose of discussion. The first group comprises nursing students. Their interactions with other nursing students (student-student), as well as interactions with other nurses (student-nurse), within the health care delivery system have certain aspects that merit separate attention. A second group comprises graduate staff nurses and their relationships to other nurses (nurse-nurse) within the health care system on the same level, that is, symmetrical relationships with other staff nurses. Staff nurses' relationships with superiors, that is, complementary relationships with head nurses or supervisors, are also discussed. In analyzing these nurse-nurse relationships, communication patterns can be clarified and better understood.

Self-awareness, which includes a knowledge of one's own identity and background, was discussed in Chapter 6 in relation to understanding nurse-client communication. A knowledge of our identity is basic to our perceptions of how we communicate with other nurses.

PERSONAL AND PROFESSIONAL IDENTITY

All communication between nurses and other nurses involves two role identities: a personal role identity and a professional role identity. A balance between these two identities is usually present. For some nurses, however, there might be an overly strong personal identity affiliation with other nurses. For other nurses, there might be an overly rigid professional role identity affiliation. Too strong an affiliation in either the personal role identity or the professional role identity can lead to an imbalance resulting in communication conflicts. In other words, nurses are expected to act in a professional manner, giving the impression at all times that they know what they are doing. At the same time, they cannot afford to be overly distant and give the impression they are insensitive to the needs of clients. Balance between personal and professional role identities is not easy to attain.

Personal Identity

If one thinks about what one really has become since beginning a career in nursing, it might well be agreed that two identities have emerged, personal and professional. The personal identity includes the emotional style, as well as the norms and values shaped by the family, schooling, religion, and friends. It is what makes one unique and different from others. Personal identity includes: feelings, expectations, life experiences, sense of physical self (body image), knowledge, and sense of self-worth.

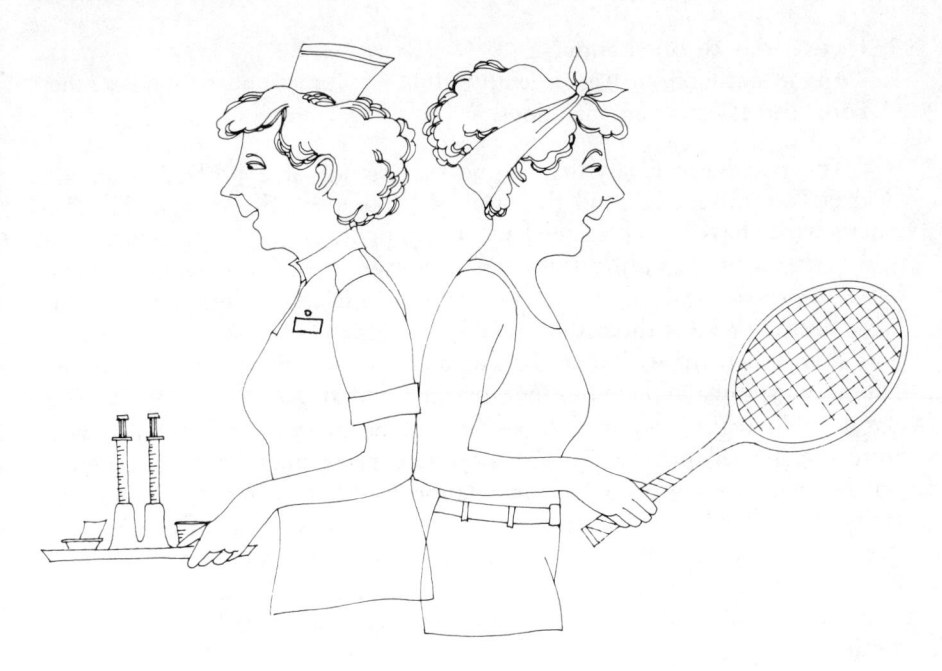

Professional Identity

Professional identity encompasses those characteristics that relate to the profession of nursing. One shares these characteristics with other nurses, as well as common beliefs about nursing and one's role within the system of nursing. One also can be identified as a professional by one's way of dressing (uniform or lab coat), which serves as a visible sign of professional group identification.

Schein (1972) defines professionals, as well as professional tasks and values, as follows. Professionals:

1. Have a strong motivation or calling to their chosen profession,
2. Possess a specialized body of knowledge and skills,
3. Make decisions on behalf of a client,

4. Have a service orientation,
5. Demand autonomy of judgment, and
6. Form professional organizations.

The two basic ideals that define the essence of a profession are the ideal of "social service" and the ideal of "expertise" (Kellams, 1977). The criteria which have been presented above are applicable to *all* professions. That is, the criteria are *interprofessional*. An important issue for nursing is whether nurses as professionals fulfill the above criteria in relation to other professions. Most nursing leaders think that nursing has attained the status of a profession. Yet others have stated that nursing is only in the process of becoming a profession and has not reached the status of full professional maturity. In reality, all professions are in the process of becoming more professional (Kellams, 1977). The most important single issue determining whether nursing is a profession in relation to other professions is centered around the profession's relationship to clients and whether it can respond directly in an autonomous way to client's needs (Marram, 1979).

Review the criteria which is presented in the preceding paragraphs once again. Weigh each criterion carefully and then ask yourself the following questions:

1. Are nurses' behaviors and actions professional in relation to the criteria?
2. Is nursing *more* or *less* professional than medicine, the law, or engineering?
3. Do you see any problems in becoming "overprofessionalized?"

So far the discussion has centered around interprofessional criteria and behaviors. What about *intraprofessional* behaviors? Are there certain behaviors that are characteristic of nurses within the profession itself? Mauksch (1975) has identified four such behaviors:

Accountability
Risk taking
Assertion
Autonomy

How would nurses rate themselves on each of these behaviors? One might use an imaginary low-to-high scale to rate oneself. Students might not rate themselves high because they are in the process of becoming professionals. As they gain more experience in the health care setting, they begin to shift from a personal role identity to a professional role identity. This is not to say that nurses should assume totally the professional role identity; rather, nurses need to learn to integrate both personal and professional identities. Nurses need to be personal to emphasize the human aspects of nursing; they need to be professional to carry out the role of administering competent care to clients. They can be competent nurses and still be warm, empathetic human beings.

Exercise in Personal Versus Professional Role Identity

1. Break up into pairs.
2. Look at the following list of statements in Column 1 (personal identity) and Column 2 (professional identity) and rate yourselves [using a scale of 1 (low) to 5 (high)] on your attitude about yourself in reference to each statement:

Column 1 (Personal Identity)	Column 2 (Professional Identity)
"I am usually happy."	"I have a strong desire to help others."
"What others think about me doesn't affect me."	"I like new experiences."
"I am easy-going."	"I like all types of people."
"I have lots of patience."	"I find satisfaction in hard work."
"I am open and sincere."	"I like to feel needed."
"I have high expectations."	"I am committed to my chosen career."

3. Discuss the similarities and dissimilarities between yourself and your partner with reference to each column. Did you find more or less mutual agreement with the statements in Column 1 or Column 2?
4. Discuss the following: When do personal and professional identities clash? When do they fit together? What kinds of communication occur in each case?

STUDENT-STUDENT COMMUNICATION

The major purpose of students communicating with each other is to socialize, establish rapport, and learn from each other. Often in beginning clinical experiences, students find mutual support in talking with each other and fostering close ties through the sharing of their experiences about their clients with each other. Initial clinical experiences, such as the "first" injection or the "first" bed bath, are always accompanied by a high degree of anxiety. In sharing these experiences with each other, students are often able to minimize the stress of the experience as well as the anxiety they feel. Through the interchange of experiences and ideas, students share each other's situations with clients in the clinical area as if it were their own. Their communication patterns are similar; they talk the same language. One form of language is called the "language of caring" (Purtilo, 1978). This language relates to clients' problems, prognoses, and progress. Another form of language, "technical language" (Purtilo, 1978), constitutes all the modern medical terminology that is specific to nursing and which few outside of nursing, including the client, would be able to understand.

In other words, experiences in client care which students share with other students become a common bond between them, as well as an important outlet for self-expression. Pre-and post-conferences also provide the setting for individual client-care situations to become the "common property" of all the group.

Communication between students is *peer* communication. There is a symmetrical relationship of two partners of equal status that is often characterized by a high level of trust. What is told to a classmate is different from what is told to a staff nurse. The former involves a trust that is specific, that is, trust in a specific individual, the classmate.

Student nurses assume primarily personal identity roles when communicating with each other. However, in hospital or community health settings, they begin to be increasingly conscious of their professional role identity over time. They often find themselves in situations where these two identities conflict, as in the following situation:

> A female student nurse was caring for Mrs. Hall, a burn patient. Mask and gown isolation precautions were ordered to prevent infection. Her classmate walked into the room and neglected to put on an isolation gown. The student nurse's professional identity role would be to tell her classmate to put on the gown. Her personal identity role might question whether she is jeopardizing her friendship with this classmate by telling her she should put on the isolation gown. An experienced nurse would probably not have found this a conflict between identities since she would have assumed a stronger professional role identity.

STUDENT–NURSE RELATIONSHIPS

Student nurses do not have a common base of current experience with staff nurses in the clinical setting. The student and the staff nurse are at different stages of development in the nursing system, both in terms of experience and professionalization. These differences in stages of development can lead to communication problems. In addition, the differences in stages of development also influence how each group perceives the other. The perception of the other group is influenced by a variety of factors that can be categorized as being either internal (to the individual) or external (to the setting).

Internal factors

Internal factors refer to views or perceptions held by the nurse or student. They include the following four perceptions:

The student nurse's perception of self
The graduate nurse's perception of the student nurse
The graduate nurse's perception of self
The student nurse's perception of the graduate nurse.

Nursing interactions in which the student nurse and the graduate do not agree about the four internal perceptions precipitate communication breakdown and lead to conflict. The following two examples serve to demonstrate this point:

> *Case 1.* Miss Taylor, the head nurse on the surgical unit in a community hospital placed high priority on high-visibility tasks. The unit she managed was run at peak efficiency. She always made sure that her clients' physical needs were met. When students came to the unit, Miss Taylor conveyed the attitude they had much to learn and she doubted whether they could assume responsibility for client care without her direct supervision. A student was assigned to Miss Taylor's floor. The student was to care for a colostomy client who was having daily irrigations. The student had looked forward to having this experience and had studied about colostomy clients and treatment before coming to the unit. Miss Taylor's comment to the student, however, regarding the colostomy irrigation was:

"Oh, you could never do that!"

Can you analyze this sequence of events using the concept of internal perceptions?

> *Case 2.* Mr. Morse had just been admitted to the medical unit of a community hospital after having been found drunk and suffering from frostbite. He was found in the poorest section of the community. Mr. Morse had had four previous admissions in the same physical state—dirty, unkempt, and with an attitude of indifference concerning his health. The nurses on the unit had worked with this man, but after four previous admissions were disgusted. One of them commented:

"Let the students clean him up. We've had it!"

In the first example, a difference exists in the way the student nurse perceived self and the way the graduate perceived this same student. The student felt he or she was capable of assuming more responsibility in client care than the nurse did. There was a lack of reciprocity in the dimension of the task; the task being the colostomy irrigation. In the second example, the nurses allowed their personal identities and values (cleanliness, concern for one's own health and welfare) to block their motivation to care for the client. They perceived the students as serving their needs first and thus gave them a task which the graduate nurses did not wish to carry out.

In both examples, an opportunity to share feelings in an environment of mutual trust would have helped both nurses and students to understand each other. The staff nurses might be surprised at how they come across if they were to obtain direct feedback from the students. Clinical instructors are often called upon to facilitate this mutual sharing.

External factors

External factors that influence student-nurse relationships include all aspects of the work setting that influence both groups. External factors in the student-nurse interactions contribute to an even larger share of communication barriers than internal factors. Again, differences in the perception of external factors between students and nurses contribute to these barriers.

One external factor in the larger health care environment is the setting in which students and nurses find themselves working together. Students are usually working in "foreign" territory; that is, they may be unfamiliar with the members of the system, as well as the communication patterns. The spontaneity and sense of equality that prevailed in the classroom or nursing arts laboratory setting is supplanted by a climate that is uncertain and controlled by others. Students in the clinical setting often do not know where specific equipment is kept or what some of the routines are. In a community agency, they are unsure of the record-keeping procedure or the geographical locations of their clients.

In addition, students are part of an "out-group" in the clinical setting. The nurse may look at students as outsiders and not share personal information. Students may feel alienated and confused; they will not know what their functions are. Hopefully, the instructor acts as an interpreter in such situations to guide and answer questions so that students can become aware of role tasks and can function appropriately.

On the other hand, graduate nurses perceive their work environment as familiar territory. They know the routines and standard paper work. They are working with other members who mirror their professional images in the same manner that the student co-worker mirrored the image of the student. They wear the same uniform and speak the same caring and technical languages. They have a sense of trust in other nurses, and respect the performance levels of their co-workers.

Another external factor is time. For example, students usually find themselves on fixed time schedules. Not only are they concerned with how they are interacting with the staff in the clinical setting, they are concerned with whether they will finish their assignments on time. Chances are that their clinical schedule is set up around their class schedule, and no extra time is allotted for accomplishing their set tasks. Hall (1969) describes two contrasting ways people handle time: monochronic and polychronic. Monochronic characterizes people who tend to focus on the task (rather than the person) and who have low involvement with others. These people schedule one thing at a time and become "rattled" when too many things are happening at once. Polychronic, on the other hand, characterizes those individuals who tend to focus on the person and who have a sense of deeper involvement with others. These people can handle several activities simultaneously. That is, they tend to "juggle" time. Often, students are placed into situations where they feel an obligation to concentrate on the task. They have a sense of feeling rushed, of being time-bound. They find they do not have time to share feelings or even pertinent information with staff nurses.

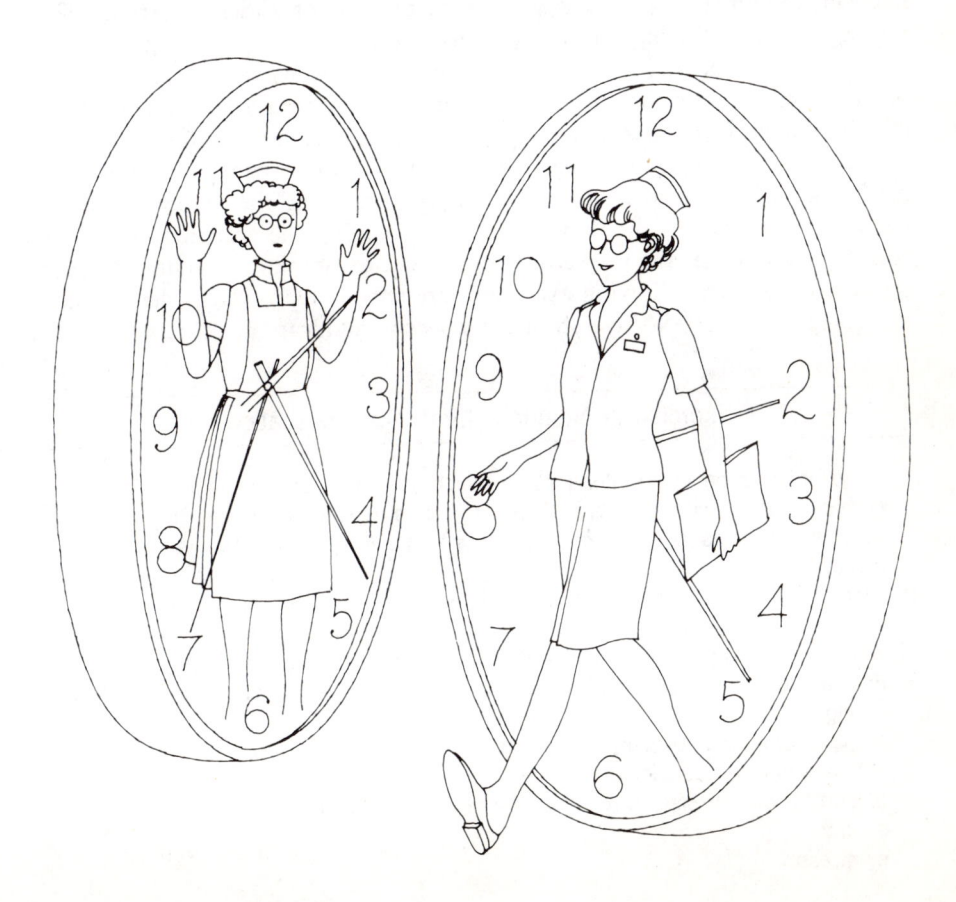

We all live in the here (space) and now (time); therefore, time becomes valuable. In our role as nurses, it is always possible that we will not be able to finish assigned tasks within the time period afforded them. Often, it is difficult to take time to communicate to students. Time restrictions limit relationships not only between nurses and clients, but also between nurses and other nurses. How nurses prioritize their time is an expression of their feelings about what is important to them. If a nurse is willing to spend time with a student, it is reasonable to assume that the nurse places a high value on the communication interaction. Some nurses become skilled in utilizing time spent in communication to good advantage. Others may assign students a low priority in their minds and not spend much time communicating with them.

Differences in perception of the hospital setting and in the concept of time, as well as the internal factors of self-worth and varying degrees in ability to perform nursing tasks, can lead to defensive communication between student and staff nurse. The result will be placating, blaming, superreasonableness, and irrelevance. Defensive behaviors tend to promote "distancing" (Purtilo, 1978) rather than a relationship of intimacy in which feelings are shared and communication is open, with both partners listening, understanding, and accepting differences and criticism from each other. Defensive communication patterns are characterized by incongruency: nurses who are busy and harrassed may smile at the students; nurses who are upset with very ill clients can appear over-worked and have no time for student questions. The messages are conflicting and difficult to interpret.

Given the possibilities for closed communication—as well as ones for open communication that is efficient, congruent, and raises self-worth—how can the student learn to communicate effectively in the various clinical settings that are encountered? The usual answer is "through trial and error plus modeling the instructor." Also, the more congruent the response of the student, the more able he or she will be to pick up the accepted "style" of communication that fits the setting and to decide how to communicate on a sensible basis. The following exercise represents a step towards determining the components of effective student-nurse communication:

Exercise in Student–Nurse Communication

1. Write or describe three situations in which you, as a student, were effective in communicating with a nurse. That is, the message sent was the message received, the message was congruent, or that self-worth was maintained on both sides.
2. Now, write or describe three situations in which your communication was ineffective with a nurse. That is, the message sent was *not* the one received, you were incongruent, or that self-worth was lowered by the message.
3. For each of the three messages in Step 2 above, make a guess as to what "went wrong":
   a. no understanding of other's words
   b. "personality" (conflict of styles)
   c. conflict of channels (e.g., one visual, one auditory)
   d. time
   e. stress

f. lack of trust
g. differences in perception of abilities
h. difference of opinion.
4. In the large group, discuss how some of these could be rectified. What can you do to change the patterns?

In addition to the internal and external factors that influence student-nurse communication, there are three common difficulties that students encounter in communicating with nurses.

1. *High expectations.* Most students begin their clinical experiences expecting to know all the answers, as well as to administer client care with little or no difficulty. Many students expect to be all things to all people. These are unreal expectations.
2. *An inability to define the problem.* The most difficult step of the problem-solving model presented in Chapter 6 (see p. 155) is pinpointing the problem. A pertinent question to ask is, "Who owns the problem?" Once the problem is identified in clear, meaningful behaviors and the "who" identified at each step of the problem-solving model, the corner has been turned towards solving the problem. An inability to define the problem is a difficulty for both students and staff nurses.
3. *The reluctance on the part of nurses to express feelings and emotions.* Nurses, students, and graduates are no different from people in general. Many people hide their true feelings, that is, they tend to act differently from the way they feel. The environment in which nursing care is administered encourages the masking of real feelings. The concept of the "good nurse" leading to a professional bedside manner fosters a stereotype of a nonlistener who interacts with people on a superficial level. Some nurses can be described as stoic or overprofessional; they are afraid of showing their feelings, of being sad and crying, or of becoming angry. They are in control and avoid all emotional involvement. Their emotions are camouflaged in an aura of superreasonableness and distraction.

These three potential student-nurse communication interaction problem areas are relevant to interactions between all categories of nurses, students, and graduates as well.

NURSE-NURSE RELATIONSHIPS

Nurses are seldom aware of the complex communication skills that are required in working with other nurses. The authors of this text asked a group of graduate nurses to describe situations which were sources of communication difficulties between nurses. The situations they described were ones in which there was a lack of reciprocity in relation to the nurse's work role. Two examples of these conflicts follows. As you look at each example, place yourself in the nurse's role and try to imagine how you would respond.

> Your supervisor calls you and asks you to work overtime because no one else is available. You have made other plans for your day off.

> You are working with a client and need some immediate help from another nurse. You see Mrs. Lee, who is sitting down having her fourth cigarette since she came to work.

In each of the two examples presented, the nurse is either judging or being judged by others. While there is no panacea for dealing with internurse conflict, there are some guidelines that can be followed.

Dealing with Stress

Stress is an expected part of any relationship. An understanding of the causes of stress, of how people react to it, and of the resulting communication barriers is also beneficial.

In the hospital, clients are ill, in pain, or helpless. In the community setting, clients are often poor and have many unfulfilled needs. Nurses work with atypical populations, namely, sick individuals. As a result, they can feel stress and helpless. New students have been known to generalize the illness concept to the total population during the intitial clinical experiences, never realizing that the vast majority of the population is well, or perhaps mildly unwell, and are able to function at high levels of wellness.

Donnelly (1980) refers to two ways of dealing with stress: reactive and active. In reacting to stress, one experiences the fight-or-flight syndrome as the only recourse. One chooses to fight the stressful situation through the use of aggression or by using defensive behaviors ("it's not my fault"). One copes by turning the stress inward and finding satisfaction in other ways: eating, drinking, smoking, sleeping, or becoming depressed (Scully, 1980). Active ways of dealing with stress are, first, to identify the *signs* of stress and then to locate the *sources* of stress. Having done this, one can learn to control his or her behavior through the utilization of exercises or relaxation techniques or by increasing a sense of "nursing self" (Winstead-Fry, 1977).

Dealing with Conflict

People tend to deal with conflict in different ways. Blake and Moulton (1964) have proposed five approaches to handling conflict:

1. Avoid situations that provoke controversy or disagreement.
2. Smooth it over by false reassurance, thinking that everything will be OK.
3. Overpower it in an authoritarian manner.
4. Bargain and reach a compromise solution.
5. Identify the underlying causes and through understanding, work out a solution—the problem-solving approach.

We are able to characterize how we react to conflict by identifying with one of the above approaches. Identifying the reasons for the conflict and attempting to resolve the underlying causes (statement 5) is the most effective approach in dealing with conflict situations. It also involves utilizing the problem-solving approach, and as previously stated, once the problem is identified, the resolution of the problem is not as difficult as it was before the problem was pinpointed.

While there are some "artful dodgers" (as in statement 1 above) who constantly avoid stress in order to survive, this is not a response that promotes psychological growth. Again, the "peacemakers" (statement 2) do not get at the heart of the problem. Statement 3, which on the surface appears to be a solution for conflict, does not probe at finding the reasons for the stress. Statement 4 internalizes the conflict, an approach that involves the risks of ulcer or high blood pressure or depression.

When conflicts do occur, some nurses utilize defensive communication patterns in which they spend most of their time and energy defending themselves. Because they have perceived themselves as being threatened, they do not listen to others but concentrate on the impact of their behavior on others. It is possible to learn to anticipate these defensive behaviors and recognize the attacks are not directed toward one's self-worth, thus depersonalizing the conflict. In the resolution of the conflict, usually both sides have to give. The skills concerning use of channels, assertion, and empathy that have been presented in other sections of this book are helpful in conflict resolution.

There are situations in which nurses are under such stress that they have little sense of self-awareness. Working with such a co-worker over an extended period of time using a behavioral approach is perhaps the only way to deal with this type of conflict. This sort of approach suggests that behavior can often be controlled by its consequences. People will most likely engage in desired behavior if they are rewarded for doing so. In other words, by creating pleasing consequences to specific forms of behavior, we can increase the frequency of that behavior (Skinner, 1953). In this way, nurses can modify the behavior of others. Ideally, the behavior they choose to reinforce is the opposite of the behavior they are trying to discourage. By ignoring the "bad" behavior and reinforcing the "good" behavior, it is possible to see some positive changes over a period of time (Wiley, 1979).

We all find situations in which certain personalities do not mesh with ours. Perhaps we are too much alike or the person might remind us of someone with whom we had a negative experience in past years. Nurses are cautioned not to place too high expectations on themselves nor should they feel that they will be able to relate to all other nurses equally well. There will always be some nurses with whom we can relate more effectively than others.

CONCLUSION

Nurses must be individuals as well as nurses. That is, they have personal as well as professional roles. Students, who are at the beginning of their nursing careers, are in the process of being professionalized. That is, they are learning certain prescribed behaviors which will facilitate their participation and performance within the profession (Hardy and Conley, 1978). Thus, students are undergoing a process of transformation from personal into professional roles. This transformation has an influence on the way they communicate with other students.

One of the greatest sources of stress for students when they communicate with staff nurses is that they hold unrealistic expectations for themselves in terms of what they can accomplish. This can be a source of incongruent messages in that the student may communicate things that are different from what they really feel. Students and graduates alike can learn to deal with stress by identifying the sources of their stress and learning how they confront conflict. These skills are necessary in order for all nurses to cope with the difficult communication problems that can arise between nurses in the clinical area.

BIBLIOGRAPHY

Blake R. & Moulton, J. *The managerial grid.* Houston: Gulf Publishing, 1964.
Donnelly, G. F. Why you just can't take it anymore! *RN,* May 1980, 34–37.
Hardy, M. & Conley, M. *Role theory: perspectives for health professionals.* New York: Appleton-Century-Crofts, 1978
Hall E., *The hidden dimension.* Garden City, N.Y.: Anchor Books, 1969.
Kellams, S. Ideals of a profession: the case of nursing. *Image,* 1977, 9 (2), 30–31.
Marram, G., Barrett M. & Bevis, E.O. *Primary nursing* (2nd ed.). St. Louis: C.V. Mosby, 1979.
Mauksch, I. Sybil Bellos Palmer Lecture delivered at Yale University School of Nursing, April, 1975.

Northhouse, P.G. Interpersonal trust and empathy in the nurse-nurse relationships. *Nursing Research,* 1979, *28,* 365–368.

Purtilo, R. *Health professional patient interactions* (2nd ed.). Philadelphia: W.B. Saunders, 1978.

Schein, E. *Professional education: some new directions.* New York: McGraw-Hill, 1972.

Scully, R. Stress in the nurse. *American Journal of Nursing,* 1980, *80,* (5) 912–914.

Skinner, B.F. *Science and human behavior.* New York: Free Press, 1953.

Wiley, L. The problem co-worker. What to do when you can't ignore her (him) anymore. *Nursing 79,* June 1979, 74–77.

Winstead-Fry, X. The need to differentiate a nursing self. *American Journal of Nursing,* 1977, *77*(9), 1452–1454.

SECTION III

COMMUNICATION AND THE PRACTICE SETTING

The third section of this book addresses communication between nurses and other members of the health care system within the context of the practice setting. Nursing has traditionally been practiced in two settings: the hospital and the community. With the advent of complex medical and nursing technology, hospitals have been organized into specialized settings, such as those for acute and chronic illness; short- and long-term illness; or acute and highly acute illness (intensive care, coronary care, renal dialysis). And the environmental structure has been organized into subunits for which particular nursing functions and activities have been delegated. In each setting, nurses have a specific set of role behaviors. Thus, nurses in a chronic disease unit of a nursing home will find themselves placing priorities on a different set of tasks than nurses in a visiting nurse association.

The concept of the practice of nursing as a system and nurses as functioning members within a system is not necessarily new. The phrase "health care system" is frequently used to describe health care in its totality. What is new is the concept of levels of nursing practice, each constituting a separate system in which individual members interact with each other in various combinations. The content of this section of the book provides the answers to such questions as: What constitutes a nursing system? Who are the members that make up the system and what behaviors pertain to the system?

A system is not only composed of interrelated parts; it has a specific goal. The goal of the nursing system is promoting client health. Systems of nursing practice are composed of groups whose members interact in such a way that when something affects one member of the group, all members are affected. System components parallel communication components in many ways: they are characterized by "inputs" (senders), "throughputs" (channels), and "outputs" (responses) that affect the system as a whole. Systems are also characterized by feedback, which acts in an evaluative way to insure that the specified goal is achieved. An application of Satir's description (1972) of a system is applied to a nursing systems model in Chart III-1.

CHART III-1
A Model For Nursing

Component	Nursing Model
Purpose or goal (why does the system exist?)	For the improvement of client care
Essential parts	Nurses, clients and families, physicians, and all other health care personnel
An order to the essential parts	Standard procedures, communication between the members, rules and regulations
Impetus for system's existence	The need for improved communication for optimum health care within the hospital community
Maintenance of system's functioning	The interactions of the members of the health team with the client
Adaptability to environmental changes	New procedures, new members, new nursing technologies

Systems can be characterized by their degree of openness. Open systems are adaptive: they respond to change and outside influence. The behavior is dynamic and ongoing. An open system is in a state of equilibrium;

that is, it will regain its balance after changes are made. Closed systems are not amenable to change: they have walls of resistance to ward off outside influence. There is no feedback. Members of closed systems are governed by a set of rigid rules and regulations. Closed systems are in a state of disequilibrium; that is, changes weaken the system and put it into a state of imbalance.

Can you give examples of open and closed systems? Do you consider the clinical area to which you are currently assigned an open or closed system? Keep in mind the following questions as you determine whether you are working in a closed or open system.

1. Do you know what your specific tasks are as you work within this system?
2. To what degree does this system receive inputs (suggestions, new ideas, new procedures) from outside the system and adapt them to the system?
3. Is there a hierarchy among the members of the system with differing levels of authority?
4. Do you feel you belong?
5. Are communication relationships with members of the system symmetrical or complementary?

In the following chapters, the structure of nursing practice is defined in relation to three systems. Communication patterns and how they interact within each system are described. Each of the three systems has been formulated using the framework initially proposed by the Southern Regional Educational Board, a group of nurse educators in the South who met over a period of 2½ years and made specific recommendations about the future of nursing and nursing education.

Systems of nursing practice. There are three systems of nursing practice: secondary, tertiary, and primary. In the secondary system of nursing practice, nursing care is directed towards those clients who are experiencing common and well-defined acute or chronic illnesses (Haase et al., 1976). Nurses who work in the secondary system of nursing practice assume the "more traditional staff nurse roles" and work in widely distributed community hospitals. Their tasks are the more routine and less complex tasks usually given under the supervision of an experienced clinician or supervisor. New graduates most often work in a secondary system of nursing practice.

Tertiary care is associated with large urban hospitals and medical centers. Nurses working in tertiary care settings deal with rare and complex illnesses, often in association with experimental and clinical research. Tertiary care facilities are less widely distributed than secondary care systems and are most often located in a university or research institution.

Nursing in a primary health care system is directed towards clients in outpatient or community settings. The emphasis of primary care is on health maintenance and health promotion. The term "primary care" designates the client's first contact with the health care system. It is not to be confused with "primary nursing," which implies responsibility for the nursing care of the client over a 24-hour period. (Nursing behaviors in the primary system of nursing practice focus on assessment skills such as history taking and nursing diagnosis.)

Examples of how nursing contexts can be characterized within the three systems are as follows:

> Secondary system: Community hospitals—medical, surgical, pediatric, obstetric, and operating room units; geriatric care settings.
> Tertiary system: Oncology units, intensive care units, coronary care units, neonatology units located in university settings.
> Primary system: Public health, occupational health, school nursing, primary care units.

Each of the three systems can be identified by examining two specific variables: the level of wellness or illness of the client and the setting in which the nurse–client interaction occurs. Chart III–2 summarizes the main aspects of each of the three systems of nursing practice.

CHART III–2
Secondary, Tertiary and Primary Levels of Nursing Practice

System	Level of Illness-Wellness	Major Setting
Secondary	Moderately ill	Community hospital
Tertiary	Acutely ill	University hospital
Primary	Well	Outpatient community

Exercise in Identifying Secondary, Tertiary, and Primary Systems of Nursing Practice

Identify the system to which the following settings and levels of client wellness-illness belong. Answers are given on the right side of the page.

Setting/Level	System
1. Teaching a teenage client with diabetes to administer an insulin hypodermic in an outpatient clinic.	Primary

2. Caring for an acutely ill client in the intensive care unit who has had a stroke. — Tertiary
3. Caring for a postoperative patient in the hospital who has had a cholescystectomy. — Secondary
4. Administering a medication for a headache to an elderly client in a geriatric care setting. — Secondary
5. Caring for a postoperative client in the coronary care unit who has had a three-way coronary bypass operation. — Tertiary
6. Assessing the psychological status of a client who is in remission for rheumatoid arthritis in an outpatient clinic. — Primary

BIBLIOGRAPHY

Haase, P., Smith, M.H., & Reitt, B. A proposed system for nursing: theoretical framework, part 2. In *Pathways to Practice* (Vol. 4). Atlanta: Southern Regional Education Board, 1976.

Satir, V. *Peoplemaking*. Palo Alto, California: Science and Behavior Books, 1972.

Chapter 9
Communication in secondary nursing practice

BEHAVIORAL OBJECTIVES

By reading this chapter, students will be able to:

1. Describe a system of secondary nursing practice
2. Describe the three dimensions of structure and how they relate to a system of secondary nursing practice
3. Relate five nurse-client communication barriers to secondary nursing practice settings
4. Describe concepts of personal space, territorial space, and the characteristics of a bureaucracy
5. Distinguish between team, functional, and primary nursing staffing patterns
6. Understand how the concepts of stereotyping the client, multichannel communication, and triadic communication affect communication interactions in the secondary care setting.

SECONDARY NURSING PRACTICE

Secondary nursing care takes place in a community hospital (Haase et al., 1976). Community hospitals vary in size but are generally from 50 to 300 beds. Clients have illnesses that can be described as single acute episodes such as a gall bladder attack or an acute myocardial infarction. Also clients have illnesses that are characterized by exacerbations associated with many chronic diseases such as cerebral vascular accident or rheumatoid arthritis. A secondary care system would include those illnesses that commonly recur and are even routine (Haase et al., 1976).

Nurses who work in a secondary system of nursing practice can be described as functioning in the more traditional role of the staff nurse. They are not highly specialized in relation to nurses in other systems of nursing practice. They are "generalists," that is, they have a broad base of fundamental knowledge that is applicable to a variety of nursing situations in which the nature of illness is not complex but is usual and expected. Secondary care nurses often work under the direct guidance of more experienced specialized nurse clinicians or nurse practitioners or staff workers.

An analysis of the structure of the system of secondary nursing practice provides a means for understanding some of the communication patterns that are characteristic of this system. Lewis (1975) defines structure in terms of three dimensions: the physical setting in which the practice takes place; the organization of activities in this setting; and the expectation of the members of the system (role). In this chapter, we use these dimensions to analyze communication in the secondary nursing system.

The Physical Setting

The first dimension of secondary nursing practice is physical setting. The concept of physical setting, according to Lewis's definition, refers to the available medical equipment, space, and means of communication (Lewis, 1975).

Often, the physical setting of the hospital itself contributes to clients' reluctance to express feelings. That is, certain characteristics of the hospital environment create communication barriers. Five barriers are:

1. The use of technical language
2. The rigid routine
3. Noise level
4. Uniforms
5. "Busy" atmosphere.

The Use of Technical Language. The use of technical language inhibits the communication process. Hospital personnel who are accustomed to the clinical setting often forget that many clients do not understand medical terminology as well as "in-house" jargon.

Examples such as "Mrs. Thompson is due for her p.o. med. stat!" or "Did you send Mrs. Thomas's cath spec to the lab?" are often spoken in the presence of the client. One study that involved 200 patients, 85 percent of whom had a high school education or better, revealed that 51 percent did not understand what the word "benign" meant (Blondis and Jackson, 1977).

Another study demonstrated that most clients in the study thought "force fluids" meant forced urination, even after they were made aware that drinking was involved (Cosper, 1977). Both studies conclude there is considerable lack of understanding for many of the commonly used hospital words. Cosper gives some guidelines to use when talking to clients in the hospital:

Use simple language when talking to the client.
When it is necessary to use hospital terms, explain to client.
Key the explanation to the intellectual level of the client.
Watch clients who are "first admissions."
Ask for feedback.
Guard against use of "hospital jargon" with co-workers within hearing of clients. (Cosper, 1977).

The use of words that the client is unable to comprehend serves to foster complementary relationships.

Rigid Routine. Clients are overtly and subtly encouraged to conform to the hospital environment. If baths are given in the A.M., the client receives the bath in the A.M., whether or not he or she feels it is needed. Meals, naps, temperatures, other procedures and doctors' visits are all routinized in the hospital environment. Clients will also conform to routinized and sanctioned "times to talk" and may become "good patients" when it is not the "correct time to share," such as when the nurse is tending to another client in the same room.

Noise Level. Despite signs to the contrary, the hospital is a noisy place. Many people go in and out of rooms with carts, charts, medications, and meals. It may be difficult to find a quiet place to talk privately to a client.

Uniforms. Uniforms have several purposes. They serve to identify staff position to the client. They also identify staff position to other staff. The uniform can provide a sense of security to clients.

At the same time, uniforms can act as a barrier to therapeutic communication. The client may assume that the nurse in uniform is "impersonal" or only interested in medical facts, not feelings. The uniform can serve to distance clients from the nurse and implies a complementary relationship.

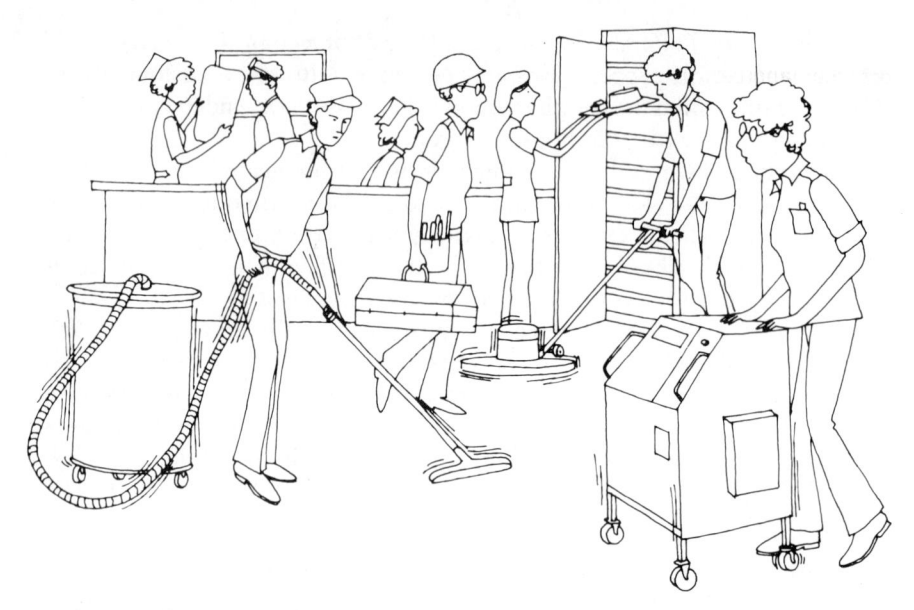

At the same time it should be repeated that the uniform represents an identity and may be a source of security to clients. Uniforms are not necessarily good or bad, but they *can* inhibit certain communication.

"Busy" Atmosphere. This is an intangible aspect of hospitals that can influence nurse–client communication. At times, clients feel that there is a sense of urgency in what nurses are doing and that their own concerns are too small to be important. They do not want to take up the nurse's valuable time talking about feelings.

Similarly, nurses may feel that they are too busy to take the time to give therapeutic care. This may be due to task realities, the nurse's own discomfort talking to clients, or a sense that this is not "the right place" to spend time talking. The nurse who continually senses this is "not the right time" has allowed the "busy" atmosphere to interfere with effective nurse-client communication.

Exercise in Developing Strategies to Handle Communication Barriers in the Hospital Environment

1. Divide into groups of three.
2. Each group will either pick or be assigned one of the following communication "barriers" within the hospital milieu:

Roommates
Technical language
Uniforms
Noise level

Busy atmosphere
Change of routine in different shifts
Fragmented nursing care

3. Each group will then think of one additional barrier *not* on the list.
4. For its two barriers, each group will come up with three ways of decreasing the impact of the barrier on effective nurse-client communication.
5. Share your strategies.

The Concept of Space. An important aspect of the physical setting is the concept of space. There are two dimensions to this concept: physical space itself and a sense of space in the abstract sense, referred to as personal space.

Physical space can directly influence the pattern and level of communication interaction in a nurse-client dyad. For example, if a client wishes to share feelings of anxiety with a nurse and finds herself in a four-bed unit where her roommates can overhear, she will not be able to share her fears and anxieties easily.

In addition, the everyday "hustle and bustle" atmosphere of the average hospital setting does not lend itself readily to effective and meaningful communication between clients, nurses, and other health professionals. Some of the most effective communication occurs during the evening and night shifts when there are fewer health professionals present and a more relaxed atmosphere prevails.

Personal space is that sense of space which is fluid and mobile; it includes the "internal territory of the self" (Yura and Walsh, 1978). One's body is the center of this personal space.

All people have a need to acquire symbolically, and defend physical territory. They have a desire to call certain territory "their own," whether it be "their car" or "their yard." Clients in hospital settings think of the room to which they are assigned as their room and attach importance to objects surrounding the bedside, such as the bedside table. Nurses who are effective in nurse–client communication have developed a sense of respect for the client's sense of personal space. Knocking before entering the client's room, standing at the foot of the bed while talking to the client, and calling the client by name are ways of giving the client more personal space. Nurses who approach clients without first assessing if the clients wish to have them come close are not respecting the clients' sense of personal space.

Nurses, as well as clients, possess a sense of personal space. In their professional role, they would prefer a sense of territory in which they feel secure. However, the physical dimensions of a nurses' station prohibit a sense of territory. In addition, the nurses' station is often used by a number of other professionals. Thus, the nurse's territory is often reduced to a locker in a cloakroom or perhaps to a small cubicle where group meetings are held. Thus there is no desk or physical space that nurses can identify as their "turf." This can lead to frustration in communicating with other professionals because of the lack of privacy.

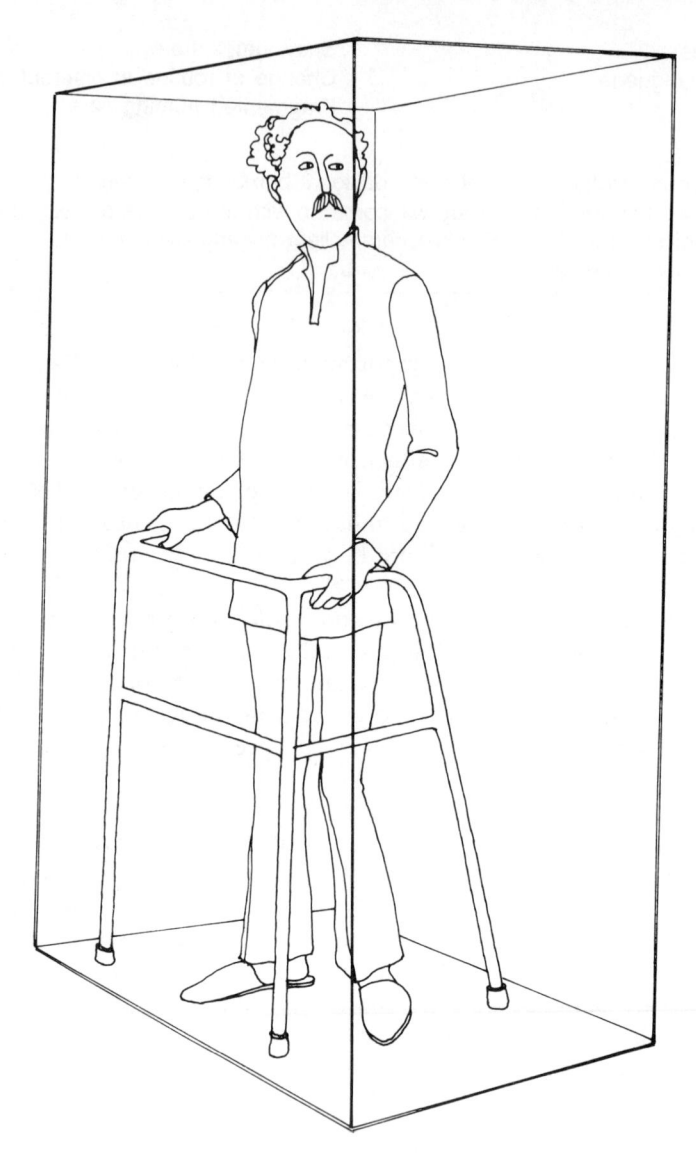

Organization of Activities

A second dimension of structure is organization of activities, which Lewis defines as the daily routine of the setting and "who nurses whom" under what conditions (Lewis, 1975). The organization of activities in a community hospital setting is bureaucratic. A bureaucracy has four major characteristics (Skipper and Leonard, 1965):

1. Specialization: In the hospital there is a clear division of labor, and activities are distributed among members who perform or are responsible for only those tasks they are assigned.
2. Hierarchy of authority: All positions are arranged in a hierarchy. There are designated superior and subordinate positions; the superior initiates the action and the subordinate is the recipient of action. Each person is held accountable to a superior.
3. An explicit set of policies: There are standard operating procedures that define and regulate all behavior.
4. An impersonal attitude: Each member conducts his or her work in an efficient manner with an attitude of personal detachment.

Bureaucracies are closed systems; they do not easily adapt to change. Bureaucratic hospitals are supposedly models of efficiency in that many tasks are accomplished, but what is gained by being efficient may be lost in poor communication patterns. The four major attributes of a bureaucracy affect nursing communication in the following ways:

Specialization. In secondary nursing practice, there is much contact with other health professionals, yet there is little or no communication among health professionals at a departmental or interdepartmental level. Nurses communicate primarily with other nurses; physicians share a greater sense of collegiality with other physicians than with other professionals. While it can be assumed that this is a natural tendency, the high level of specialization present in the hospital encourages little or no communication among subspecialities of these professions. That is, operating room nurses communicate primarily with other operating room nurses, and pediatric nurses tend to communicate with other pediatric nurses.

Interdepartmental communication is often a problem in the bureaucratic structure of the hospital. Other departments do not have the same set of priorities as the floor unit. For example, a nurse calls the surgical supply department to order a tracheostomy set and is told by the receiver of the call that the old set must be returned before a new one can be sent to the floor. The nurse's top priority is to get the tracheostomy set as soon as possible because of a crisis situation; the technician in the surgical supply department has different priorities, ones given by the supervisor.

Specialization encourages written memos and directives on printed forms. Person-to-person contact is limited, leading to a sense of isolation and alienation of individuals working or receiving nursing care in the system.

Hierarchy of Authority. The second characteristic of bureaucracy implies levels of authority in which one is responsible to a superior but at the same time has control over a subordinate. For example, a staff nurse reports to her head nurse but at the same time she supervises the licensed practical nurse. Hierarchy of authority is most evident in two patterns of staffing in community hospitals: team nursing and functional nursing.

TEAM NURSING. In team nursing, the nursing staff (RNs, LPNs, nursing assistants, and aides) is divided into teams and each team is assigned to a specific location in the hospital. The team is responsible for a designated group of clients. Acutely ill clients are usually assigned to the most capable and experienced members of the team. The team leader assigns the duties to the team members on an *ad hoc* basis during each shift and reports directly to the head nurse. There is a clear hierarchy of authority. Communication follows the same lines. The team leaders report to the head nurse, who reports to the supervisor, who reports to an assistant or the director of nursing. The team leader can also communicate "down" to the RN on the team, who communicates to the LPN, who communicates to an aide.

Team nursing places the nurse in a "middle management" position; one in which the nurse is giving and receiving communication from both "above" and "below." When messages conflict, highly stressful situations result. The team leader may find him- or herself in a "double-bind" position of receiving conflicting messages from above and below. While the first priority is the client, who is at the bottom of the hierarchy, there is a natural inclination to obey orders from above.

HEAD NURSE to team leader: "Ambulate Mr. Jones today."
TEAM LEADER to staff nurse: "Ambulate Mr. Jones."
STAFF NURSE to team leader: "Mr. Jones will not get out of bed. He is threatening to call his doctor if the nurses do not leave him alone."

In this situation given, the team leader has some options:

1. Order the staff nurse to go back and ambulate Mr. Jones.
2. Tell the head nurse Mr. Jones will not get out of bed.
3. Go to Mr. Jones directly and explain to him why it is important for him to ambulate.

The team leader is also the coordinator of total client care, a role in which he or she coordinates communication from several departments (pharmacy, dietary, X-ray, laboratory, etc.). As such, the team leader is held accountable for the smooth functioning by a variety of sources, placing the leader in highly stressful situations.

In communicating down, it is usually not necessary to legitimize one's message. Nurses do not have to explain or apologize to orderlies when they are asking them to clean the floor. Opportunities for educating those at the lower levels of the hierarchy are often missed because of the nurse's perceived need to comply only with messages from above. However, if a nurse finds it necessary to initiate communication with a person on a higher level of authority, such as waking a physician up in the middle of the night to ask him to renew a pain medication for a client, the nurse often tries to legitimize the message, even occasionally using defensive communication:

"I'm sorry, Dr. Smith, but..." (placating)
"I know you don't like my waking you, but..." (blaming)

FUNCTIONAL NURSING. Functional nursing differs from team nursing in one respect: in the functional nursing approach, nurses perform specialized duties throughout the shift, usually serving clients who are assigned two or more teams. One nurse may pass out medications for the entire floor; the LPN may take vital signs, and the aide may take temperatures for all clients. All the responsibilities of the unit are assigned to selected people in accordance with their expertise. The head nurse has ultimate responsibility for the client. The functional team nursing staffing pattern also has bureaucratic organizational characteristics. Both functional and team nursing result in "fragmented" care for clients. Different people are caring for one particular aspect of the client's needs. The client is bathed by the nurse; given medications by another "med" nurse; temperature is taken by an aide; and the client is transported to X-ray by the orderly. Each care taker relates to the client in his or her idiosyncratic way. Student nurses, who are traditionally assigned to the client's total care, often pick up errors related to nursing care due to this pattern of having many people caring for single aspects of a client's health.

An Explicit Set of Policies. Rules and policies, the third characteristic of a bureaucracy, in a community hospital tend to foster rigidity, as well as enforcing a closed system. There are standard procedures for all nursing behaviors, and these discourage suggestions or creativity from outside sources. Most nursing systems have explicit written procedures to insure client safety and cost effectiveness within the hospital. Gross violation of rules and procedures in the hospital could be threatening to client care. At the same time, these rules and procedures contribute to overly rigid boundaries. Such boundaries of a system are referred to as "disengaged"; the other extreme, in which boundaries are blurred, is called "enmeshed" (Menuchin, 1974).

An explicit set of policies is necessary in an organization such as a hospital in order for its members, which includes *all* the people who work in the hospital, to have a course of action for dealing with events and situations. Clearly, it is important that these policies exist, but it is necessary, too, that they undergo examination periodically to insure that they are not outdated. For example, many hospitals have policies regarding the exact time of visiting hours. These policies are reviewed often in order to provide the client support from friends and family members, as well as to provide the best care. If the policy obstructs rather than helps the client, the rules need revision.

An Impersonal Attitude. The fourth characteristic of a bureaucracy is an impersonal attitude. Nursing behaviors in a nurse-client interaction can be broadly grouped into three major components:

Cognitive—thinking component
Affective—feeling component
Psychomotor—doing component.

Bureaucratic systems value the psychomotor, doing component. The nurse who is task-oriented as opposed to person-oriented is also more highly rewarded for visible accomplishments. Remember, the greatest asset of a bureaucracy is its efficiency. It is logical that high-visibility tasks would be rewarded, since they can be evaluated easily and judged in terms of efficiency.

A concept that has been used in attempting to counteract this efficiency focus on task is that of primary nursing. The primary nurse assumes 24-hour responsibility for a limited number of clients (4 to 6). Clients are assigned to a primary nurse until they are discharged or transferred, and he or she directs the overall care of the client on a 24-hour basis through orders that are written on the kardex, as well as through other channels of communication when the nurse is not on duty. The primary nurse has the authority and autonomy to plan and implement care. He or she communicates directly with the physician and the client. In primary nursing the head nurse assumes a broader role, that of client-care coordinator; and she or he is responsible for communication between the staff nurse and the physician. Also, the head nurse serves as a resource consultant to all nurses concerning problems in client care.

The advantages of primary nursing in facilitating communication are obvious. By having total responsibility, the nurse can focus on emotional as well as physical needs when they arise. The nurse also serves as a direct link to the client at all times. In one study, clients who had a primary nurse stated that "nurses tried to reduce their worries about hospitalization, kept them informed about what was happening to them and gave them a chance to talk about their problems, asked questions or sought help" (McCarthy, 1978). Clients feel they are better prepared through communication for the experience of hospitalization with primary care nursing (Marram, 1976).

One purpose of primary nursing is to develop better systems of communication with agencies following discharge (public health or nursing homes, for example). While the advantages for the client of greater continuity and effectiveness of care resulting in closer client–nurse relationships outweigh the disadvantages, there are drawbacks for the nurse. Primary nurses are isolated from their colleagues. Nurses' stations are often lacking, resulting in yet a further loss of territoriality. In addition, no allowances are made for group planning of client care. Thus, while the client focus and communication may be improved, primary nursing has to grapple with these new barriers to effective interstaff communication.

Expectations of Participants

The final dimension of the structure of a system is how the members of the system view each other in relationship to roles. Each participant in a system has certain expectations of the other's performance. These expectations will determine role and communication behaviors. For example, in one hospital, nurses and physicians might work collaboratively in making decisions about clients. This is the expected role. In another hospital, physicians might communicate almost exclusively with the head nurse. In this situation, collaboration between physicians and staff nurses would be impeded because the expectation is that nurses do not normally communicate with physicians.

In examining the expectations of us as nurses, we can learn about our own system's values and priorities. Is there a higher priority on "doing" rather than "thinking" or "feeling?" Are nurses expected to be able to communicate therapeutically and take nursing histories? Answering these questions helps us to understand our own system more clearly.

Nurses develop an internal set of expected role and communication behaviors, which is determined in part by the expectations of the other members of the system (clients, peers, and other health workers). While a nurse interacts therapeutically with a client to assess the extent of the client's pain, a different kind of communication is necessary to obtain the physician's order for the pain medication. The expectations of the nursing role include not giving medication unless an order is written by someone else. However, some expectations are not clear-cut. If the client asks the nurse for specific information about his or her condition, diagnosis, prognosis, or exact teaching needs in relation to the diagnosis, it is not always clear how the nurse should answer. Each secondary care setting will be slightly different. Nurses who have experience and are familiar with the specific setting are aware of their own expectations of the behavior of others, and they are also aware of what the other members expect of them. Like characters in a well-rehearsed play, they know their part and how that part influences their nursing actions.

When internalized expectations of role are incongruent with external expectations, conflicts occur. Consider the following situation:

> Mrs. Richards, a new staff nurse working on a medical unit of a community hospital, had several years' experience as a staff nurse in a large urban university hospital. When an ECG was ordered for her client, she assumed part of her expected role was to teach the client about the ECG and what the various waves on the recording signified. When the supervisor of the particular community hospital noted her behavior, she was informed in an abrupt manner that clients are not instructed about ECGs.

In secondary care settings, nursing priorities vary as well. One of the purposes of this book is to have you place a high priority on therapeutic communication. If you make this a high priority, you might find that you will be in conflict with expectations of your head nurse. The head nurse's top priority might be to see that the tasks are completed. (See the section on assertion in Chapter 8 for ways to handle this conflict.)

Nurses often place unrealistic expectations on themselves. An example of this would be if a nurse expected to have a significant influence on all his of her clients' lives through short-term therapeutic interactions. Such an expectation is probably unrealistic for clients with routine and recurring illnesses who remain three to five days in the community hospital (Norris, 1977).

Is it reasonable to assume that nurses can be empathetic for large numbers of clients given all of the outside influences also at work? After all, time, stress, and bureaucratic settings can be counterproductive to empathetic relationships. Nurses should not think of themselves as all things to all people. Each nurse has to answer the question of how to juggle time, task, and multiple client relationships for him-or herself. Determining how to be a caring and competent nurse in the health care system is a crucial issue for the nursing profession in the 1980s.

THE SECONDARY PRACTICE SETTING AND COMMUNICATION

Three concepts that affect communication patterns in the community hospital setting are stereotyping of the client role, multichannel communication, and triadic communication.

Stereotyping of the Client Role

Everyone has preconceived ideas about people based on past experiences. When these expectations become categorized or polarized, stereotyping occurs. It is difficult for nurses interacting with clients not to fall into the habit of stereotyping, which means that the client is prejudged rather than assessed and treated accurately. Stereotyping usually takes place with people who are "different"—be they poor or of a different culture, ethnic group, or race. Stereotyping clients by race and culture is antithetical to effective nursing and therapeutic communication. One specialty area where this is particularly true is the area of geriatric care.

Who are Geriatric Clients? This question may seem silly to some readers. "After all," they might answer, "they are just old people who are sick." If by chance these readers were questioned further, they might add that they think most older people are sick anyway, that they are hard to talk with, that they are senile and confused.

Many nurses are faced with this problem. There are many older people receiving care, but it seems hard to relate to them and the nurses aren't particularly thrilled about working with the elderly.

There are two important aspects to the problem. First, many nurses do not have accurate information about older people and the effects of disease and hospitalization. Second, many nurses (and other health providers) have prejudgments about the elderly that prevent good communication and information gathering.

Disease is a common occurrence with the elderly. Eighty-six percent of all older people have a chronic illness of one sort or another (Butler and Lewis, 1973). However, many of the illnesses, such as diabetes, are controllable. Only 5 percent of the elderly are in an institutional setting at any particular time (Burnside, 1976). Thus, while there is more illness with old age, most older people manage their own lives with a good deal of independence. When they are faced with an illness, it can be quite upsetting *because* the independence for which they have fought for so long is now threatened by the dependency of the client role.

At the same time, many nurses encounter the elderly *only* when they are ill and form their impressions of what to expect from the elderly based on such clients. Thus, the nurse may subtly *slow down* recovery by reminding a client that she's "pretty old to try this" rather than encouraging a return to the client's highest possible level of functioning. In addition, while nursing has always played an important role in the care of the elderly, nurses who have worked in nursing home settings have often been looked down upon by other nurses. Thus, there is low status in working with the aged.

Some common stereotypic thoughts nurses have about the elderly are:

1. They're hopeless.
2. They're going to die (so why help?).
3. They're all senile.
4. They're chronic complainers (so why listen?).
5. They're sexless.

The problem with stereotyping is that it distorts the unique information presented by a client. The nurse who has decided that the elderly are all chronic complainers will not be able to listen *well* to an older client's concern. Remember, the older client you see today is *you* 50 years from now. Treat them as you hope you will be treated if you are ever in the same situation.

The answers to the above myths can be called the "five truths about the elderly" (see Palmore, 1976, for more information on myths and facts about aging):

1. No one is totally hopeless.
2. A client may be terminal, but much can be done for him or her *now*.
3. Only 15 percent of the elderly ever exhibit signs of organic brain syndrome. Many, if treated properly, can be cured.
4. Some older people complain extensively. Others don't complain enough.
5. Like all other adults, the elderly have sexual interest and feelings of personal intimacy.

Multichannel Communication

Many people use a predominant channel of communication when interacting with others. The environment in which one interacts with others often influences which channel or channels of communication are used. In the secondary nursing context, it is obvious that answering the telephone requires the auditory channel; reading a chart necessitates using the visual channel, and interacting with a client requires auditory, visual, and even kinesthetic channels. The hospital environment is one in which, at times, all channels (visual, auditory, kinesthetic, olfactory) are utilized. Thus, the nurse responds to a multistimuli environment.

The simultaneous use of more than one channel is necessary in order for the nurse to adequately respond to the hospital environment. Many events, the majority of which are stressful, are occurring at the same time, both from the standpoint of the nurse who is caring for a number of clients, as well as from the standpoint of the client, who perceives a number of events taking place. The frenetic pace of the floor or hospital wing is obvious. Nurses strive to maintain an outward placidity, especially when they are interacting with clients. When nurses go from busy hallways into quiet interiors of acutely ill clients' rooms, they are required to shift gears and readjust communication behavior, as well as their level of cognition. When seeking information from clients, nurses must initiate the communication process by briefly encapsulating what is being asked and why. Clients do not possess the shorthand skills that nurses have, and this mandates that nurses must be explicit when seeking information with clients, that is, starting with one detail and focusing on one specific problem.

In addition, there is a tendency to view the client as "being one of us." Almore (1979) refers to this as "assumed similarity"; that is, nurses tend to assume clients will think, act, and communicate like a member of the nursing community, and their perceived failure to do so can create a psychological barrier that can impact on the nurse-client relationship.

If the purpose of nurses is to enable clients to share feelings, they must be adept in the precise timing and framing of their communication interactions with clients, utilizing the skills needed for nurse–client therapeutic interactions and information gathering. (see Chapters 4 and 5). It is important for students and new staff to recognize that becoming more adept at sorting out multisource messages depends on nurses' becoming more familiar with their role. Clients do not have this familiarity with the setting. Because of this, they are often "paced" by the multistimuli environment; that is, they let the pace of the events affect their communication behavior. Nurses who are not familiar with the environment often let either the client or the environment "pace" them as well, as is shown in the following situation:

> When the nurse went to give Mr. Johnson his A.M. care, he (Mr. Johnson) was visibly upset over the disappearance of his pajama bottoms. The nurse looked everywhere in his bedside unit and immediately reported the loss to her team leader, who informed the head nurse. After the head nurse called the laundry and no pajama bottoms were found, the problem started to escalate until the entire staff was either commenting on Mr. Johnson's loss or actively looking for the bottoms. Finally, Mrs. Brown, an instructor for the nursing students, came to the floor, entered Mr. Johnson's room and asked:
> "When was the last time you saw the pajama bottoms?"
> Mr. Johnson replied:
> "When the night nurse removed them because I perspired with a high fever."
> Mrs. Brown, thinking that perhaps the night nurse might have rinsed them out, looked in the bathroom adjoining Mr. Johnson's unit and found the bottoms drying on a towel rack.

The nurse (and others) in this situation let the client's anxiety put them into a high state of activity rather than attempting to solve the problem at a more appropriate pace.

Oftentimes communication problems arise due to timing as well as pacing:

> Mrs. Hayes, a 70-year-old diabetic, had doctor's orders to have her 7 A.M. insulin after she had eaten her breakfast. The aide told the medication nurse that Mrs. Hayes had eaten and her tray was removed. The aide also gave the same information to the student assigned to Mrs. Hayes. The medication nurse prepared the insulin and gave it to Mrs. Hayes. She did not record it immediately on the chart or kardex. Within 5 minutes the student nurse prepared the *second* insulin injection and, under the supervision of her instructor, administered the injection.

Simultaneous messages in the above situation created a serious error. The error was created because of lack of communication in the following ways:

1. The aide informed two nurses, both of whom assumed they would be the one to give the medication without checking with each other.
2. The medication nurse did not record the medication immediately.
3. The client did not inform the student she had already had the injection.

Triadic Communication

> A doctor and a nurse are talking to each other in a client's room in the hospital. The client had a hernia operation and the doctor is questioning the nurse about the client with reference to her order, "Ambulate twice a day." The client is listening to the conversation between the doctor and the nurse, shifting her eyes from one to the other as they converse. How many people are there in this conversation?

Up to this point, dyadic communication has been the basis for discussion of communication interactions. Dyadic communication involves two people in a face-to-face interaction. However, many communication interactions involve more than two people and are referred to as triadic communication. A triad is a social system composed of three people transacting in a face-to-face situation (Wilmot, 1975). Many forms of triadic communication exist in nursing. If one were to analyze the communication interaction between nurse and physician, as in the above situation, one could conclude that the majority of nurse-physician interactions are essentially *about* the client. The client might be present during the interaction (as in this situation). Thus, the client becomes a third member in the interaction even though nothing is contributed to the communication by him or her. He or she functioned in the above example as a listener.

Think about the situation between the doctor and nurse with the client physically present again in terms of hierarchy of authority. Who, in the example given, has the ultimate authority? The physician (A) has written an order that the nurse (B) is carrying out. The client (C) is the recipient of the order. In this particular situation the physician has the greatest authority, the nurse less than the physician, but greater than the client, and the client the least. The situation is diagrammed in Figure 9–1.

Interactions that are three-way, as above in the figure, have tendencies to cause the formation of coalitions; that is, two members will pair up in opposition to the third. Even more revealing is the fact that these coalitions can be predicted with considerable accuracy if the relative power of the three members is known (Caplow, 1968). In this siuation, it can be predicted that the nurse (B) will probably form a coalition with the client (C), depending on the amount of authority that the physician (A) chooses to use. If A is threatening, B and C will become mutually supportive of each other in order to protect themselves against the superior authority of A. While this is not the outcome in every situation of this type, a tendency toward the coalition of B and C is often felt in situations such as the one presented, and the B and C coalition should result more frequently than by chance alone.

If A does not display authority and works in partnership with either B or C, the chances of A forming a coalition with either B or C are much greater. In other words, a display of less authority puts her (the physician) at an advantage, just as a display of authority had been a handicap. The physician controls the balance of the triangle depending on how much authority she wishes to wield.

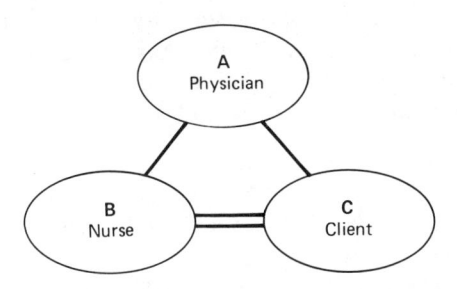

FIGURE 9–1. A communication triad with B (nurse) and C (client) forming a coalition against A (physician).

Consider the following situation:

> A nurse is in Mrs. Scott's room performing health teaching with a client who is going to have a cardiac catherization. The client has told the nurse that she knows nothing about what is going to happen to her. The client's doctor enters the room, observes what is going on and turns to the client and says:
> "I will perform your catherization tomorrow. I've done many of these procedures before, so don't worry about it."
> He turns to the nurse and says, "Have Mrs. Scott ready at 10 A.M." and leaves the room.

In this situation, the physician's use of authority has increased the affiliation of nurse and client. They both feel a sense of helplessness due to the physician's approach and they may join forces for mutual support. Contrast this with an approach on the part of the physician in which he addresses the nurse by name and acknowledges the teaching she is providing the client and also addresses the client, asking if there is anything she does not understand. The tendency towards a coalition between the client and nurse is considerably lessened, and all three parties are more likely to have open communication with each other.

Triads are omnipresent in the secondary health care setting. The above situation could be replicated using a head nurse (A), a staff nurse (B), and a client (C) or a staff nurse (A) an aide (B) and a client (C). Staff nurses have more authority than aides, who have more authority than clients. Are there situations in which the aide forms a coalition with the client to counteract the authority of the staff nurse? An experienced staff nurse could undoubtedly cite many situations.

It has already been established in an earlier section of this chapter that the community hospital is a bureaucracy, and as such, a hierarchy of authority exists among its members. Each member in the organization has a rank. Thus, in organizational triads, the superiority, equality, and inferiority of the members who are interacting with each other has already been established; the balance of power is not evident (Caplow, 1968).

pediatrics. Consider the following example:

> Sally Leighton is a new admission with a diagnosis of juvenile diabetes. Because she is only 8 years old, her parents have taken turns staying with her throughout her hospital stay. The nurse has prepared an injection of insulin that was ordered:
>
> NURSE (to Sally): I have your insulin injection, which I will give to you in your thigh. Tomorrow, when you feel better, we are going to teach you more about your diabetes.

MRS. LEIGHTON (to the nurse): Is that a large amount of insulin? The doctor said she would only need a little.
NURSE (kindly): This is what the doctor ordered.
MRS. LEIGHTON (to Sally): Let the nurse give you the shot. It won't hurt!

In the above example, the parent, Mrs. Leighton, interacts with the nurse on behalf of her child, Sally. A communication triad exists. Brink (1972) has described this type of triad as a "natural triad." It can be diagrammed as shown in Figure 9–2.

This type of triad involves three categories of persons in the communication interaction (Brink, 1972):

1. A person of high status who is considered an authority in the relationship (the nurse)
2. A person of lower status who is considered subordinate to the authority figure (the client)
3. A person of higher status to the subordinate but not necessarily equal to the authority, who serves as a friend or, in this example, parent to the subordinate.

There are three dyads present in the example presented:

Nurse–client. This relationship is one of distance and possible fear and is designated as negative.
Client–parent. This relationship is one of closeness and nurturance.
Parent–nurse. This relationship is one of formality, distance, and respect and is negative.

Certainly in the case of Sally and the nurse, the relationship is one of distance, and even possibly fear, because the nurse is viewed as an authority figure, someone who might not be trusted, especially if the nurse disagrees with

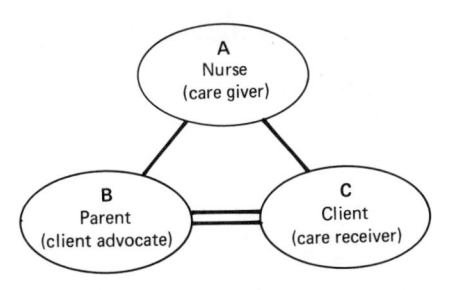

FIGURE 9–2. Communication triad with B (parent) and C (client) forming a coalition against A (nurse).

Sally's mother. Sally will do what her mother says, and the nurse might find herself in the position of being the adversary with regard to these two. The nurse, in order to establish a trusting relationship with Sally, must communicate with the parent, who is serving as the child's advocate as well. If the child is too young to communicate, the parent will intervene for the client, which not only serves to assist the nurse in her plan of care, but is more therapeutic for the client.

One final word about communicating with pediatric clients is that the hierarchy of authority is not always evident given the nature of the clients. Communication is more open in the system of secondary pediatric care. Rules are more flexible, and the hierarchical arrangement of staff positions is not as obvious as in other specialties, such as surgery or medicine.

CONCLUSION

A system of secondary nurse practice can be described in relation to three dimensions of structure: the physical setting, organization of activities, and expectation of participants who function within the system. Communication patterns within each of these dimensions were presented.

Three concepts that affect communication patterns in a system of secondary nurse practice are the stereotyping of the client role, multichannel communication, and triadic communication. Nurses who practice in these settings have the opportunity to relate the concepts presented here to their interactions with clients and other staff.

BIBLIOGRAPHY

Almore, M.G. dyadic communication. *American Journal of Nursing*, 1979, 79 (6), 1076–1078.

Blondis, M.N. & Jackson, B.E. *Nonverbal communication with patients: back to the human touch*. New York: John Wiley, 1977.

Brink, P. The natural triad in health care, *American Journal of Nursing*, 1972, 72 (5), 897–899.

Burnside, I. *Nursing and the aged*. New York: McGraw-Hill, 1976.

Butler, R. & Lewis, M. *Aging and mental health: positive psychosocial approach*. St. Louis: C.V. Mosby, 1973.

Caplow, T. *Two against one coalition in triads*. Englewood Cliffs, N.J.: Prentice-Hall, 1968.

Cosper, B. How well do patients understand hospital jargon? *American Journal of Nursing*, 1977, 77 (12), 1932–1934.

Haase, P., Smith, M.H. & Reitt, B. A proposed system for nursing: theoretical framework, part 2. In *Pathways to practice,* (Vol. 4). Atlanta: Southern Regional Education Board, 1976.

Lewis, J. Structural aspects of the delivery setting and nurse practitioner performance. *Nurse Practitioner,* 1975, *1*(x), 16–20.

Marram, G. The comparative costs of operating a team and primary nursing unit. *Journal of Nursing Administration,* 1976, *6,* (4) 21–24.

McCarthy, D. & Schifalacqua, M.H. Primary nursing: its implementation and six month outcome. *Journal of Nursing Administration,* 1978, *8,* (5), 29–32.

Menuchin, S. *Families and family therapy.* Cambridge, Massachusetts: Harvard U.P., 1974.

Norris, C. Delusions that trap nurses. *Canadian Nurse,* 1973, *69,* 37–40.

Palmore, E. Facts on Aging. *Gerontologist,* 1977, *17,* 315–321.

Skipper, J. & Leonard, R. *Social interaction and patient care.* Philadelphia: J.B. Lippincott, 1965.

Wilmot, W. *Dyadic communication: a transactional perspective.* Reading, Massachusetts: Addison-Wesley, 1975.

Yura, H. & Walsh, M. *Human needs and the nursing process.* New York: Appleton-Century-Crofts, 1978.

Chapter 10
Communication in tertiary nursing practice

BEHAVIORAL OBJECTIVES

By reading this chapter, students will be able to:

1. Describe a system of tertiary nursing practice
2. Identify the three dimensions of structure that are present in a system of tertiary nursing practice
3. Differentiate clients in systems of tertiary nursing practice in terms of internal and external factors
4. Recognize how clients in systems of tertiary care communicate in three channels (visual, auditory, and kinesthetic)
5. Interpret the effect of stressors on the nurse who works in a tertiary care setting.

The locus of tertiary nursing practice is large hospitals (300 or more beds), usually in association with university-affiliated settings. The environment in which tertiary nursing practice occurs is highly specialized. Examples of tertiary nursing care settings are the critical and intensive care, neonatology, and oncology units. The nursing care rendered is often experimental in nature and associated with research projects. Clients have acute episodes of illness presenting uncommon, complex symptomology and are critically ill (Haase et al., 1976).

Nurses who work in a system of tertiary nursing practice are specialists in their chosen field. They make clinical decisions in their area of specialization. They interact with clients whose illness outcomes are not predictable. Clients in tertiary care require significant amounts of monitoring. Nurses in tertiary care settings often function in leadership roles, directing other levels of nurses in the delivery of care to several clients. They also work collaboratively with other health care co-workers (Haase et al., 1976).

In Chapter 9, a system of secondary nursing was analyzed in terms of the three dimensions that Lewis ascribed to structure: the physical setting, the organization of activities, and the expectation of participants (Lewis, 1976). This same analysis can be applied to systems of tertiary nursing. The characteristics of structure are similar to those of secondary care but are more obvious in a system of tertiary nursing. It is evident that as the illness within a given hospital environment becomes more acute, the dimensions of the structure become more visible.

The impact of the first dimension, *the physical environment,* in a tertiary care setting is felt by both clients and staff. Settings such as an ICU or a CCU are worlds unto themselves in which it is often difficult to distinguish the client from the physical environment of tubes and life-support systems which are crowded into a limited physical space.

The second dimension, *organization of activities* in critically ill settings, is characterized by the four bureaucratic role patterns discussed in Chapter 9: a high degree of specialization, a hierarchy of authority, explicit rules and policies, and an impersonal attitude. The bureaucratic role patterns are necessary for the smooth and efficient functioning of units in which the maintenance and preservation of life is so crucial. A requirement for nurses working in critical-care units is that they have specialized roles and a sound knowledge base, as well as a high degree of clinical expertise. They know their role, both in terms of their responsibility to those above as well as those below on the organizational ladder. The activities are governed by rules and policies which define the large number of life-saving procedures for all possible situations that might occur. Nurses are expected to undertake workloads in as efficient a manner as possible with attitudes of personal detachment; that is, feelings should not interfere with work. The high value placed on human life necessitates bureaucratic behaviors. All activities and functions within the organization must be coordinated into an efficient operating unit.

The *expectations of participants* or role expectations, the final dimension of structure, are often clearly defined with reference to nursing responsibilities and procedures in policy manuals and books. Conflicts do occur, however, between professionals in the health care system when the nursing role expectations are finally implemented. The work in tertiary care nursing

Communication in Tertiary Nursing Practice 235

settings is demanding both physically, and intellectually. The work space in areas such as an ICU or CCU is limited and malfunctioning of intricate equipment can cost a client's life (Hay and Oken, 1972). All these factors lead to communication conflicts. In this chapter, we examine how and why these conflicts occur. The discussion is divided into three major sections: the first section examines the tertiary care setting and communication from the standpoint of the client; the second analyzes tertiary care communication using the concept of communication channels; and the third covers these topics from the standpoing of the nurse.

THE CLIENT IN THE TERTIARY CARE SETTING

Neither staff nurses who are inexperienced nor students are usually assigned to critical-care units. In spite of the fact that these nurses have never worked in an ICU or CCU or similar specialized unit, they have observed such areas. It is interesting to think about what we might see, observe, and hear or listen, touch, and feel in such a setting.

If we close our eyes and imagine a client in the tertiary setting we might "see" the following: machines, bottles, suctioning devices; a client who appears anxious (look at facial cues); a client who is heavily sedated; a client who requires lifting.

We might "hear": moaning and groaning; beeping monitors; suctioning; ventilators; nurses talking to physicians, other clients, or each other; clients crying; clients asking questions.

We might feel: a tension-charged atmosphere; frightened because of the severity of the client's illness; empathy or sympathy.

What might we *perceive* about a client in a critical-care setting? We might perceive that clients are anxious; that they are physically, and to some extent emotionally, dependent; that they are often unable to cope with their feelings; that they are in a hostile environment; and that they feel isolated. We also might perceive that the physical status of the critically ill client impacts on emotional needs through various internal and external factors. Internal factors are factors "inside" the client; external are "outside" the person.

Internal factors

Internal factors include how the client perceives his or her immediate environment. Two examples are the "psychological aspects of illness" (reviewed in Chapter 6) and the concept of "personal space" (reviewed in Chapter 9).

Psychological Aspects of Illness. The psychological aspects of illness are extremely pronounced in clients who are critically ill. These clients are at times totally dependent psychologically, extremely passive in terms of any decision making, and have very high levels of fear and anxiety; additionally, their feelings of self-worth are low and they experience a great sense of identity loss and confusion. These psychological aspects of illness represent "person" needs such as for empathy and understanding. In addition, the acute nature of the illness is such that the client is oftentimes totally dependent on the nurse for the fulfillment of "task" needs, which include all physiological needs.

When one talks of need fulfillment, the temptation is to think of needs in terms of the basic physiological needs (air, food, oxygen, water, sleep, for example). These are the basic needs at the bottom level of Maslow's hierarchy, and they must be fulfilled before proceeding to higher level needs—psychological ones (Maslow, 1970). Unfulfilled psychological needs in critically ill clients lead to such fear and anxiety that clients can become totally uncooperative, disoriented, and even combative. Taken collectively, these symptoms are called the ICU syndrome and are present in as many as 70 percent of clients in the ICU (Noble, 1977). The loss of identity has become so acute that the client attempts to assert personhood by fighting in every way possible such as refusing medication or yelling at the nurses. While in one sense this attempt to retain identity helps to preserve life in the psychological sense, it can severely jeopardize the fulfillment of physiological needs. The interrelationship of the psychological aspects of illness with physiological needs is always present. It has also been shown that clients who are unable to express fear and anxiety before surgery are more prone to develop ICU syndrome in the postoperative period (Brunner and Suddarth, 1980).

Clients in critical-care units have shed the usual identity that they assume in healthy states and have taken on passive rather than active roles. This passivity coupled with immobility and pain affects the client physically and psychologically.

Self-rejection and lowered self-worth result from the numerous invasions of privacy by health care workers. There is a sense of depersonalization in which clients become nonpersons. The person is de-emphasized, and the task often assumes the greatest priority for the nursing staff and other health care workers. This contributes to an overall sense of identity loss and lowered self-worth.

Personal Space. The second internal factor, the concept of personal space, is also closely related to one's sense of identity. Personal space is violated repeatedly in acute illness states because of the need for nursing interventions such as giving injections, insertion of intravenous lines, and the use of monitoring devices. These numerous violations of personal space by nurses and other co-workers, especially in such instances where they do not take the time to introduce themselves or explain their purpose, often lead to heightened anxiety on the part of clients.

External Factors

External factors present in tertiary nursing care systems include aspects of the physical setting itself. The five barriers in secondary nursing care systems discussed in Chapter 9 (the use of technical language, the rigid routine, noise level, uniforms, busy atmosphere) are present in tertiary nursing care systems as well. In particular, physical space and noise level contribute to the creation of communication problems in the highly specialized area.

Physical Space. The client's sense of physical space is threatened in units such as ICU and CCU. The overutilization of small spaces, as well as the use of mechanical devices, contributes to a crowded physical environment in which clients feel a heightened sense of anxiety (Gowan, 1979). The units are closer together, and this imposes spatial boundaries that foster a feeling of constriction for both clients and nurses.

Noise Level. The noise level of ICU and CCU units is often elevated because of beeping monitors, respirators, staff communications, and noise from other clients. This increased noise level is directly related to sleep deprivation (Woods and Falk, 1974).
"If I had to say what the biggest problem for me was in the ICU, it was the other patients. I still can remember the patients on either side of me and how one was always trying to get out of bed because he didn't know what was going on and how the other was using such profanity all the time" (Bixler, 1980).
We have presented a picture of the client in a tertiary care setting, using an ICU unit as a prototype. The total impact on the client, an altered sensory environment, in which the client's behavior is affected by a combination of internal physiological, psychological, and external environmental factors, has been summarized. The influences of increased noise level, constant manipulation of the client's environment in order to carry out nursing interventions, and depersonalization contribute to "deprived states of affect, cognition and perception" (Bolin, 1974). The integration of external and internal factors provides the basis for the client's ability to perceive the total environment. How much do clients really perceive and do they remember what they perceive?

Clients in critical-care units can often recall exactly what happened even though at times they appear to be in a semicomatose state. For example, one woman recalled nurses talking to her, asking her to open her eyes. Because she was on a respirator and was having everything done for her, she asked herself why should she open her eyes, and consequently she did not (DeMeyer, 1967). She gave the impression, then, that she was totally unaware of what was going on.

Another client recalls an incident in which he suffered cardiac arrest:

> "I can hear Bill (the nurse) yell.... Now hearing fades too. Buzz, buzz, buzz. Voices serious—serious, subdued, working voices. Two main ones, others on the periphery.... The voices become clearer. The doctor asks for a syringe. I brace expecting a needle to plunge through my chest into my heart. I feel nothing.... My eyes are closed and I marvel that Dr. Bailey speaks to me. Maybe it's because he knows what it's like to be unconscious except for your ears? (Derrick, 1979, p. 281)

How much information are clients who are acutely ill able to process? When clients are conscious they are able to see, hear, and feel. However, there are levels of perception, and these are sometimes dependent on the severity of the illness. Is the client who is critically ill able to utilize channel communication on a higher level of integration: observing, listening, and feeling? And finally, is the critically ill client able to integrate all levels of channel communication and perceive what is happening? Critically ill clients may well move in and out of levels of perception within each channel and thus may not be able to integrate all three channels. Therefore, the fragmentation of information received becomes one of the biggest communication challenges for the nurse attempting to communicate in the tertiary care setting.

CHANNELS OF COMMUNICATION IN TERTIARY CARE SETTINGS

Auditory Communication

For the critically ill client, the noise level tends to be constant during the day and sporadic during the evening and night hours. Because of the constant noise level during the day, some clients are able to sleep better in the daytime hours than in the nighttime hours. Other factors that might contribute to this sleeping pattern are heightened fear and anxiety at nighttime. Substituting music for the strange and foreign noises of the tertiary care system has been attempted. In one hospital, a client used a stethoscope taped to a radio in order to replace the outside noise disturbances (Bender-Dougherty, 1980).

In spite of the intermittent loud noises or the constant high level of noise from machines and suctioning equipment, the most disturbing auditory stimuli according to clients recalling their experiences were *staff communications!* (Noble, 1979). Staff, especially nurses and physicians, in order to overcome the noise factor within the acute care environment, raise their voices and are often within earshot of the client. While the majority of these communication interactions are related to client care and treatment (65 percent), a high proportion of communication between staff is "shoptalk" and personal (Noble, 1979, p. 196). At the same time, staff rarely talk to the clients as they administer care and treatment. When they do talk to clients who are on respirators and intubated, the staff are likely to shout at clients as if their hearing and speech are impaired.

It is often difficult for nurses working in ICU and CCU units not to fall into the habit of stereotyping the clients. They assume that all clients who are semicomatose or even comatose cannot understand what is going on. Indeed, many cannot comprehend what is happening. At the same time, it should be emphasized that while the client may present an outward picture of unawareness, he or she can be well aware of what is going on. Such staff comments as, "She's really out of it!" or "He's totally nonresponsive" are liable to be repeated to the staff by the client at a later date. The auditory channel is usually the last channel to become nonfunctional in the process leading to unconsciousness, and nurses should guard against misuse of the auditory channel with *all* clients. This includes regard and respect for what the client can hear at all times!

Often clients think they are dying when they are not. One client recalls she thought she was dying when the drug she was given inhibited her respirations to such a degree that she had difficulty breathing. She was placed on a respirator, and after about 10 days stated that if only the nurse had told her that it was the drug that was causing her difficulty in breathing, she would have been far less anxious and fearful.

Visual Communication

The use of artificial light on a 24-hour basis sometimes results in sensory-deprivation reactions by clients. Crises in the ICU are as likely to occur during the evening and night as in the daytime, and often the lights are left on for 24 hours to provide for continued observation of clients. Natural light still provides the best means of sensitizing the client to the environment. One study demonstrated how the use of windows in an ICU had a positive effect on psychological equilibrim in the postoperative period (Wilson, 1972). The study compared two ICU units, differing only in the presence or absence of windows. The study demonstrated that there were twice as many patients with ICU syndrome in the windowless unit as there were in the unit with natural lighting and windows.

The use of drugs for sedation and narcotic analgesics contributes to sensory deprivation in the acutely ill client and can create visual hallucinations. One physician who was a patient in the ICU commented on how he lost track of time and every time he looked at the clock it was five o'clock. Consequently if he slept, he was convinced he had slept for twenty-four hours (Guida, 1980). It is essential to preserve an orientation to reality (reality orientation) for tertiary care clients through constant reminders of time (e.g., clock on wall) or day of the week (e.g., calendar on wall). In addition, nurses can assist clients to relate to time by reminding them who they (the nurses) are and what shift they are working. In some hospitals where nurses rotate shifts, it is impossible for clients to associate a particular nurse with time of day.

Kinesthetic Communication

Acutely ill clients, by virtue of their illness, often utilize kinesthetic channels of communication more readily than they would normally. Critically ill clients feel in both the physical and emotional connotations of the word. They feel pain or discomfort; they feel lonely or angry.

Tactile communication with clients can have therapeutic effect. Lynch (1978), for example, conducted a survey in which he measured alterations in heart rhythms during nurse–client interactions, such as taking a pulse or measuring blood pressure. He studied clients in two acute areas, CCU and shock trauma unit, and found that clients' heart rates would increase during an interaction with a nurse. He concluded that human contact seems to be desperately important to clients in these acute areas (Lynch, 1978).

Nurses can learn to develop an appreciation of critically ill clients' increased awareness of kinesthetic channels. One way is decrease the concurrent use of auditory and visual channel communication.

There are many instances in which nurses should not expect to carry on two-way conversations in which there is feedback with acutely ill clients. Clients do not always have the ability to process auditory and visual channel communication. Interactions between nurse and client in these cases should be basic and simple, such as, "Your IV is OK now," or "I'm right here." The nurse cannot assume the client knows the intravenous line is all right or that the nurse is there to support the client. Finally, clients do respond kinesthetically even when they are in pain or anxious. Observing body language or watching facial cues often provides more information about how the client feels in these instances, even if the client is unable to verbalize.

THE NURSE IN THE TERTIARY CARE SETTING

Having identified some of the external and internal factors pertaining to the client in critical-care settings, as well as discussing the three channels of communication and their impact on communication, we now turn to the nurses who work in these settings. The following discussion focuses on some of the forces which affect nurses in tertiary care and how these influence the communication process.

The critical-care setting is a stressful environment. In the literature, critical care has been called a "pressure cooker" environment (Shubin, 1979, p. 53). One can assume that nurses working in these environments find themselves under stress. Because we assume that stress is present and that stressors block effective communication, it is important that the *sources* of stress be identified.

Think of stressors you as a nurse have in your work role. What specific stressors are you able to identify? Stressors, or sources of stress, become activated by one's own sense of low self-worth. Did any of the following thoughts cross your mind as you attempted to identify the sources of stress?

"Others may think of me and my work performance as not good enough."
"I am incapable of carrying out my assignment."
"My workload will be too demanding, both physically and psychologically."
"I don't know what to do."
"My supervisor (or instructor) will not think I am a 'good' nurse."
"I have too much decision-making responsibility for clients."

The examples listed are internal perceptions nurses have about their work roles in relation to others. The internal self-worth issue can be handled through utilization of a problem-solving model with another co-worker or supervisor. Once identified, communicating about the stressors with another person who is open and willing to share feelings can help to solve some of the sources of concern.

There are also stressors which are related to specific settings. These stressors are more likely to be external stressors. Chances are that nurses have little or no control over these stressors, but an awareness of them and how they relate to communication can assist nurses tangibly in dealing with them. The remainder of this chapter is focused on assisting nurses in this way.

Several stressors that have been identified as present in tertiary nursing care systems are:

1. The overly bureaucratic nature of the setting
2. The person versus task orientation
3. The communication interactions between nurses and families of clients.
4. The sensory overload felt by nurses.

The Overly Bureaucratic Nature of the Setting

The characteristics of a bureaucracy have been reviewed in another section of this book (see Chapter 9). Tertiary care settings tend to be exaggerated forms of a bureaucracy. Bureaucracies, which are closed systems, often depersonalize both clients and nurses. All nursing systems have elements of a bureaucracy, some more than others. The bureaucratic element of a nursing system can be so strong that the client ceases to be the prime reason for its existence; rather, the system exists to perpetuate itself. Not only is such a system counterproductive to professional nursing values, but it also hinders effective communication between members of the health care system, including the clients (Oselladore, 1978).

Gruber (1980, pp. 8–9) lists some consequences of what happens to communication within a nursing system when bureaucracy goes unchecked and unmodified:

1. *Decreased morale*—lack of communication from the top to the bottom of the hierarchy.
2. *Decreased productivity*—low morale, decreased communication, sense of isolation and alienation.
3. *Lack of communication*—each specialty and subspecialty is an end unto itself. There are in-groups. Groups are isolated from each other.
4. *Lack of interest in the whole of institutional aims*—Each department is an end unto itself. There is no real interest if the whole institution survives or thrives, only if one's own specialty survives.
5. *Lack of creativity*—Aspects of the structure such as decreased morale cause decreased creativity, decreased risk taking, and increased resistance to change.
6. *Typical comments of staff*—"We against them"; some mysterious "them" in the organizational structure is responsible for hindering "our" aims.

Communication in Tertiary Nursing Practice

7. *High resistance to change*—Change is difficult for persons to handle.
8. *Low autonomy of the individual*—A common complaint is "too many chiefs" and "no Indians." Subgroups are seen as suborganizations rather than a group of unique individuals.
9. *Poor patient care*—The effects of low morale, decreased productivity, and the other factors mentioned filter down to patient care. The client senses the inadequacy of care, the overworked and burned-out staff. There is also a decrease in humanistic care, another byproduct of the dysfunctions of a bureaucratic institution.

A good discussion might center around the question: "How do you think the problem of overbureaucratization in the system of tertiary nursing care will be alleviated in the future?"

Person versus Task Orientation

Person-task orientation has been defined in Chapter 3 of this book. Some nurses may rate high on person orientation; others may rate high on task orientation; and some may rate high or low on both; in other words, it has been determined that person and task orientations are not either/or but may be found in various combinations in different individuals (Hersey et al., 1976). The tertiary care setting is a task-oriented setting. Stress is laid on procedures and the clients' highest needs are ones of survival. What happens when nurses who have "high person" orientation and "low task" orientation work in this setting? While this sounds as though it might be unusual, it has happened for a number of reasons. One reason is that the critical care units have a certain amount of prestige attached to them. In most instances, nurses who are experienced and have a sound theory base of nursing knowledge are asked to work in these units. Another reason is that there exists an "esprit de corps" in which nurses work together as members of a tightly knit team, sharing common experiences (Hay and Olan, 1972). Nurses become readily socialized into this group team situation because of the high workload demands and competencies expected of them. The pressures to assume a task orientation are great.

Experienced nurses can usually handle the demands of the task and still be able to communicate effectively by empathizing with clients. However, some nurses are not able to juggle the task-orientation demands and their own feelings of sensitivity and closeness with clients. They thus experience role ambiguity. They often impose upon themselves the concept of "good nurse" and say to themselves:

"I really should always think of the client first and not my own feelings."
"I should never be sympathetic and cry."

There are instances where it is OK to cry with the client, and it is OK to think of one's own feelings first. Nurses have a right to such feelings.

Probably the best question that nurses could ask about their clients in relation to the person-task orientation is, "Is the client as a person neglected because of the emphasis on task?" If the answer is no, then the nurse can feel less stress and more comfortable in his or her orientation with clients.

Communication Interactions between Nurses and Clients' Families

It is difficult to know what it feels like to be a member of a family of a client who is critically ill unless we have had the firsthand experience. The stress that is felt by a family member as a result of the helplessness and of not knowing what to do or what is wrong may be even greater than the stress that the nurse feels in confronting the family member.

Most often the interaction between the families of clients and the nurses in critical-care units revolves around visiting hours. Hospitals differ in their policies, but many allow five minutes every hour. The families find themselves telescoping their needs for reassurance, information, and guidance into this short space of time. They spend the remainder of the hour in the visitor's lounge comparing notes with other visitors and the cycle of anxiety-visiting period-anxiety becomes more acute.

In nurse-client-family member triads, the tendency towards the formation of a coalition between the family member and the client is often seen (shown by the double line in Figure 10-1). In such triads, nurses have the ultimate control and power, they often find themselves functioning as "gatekeeper" over the family for the visiting hour period.

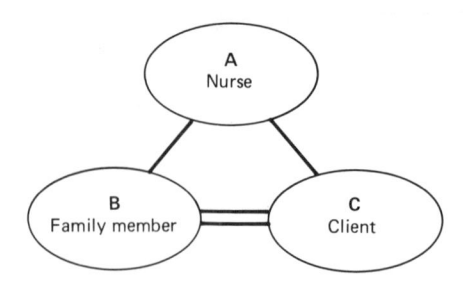

FIGURE 10–1. A coalition triad with B (family member) and C (client) forming a coalition against A (nurse).

Communication in Tertiary Nursing Practice —————————————— **245**

Family member-nurse communication is often one of the most challenging and difficult forms of interaction for the nurse. The stress surrounding the interaction is so great that misunderstanding leading to communication breakdown is not unusual. In some instances, nurses can be judged as "defiant" by family members, and, in turn, family members can be judged "abusive." Nurses can fall prey to the "good visitor" stereotype in which quiet, nonthreatening behavior can be rewarded by an extension of the period of visit: "They let my wife stay longer, because she caused the nurses no trouble and seemed to understand why they were so busy" (Bixler, 1980).

The most important technique that the nurse can utilize in family-nurse communication is the use of empathy. It is not always easy to place oneself in the other person's frame of reference, especially when one's actions are subject to misinterpretation. Keeping the family member informed at all times as to exactly what is happening will alleviate stress and anxiety.

The Sensory Overload Felt by Nurses

Critical-care nurses are prime targets for sensory overload. They work in multistimuli environments in which they are expected to use all channels simultaneously. The constant demand to prioritize which stimuli to respond to is in and of itself a stressor.

Multichannel messages are often sources of stress. A nurse in a nurse-client interaction in a critical-care unit could be involved in the following activities *at the same time:*

> Performing a treatment (kinesthetic)
> Talking to the family in the client's unit (auditory)
> Observing the client's behavior (visual)
> Listening to the head nurse give yet another physician order for the client (auditory)
> Thinking about what is going to be recorded in the client's chart with regard to what has taken place (perception—integration of all three channels).

Conflicting messages are another source of stress for the nurse. An example of this type of message is one in which the head nurse tells the staff nurse one message, "Add the 1000 cc of 5 percent glucose to the IV line," and within seconds, the physician is telling the same nurse, "Add 1000 cc saline to the IV line." The nurse should be careful to check the physician's order to see which verbal message is correct, but she or he must also be sensitive to *listening* at all times to what is being transmitted.

One way that nurses react to sensory overload is to respond by using defensive behaviors to counteract the stress. Five defense mechanisms that can often be observed in tertiary care settings are listed below. These defense mechanisms have been used by all of us when we felt overwhelmed by sensory stimuli in the hospital setting where we worked.

> Denial: the negation of an uncomfortable impulse or truth
> Projection: placing one's inner conflicts on others
> Rationalization: making up excuses or reasons to cover behavior
> Reaction formation: acting the opposite of how one feels
> Repression: forgetting or putting one's uncomfortable thoughts or feelings out of awareness

Highly stressful situations can produce group defensive behaviors. For example, critical-care nurses are constantly exposed to clients who are dying. The nurses react not only individually but as a group. Group reaction formation can be inferred from nurses' laughing or talking about the latest movie or party within earshot of clients in the unit. Indeed, they have even been observed singing or whistling (Hay and Oken, 1972). This particular set of behaviors has been termed "cheerful denial." The stress felt by nurses is often so overwhelming that they laugh instead of cry; however, once they leave the unit and return to their homes, the repressed feelings emerge and the crying begins.

Group stress is evident in critical-care units. Nurses respond as a group to experiences such as the imminent death of a young client with whom they are able to identify. They can, as a group, deny that death might be imminent, and when it occurs, they can view it as a collective failure on their part. "If only we had..." or "Why didn't we..." are thoughts that might run through their minds.

Group stress impacts on systems. When one individual member of the system is affected, other members are affected. So it is with groups; when one subgroup such as the day shift is affected, the total 24-hour staff is affected (Scully, 1978). Group indicators of stress are arguments among the staff, "good nurse" behavior, overuse of defensive styles (blaming, placating, superreasonableness, and irrelevance), and staff turnover (often higher in critical-care units than any other area).

At no time is group stress more evident than with the change of shift. Each shift represents a subsystem of the total system of nursing staff in a given unit. One of the ways that stress and defensive group behavior is evident is in "scapegoating between shifts," expressed by statements like, "It's their fault." In the process of blaming, while the group collectively defends itself, the other shift is attacked. This is not difficult to do, and a look at the three shifts in Figure 10-2 will show why.

The shift that is blamed is blamed indirectly; that is, the night shift blames the evening when reporting to the day shift and so forth, such as in reporting, "We do all the work on our shift!" The intershift report itself often becomes a release for the stress that is felt. The report can be centered around small talk rather than actual client care (Mitchell, 1976): "The one thing I remember was the change of shifts of the nurses and how the nurses talked about their personal matters" (Bixler, 1980).

Unfortunately, there is no panacea for nurses who work under these conditions. The first step, however, is to *identify* the stressors. Group meetings in which nurses can deal with their feelings and also increase their self-awareness are also helpful. These meetings can be guided by a professional in the fields of social work, psychology, or psychiatry. Whoever guides the group should be aware of the problems that exist in the critical-care environment. The use of such techniques as role playing, in which nurses assume the role of terminally ill clients, or the use of a feedback model, in which the nurse paraphrases what the client has said, lead to more effective communication patterns. If nurses paraphrase, using variation of the statement; "You feel...because...," the receiver of the message must focus on both the content and the emotions underlying the statement. This has been found to be beneficial for nursing staffs (Stillman and Strasser, 1980).

CONCLUSION

The tertiary care setting is among those with highest status in terms of nursing care. At the same time, it is one of the most stress-producing environments in health care. The depersonalization of clients and their decreased sensory awareness make the nurse's role as an effective communicator difficult but even more important. By improving communication between self and other health professionals and between self and clients, the nurse can influence the course of the client's illness.

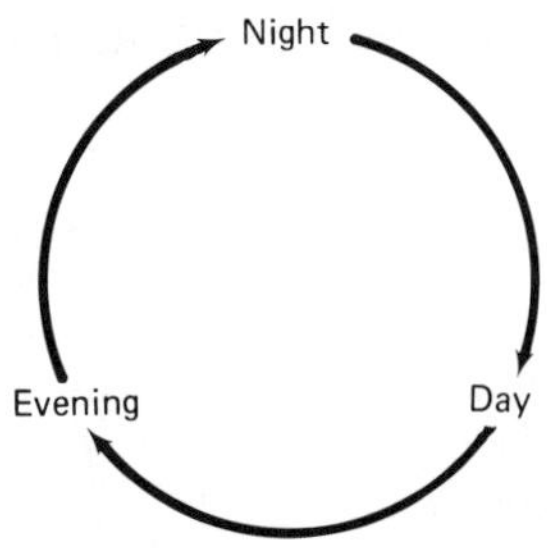

FIGURE 10–2. The cycle of day, evening, and night shifts.

BIBLIOGRAPHY

Bixler, R. Personal interview, June 5, 1980.

Bender-Dougherty, B. Personal interview, April 14, 1980.

Bolin, R.H. Sensory deprivation: an overview. *Nursing Forum*, 1974, *13*, 241–257.

Brunner, L.S., & Smith Suddarth, D. *Textbook of medical-surgical nursing.* Philadelphia: J.B. Lippincott, 1980.

DeMeyer, J. The environment of the intensive care unit. *Nursing Forum*, 1967, *6*, 263–271.

Derrick, F. How open heart surgery feels. *American Journal of Nursing*, 1979, *79*, 276–285.

Gowan, N.J. The perceptual world of the intensive care unit: an overview of some environmental considerations in the helping relationship. *Heart and Lung*, 1979, *8*, 340–344.

Gruber, S. Dynamics of health care administration for nurses, Part 2. *Health Care Horizons*, 1980, February 10, 8–10.

Guida, F. Personal interview, June 21, 1980.

Haase, P., Smith, M.H., & Reitt, B. A proposed system for nursing: theoretical framework, part 2. *Pathways to Practice* (vol. 4). Atlanta: Southern Regional Education Board, 1976.

Hay, D. & Oken, D. The psychological stresses of intensive care unit nursing. *Psychosomatic Medicine*, 1972, *34*, 109–118.

Hersey, P., Blanchard, K. & Lamonica, E. A situational approach to supervision: leadership theory and the supervising nurse. *Supervisor Nurse*, 1976, May, 17–20.

Lewis, J. Structural aspects of the delivery setting and nurse practitioner performance. *Nurse Practitioner*, 1975, Sept.-Oct., *1*, 16–20.

Lynch, J.J. The simple act of touching. *Nursing 78*, 1978, June, 32–36.

Maslow, A.H. *Motivation and Personality* (2nd ed.). New York: Harper & Row, 1970.

Mitchell, M. Inter-shift reports—to tape or not to tape. *Supervisor Nurse*, 1976, October, 38–39.

Noble, M.A. Communication in the ICU: therapeutic or disturbing? *Nursing Outlook*, 1979, *27*, 195–198.

Oselladore, Y. The nurse within the bureaucracy. *Australian Nurses' Journal*, 1978, *7*, (10), 46–48.

Scully, R. Stress in the nurse. *American Journal of Nursing*, 1980, *80*, 912–914.

Shubin, S. Rx for your stress. *Nursing 79*, 1979, January, 53–55.

Stillman, S.M. & Strasser, B.L. Helping critical care nurses with work related stress. *Journal of Nursing Administration*, 1980, *10* (1), 28–31.

Wilson, L.M. Intensive care delirium—the effects of outside deprivation in a windowless unit. *Archives of Internal Medicine*, 1972, *130*, 225–236.

Woods, N.F., & Falk, S.A. Noise stimuli in the acute care area. *Nursing Research*, 1974, *23*, (2), 144–150.

Chapter 11

Communication in primary nursing practice

BEHAVIORAL OBJECTIVES

By reading this chapter, students will be able to:

1. Describe a system of primary care nursing practice
2. Describe the three dimensions of the structure of a primary care nursing system
3. Identify the role of the client in the primary care setting and the relationship of this role to communication
4. Identify the role of the nurse in the primary care setting and the relationship of this role to communication
5. Define three barriers to effective communication by primary care nurses in their role as information takers
6. Define "linear thinking."

PRIMARY NURSING PRACTICE

A system of primary care nursing is the most all-inclusive system of the three systems in nursing practice. It can encompass the total management of chronic illness as well as of health maintenance and health promotion. The reader is cautioned not to confuse this term with primary care nursing. Primary nursing differs from primary care nursing. In *primary nursing* the primary nurse is the "chief nurse of the patient" (Marram et al., 1979, p. 3). *Primary care* usually implies the context in which the client's initial contact with the health care system takes place; also, it can imply continued surveillance of a chronic illness state in which the client's contact with the system is more sporadic, where clients are in and out of the system (Haase et al., 1976).

The focus of primary care nursing practice is on the caring aspects of nursing, rather than the curing aspects (Haase et al., 1976). These two aspects of nursing were described in Chapter 7. There are many different settings in which primary nursing care is practiced; outpatient clinics, health maintenance organizations (HMOs), physicians' offices, schools, industries, or the client's home. Consultative and referral resources are less readily available in these settings than in an acute care setting. Primary care nurses often utilize assessment skills. They also act as coordinators for *all* health services, setting priorities in order to meet the client's needs. It has been estimated that a primary care nurse in one voluntary health agency knew over 100 agencies to which client referrals were made (Fagerhaugh, 1975). Primary care nurses use innovative and less standardized means of meeting the health needs of clients—health needs which are usually less predictable and require monitoring over a long period of time (Haase et al., 1976).

The changing roles of client and nurse (discussed in Chapter 6) have shifted the emphasis in health care from illness to wellness. It has been estimated that 88 percent of all health care needs are primary care needs (Lysaught, 1975). A major goal of nursing is to provide better and more comprehensive health care to all people; it is likely that primary care nursing will be the mode of nursing in the future.

It is highly probable that nurses graduating from schools today will be practicing nursing well into the 21st century. One of the major trends that continues to foster a reorientation in health care is the impact that certain factors relating to the environment seem to have on the health of individuals. Several of these are presented in the Chart 11-1. In examining the chart, it appears that many of the health problems present today are in part due to environmental factors. Examples include lung cancer due to smoking, and chronic heart disease due to poor diet and/or a stressful life style. The incidence of these chronic disease conditions will disappear only over an extended period of time. Solutions will not come overnight. What is emphasized here is that the answers to these chronic conditions will constitute one focus of nursing in the future.

Greater emphasis is placed on the nurse's role in the management of chronic illness in the community setting rather than on the nurse's role in health maintenance in a clinical setting such as a community health clinic. This is because students are more likely to have experiences in community health

CHART 11-1
Environmental Factors Leading to Chronic Conditions

Environmental Factor	Chronic Condition
Maldistribution of health care delivery systems in the United States	Inadequate delivery of health care to more than 45 million Americans (Shorr, 1976)
Chemical pollution of the environment	Increased incidence of certain forms of cancer (Harvey et al., 1976)
Increased longevity	Increased incidence of chronic illness (longer than 3 months) (Yurick et al., 1980)
Stressful life styles	Obesity, smoking, coronary heart disease (Strain and Grossman, 1975)

settings; although many will spend time in health clinics. Both roles have been included in this chapter. One goal of this chapter is to familiarize the student with the role of the nurse in a primary care setting and to provide a foundation to the more specialized learning that will follow at some future point in time. The chapter will first cover the structure of a system of primary care nursing, using the framework of the three dimensions proposed by Lewis (1974). The relationship of these three dimensions to specific communication patterns between the nurse and the client is also covered.

The Physical Setting

The first dimension of primary care nursing practice is physical setting (Lewis, 1974). Consider the physical setting in the following two cases:

Case 1. Mrs. Garcia is Puerto Rican and lives in the Puerto Rican section of a large city. The health of her baby is being assessed by a nurse practitioner in the well-baby clinic located in the basement of the school near her apartment. Mrs. Garcia's four-week-old baby is being seen by the nurse for a first regular check up. Mrs. Garcia has some questions about the baby's diet and sleeping habits. She is anxious, since she has lived in the continental United States for only a year and finds it difficult to understand English. A bilingual nurse is usually present when Mrs. Garcia sees the nurse practitioner.

Case 2. Mr. Booth is a 75-year-old widower who lives alone. His sole income is from Social Security. Mr. Booth has diabetes complicated by peripheral vascular disease. His visual acuity is poor. The VNA nurse is making a home visit in order to change the dressing on an ulcerated area on Mr. Booth's leg. Mr. Booth feels lonely and isolated, and his knowledge of community resources is limited.

In Case 1, the physical setting is a primary care clinic. Clinics can be related to a specialty area such as a pediatric well-baby clinic. The emphasis in this clinic is on health teaching. It is not necessarily disease-oriented or diagnostic.

In Case 2, the primary care setting is the client's home. The illness can be chronic, and the client needs ongoing guidance to assist him in the development of a regimen that will reestablish a state of health equilibrium.

The two cases presented serve as a means to conceptualize two major primary care settings: the first case closely parallels a physician's office and the second is in the home setting.

Physical Setting and Communication. The physical settings in primary care nursing systems often lend themselves to different client approaches by nurses. The client, especially in the home setting, is not usually seen as a single individual: rather, he or she is viewed within the family context. Thus, in the home setting, the nurse is exposed to family members as well as the client. The nurse-client interaction can be triadic in nature and is diagrammed in Figure 11–1.

As illustrated in Figure 11–1, the family member often serves as the interpreter for the client. The family member could be a husband or wife, a child, a relative, or even a neighbor. The physical presence of the family must be recognized by the nurses if they are to be effective in communication with clients. Nurses find themselves in the home setting on the clients' terms; they are "guests" in the clients' physical territory, and they cannot assume they

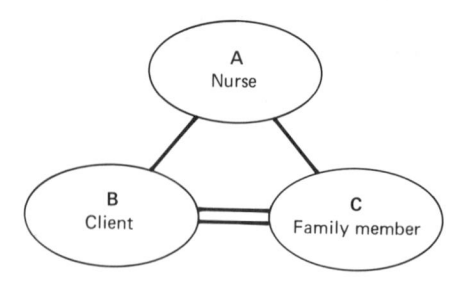

FIGURE 11–1. A communication triad with B (client) and C (family member) forming a coalition against A (nurse).

have the right to ask family members to leave. At the same time, the nurse still controls the interaction. There still is a tendency for a coalition to form between the family members and the client. The nurse, in order to interact with the client, must determine who the pivotal person is in terms of decision making within the family context. In some instances, decisions are made for the client by the total family group (Bernstein and Bernstein, 1980); in other instances, one spouse may make the decision for the other. Thus, if the community health staff nurse decides to teach basic methods of contraception to the mother of eight children and to ignore the husband, who happens to be the decision maker and who happens *not* to approve of contraception, the nurse may only add to the mother's anxiety and guilt feelings rather than provide effective health education.

Development of Trust. A key concept in the nurse-client relationship is the development of trust. The three phases of a level of trust are described in detail in Chapter 6. In the nurse-client relationship, especially in the home setting, where the illness is chronic and long-term, a high level of trust may be readily established due to longer duration of the working phase of the process of developing trust. The nurse, exposed to the client and family over extended periods of time, can progress from superficial to in-depth levels of communication. These communication interactions will tend to be symmetrical because the client has more independence and is more in control of his or her total environment. The nurse's major purpose in client interactions in the primary care setting is the promotion of the client's well-being. The challenge is to enable the client to understand the "why" associated with a particular health care regimen.

The fact that nurses are not physically present at all times to enforce the health regimen, such as when to take a medication, means that clients and family members have to understand *why* the medication is being given in the first place. In other words, the clients have a high degree of freedom of choice in complying with their regimens. If high levels of trust and understanding have been established, then the likelihood is greater that the client will comply with the medical and nursing regimens that have been recommended than if they are low.

In one sense, it is easier for the client to build a level of trust in the nurse-client relationship than it is for the nurse. This relates to the client's familiarity with the physical setting. The barriers that exist for the client in the inpatient hospital setting are not present. At the same time, the nurse does not have the security of the hospital environment (presence of co-workers and peers, uniforms, and control). The primary care setting is not the nurse's home territory.

Organization of Activities

The second dimension of the structure of primary care is organization of activities. Many primary care settings can be described as nonbureaucratic in nature. An examination of the four characteristics of a bureaucracy will demonstrate why this is so.

Specialization. The degree of specialization relative to the nursing staff is limited in primary care settings. Most nurses who work in primary care settings would probably describe themselves as "generalists." It should be noted that there are "specialists" as well, for example, pediatric nurse practitioners in child health clinics. Nurses who are generalists work with client problems that are broad and varied, as shown in the following case situation:

> Mrs. Brainard is a 60-year-old diabetic who had a below-knee amputation 6 weeks ago. Mrs. Brainard lives by herself in a second-floor apartment. The nurse is making a home visit to ascertain her physiological status and check on administration of insulin and other medications, adherence to diet, and sleeping and exercise patterns. In addition to this the nurse has assessed the following:

1. The safety of the environment: Mrs. Brainard's ability to move about, especially with regard to cooking for herself and if she is able to go up and down stairs.
2. Her ability to obtain transportation to the outpatient clinic to see the doctor and physical therapist.
3. Mrs. Brainard's socialization status with reference to her immediate and extended family as well as significant others.
4. Mrs. Brainard's financial status and how she is currently paying for her medications and special equipment.

These problems are only the initial ones. This is only a beginning. Clients may present additional problems over time, some of which require ingenuity and creative thinking in order for the nurse to enable the client to cope.

Within the nonbureaucratic structure of the primary care nursing setting, nurses often find themselves on their own and unable to rely on peers or co-workers for mutual support. They communicate on a collegial level largely by making referrals to other professional health workers, but these co-workers are not physically present in the field.

One area where specialization is evident in systems of primary care nursing is in written communication. Nurses are expected to keep records of client visits as well as reports relating to insurance, Medicare, and Medicaid. The amount of paperwork is voluminous, and nurses sometimes take portions of it home to complete at night in order that they might have more time during the day for "short calls" on their clients (Fagerhaugh, 1975). Orders are usually transmitted as written orders. At the same time, any change in an order is usually communicated by the physician to the nurse over the phone. Thus, while nurses working in primary care nursing settings primarily use auditory communication such as the telephone with other professionals, they also utilize visual channels of communication through numerous written reports and memos.

Hierarchy of Authority. The hierarchy of authority, the second characteristic of a bureaucracy, is the least obvious in the home-setting. The client does not always perceive him or herself as one-down when interacting with the nurse. Within the community health agency itself, the staff's line of authority is from the director to the supervisor to the staff nurse in a downward direction. The staff nurse and the supervisor work together in a relationship which is primarily symmetrical. They have conferences in which they develop patterns of health care for families mutually. The supervisor functions in a role consonant with the root meaning of the word *supervisor*, that is, one who oversees or has a broader vision. It is recognized that the supervisor has more expertise and the nurse utilizes his or her resources. There is planned supervision of the staff nurse by the supervisor in the form of a periodic evaluation, usually on a semiannual or annual basis. The supervisor also covers the staff nurse's caseload while the staff nurse is in the field. This requires answering questions from physicians or any other health professionals who might call in during this time. The reporting of information by staff nurses to their supervisor is done primarily from the vantage point of the nurse; that is, they report what *they* wish to report, what *they* have seen, heard, or felt.

In primary care settings, nurses do not usually communicate with physicians in face-to-face interactions. They request written orders or a written summary of what the client needs from physicians. If nurses have questions, they usually communicate by phone. This can present the challenge of determining what is the most effective way to communicate with a particular physician. One physician might prefer that nurses not request specific orders, while another appreciates this approach. One barrier to effective nurse-physician communication can be the physician's office nurse, who usually protects the physician from outside calls. It can be as frustrating for nurses as it is for clients to communicate directly with a busy physician. It is best to find out when the physician is in his or her office by asking the secretary *when* to call. Staff often sit down and write ahead exactly what they are going to ask or discuss so that they have organized their thoughts prior to the interaction.

Kelly (1978) gives two important guidelines for nurses to follow when communicating with physicians by phone:

1. Ask the right questions.
2. Never *assume* anything.

In telephone conversations with physicians or other professionals, it is important for nurses to establish *which* client, *what* the content of the message is, and *why* they are calling.

The second admonition is that you should never *assume* that you, the nurse, and the physician are speaking about the same client; always identify the client by first and last names. Also, you should never assume you understand what the physician or other professional means until you have written down the verbal message and read it back to make sure it has been understood.

The nurse-physician relationship, while more collegial than in a hospital setting, can be fragile in many instances. Nurses, aware of the delicate balance between the two professions, are careful not to offend physicians by "taking over" clients. Physicians are willing to accept suggestions more readily from nurses when clients are in the recovery phase of illness as opposed to acute phase of illness (Fagerhaugh, 1975). To avoid a confrontation, nurses play the "doctor-nurse game," as exemplified in the following telephone conversation:

NURSE: I'm calling you, Dr. Johnson, because Mrs. Reed is having a recurrence of those headaches again. She had an order for codeine and aspirin last week, which helped alleviate the pain. Do you wish to reorder this?
DOCTOR: Fine, I'll write the prescription.
NURSE: Thank you.

In the above conversation the nurse suggested to the physician what medication to reorder in such a way that the physician felt he was assuming responsibility for giving the order, although he was only agreeing with the nurse. The physician assumed a superior role in a nurse-physician complementary relationship.

An Explicit Set of Rules and Policies. The old adage that rules were made to be broken might well apply to primary care settings. The key word in relation to rules and policies is flexibility. Routine policies are often stretched to adapt to the client's (or client's family's) needs, as shown in the following case situation:

Mrs. White has multiple sclerosis and is confined to her bed. Mrs. White's husband, who assumes complete responsibility for his wife's care, works nights. Because Mr. White sleeps during the day, the community health nurse does not call at the White's house until early evening, when she knows Mr. White will be awake. The policy of daytime visits has been stretched into early evening to adapt to the needs of this family.

Nurses who have functioned in hospital settings often find it difficult to adjust to this flexibility. The set regimens and strict procedures to which nurses adhere in performing high-visibility tasks are modified according to the client in a particular primary care setting. The emphasis of communication interactions is on the total person and his or her unique physical and psychosocial needs.

An Impersonal Attitude. The last characteristic of a bureaucracy is an impersonal attitude of the staff toward clients. It is more difficult to maintain such an attitude in systems of primary care than in systems of secondary or tertiary care. As stated previously, clients are seen over extended periods of time, and nurses look at the client as a total person. Thus, nurses are encouraged to perform teaching and establish therapeutic relationships along with performing tasks.

One study investigated the topics of communication interactions between the nurse and client in home visits. The study was able to isolate 17 categories of subjects. The three most frequently talked about were (1) general health and symptoms, (2) medical care regimens, and (3) personal and family emotional problems. The least talked about subjects were assistive devices for dressing oneself, and attendant care (Mayers, 1973). In other words, the topics of communication were based on nursing content. This suggests that it is the nurse who controls the communication interactions during the home visits.

Role Expectations for Clients

The Client's Role. There is no such person as the typical client in a community health setting. Clients can range from old to newborn, from acutely ill to well, and from recent immigrants to Native Americans. In spite of the variety of clients seen by the public health or community health nurse in the primary care nursing practice setting, if one were to ask one of these nurses to describe a "typical client" (which is what we did), one might receive the following response: "the 'typical' client is elderly, often lonely and isolated, and sometimes terminal." Each of these three descriptive phrases will be covered in further detail in the following discussion. Again, it should be emphasized that the setting is the home. Other primary care settings have different populations, such as mothers and newborns in a well-baby clinic.

Elderly Clients (65+ years). Nurses who work in primary care environments, especially the home setting, often find they are working with geriatric clients, many of whom have some form of sensory impairment that can affect one or all communication channels (Burnside, 1978). By sensory impairment we mean a decline in the functioning of one or more senses, which may be caused by environmental influences as well as aging (see Chapter 10).

It is helpful for nurses to realize the impact of sensory losses when communicating with elderly clients. Clients who have a major sensory loss in one channel are often forced to compensate with other functioning channels. For example, a client may switch to increased use of the auditory channel because of poor vision. There are clients who have sensory deprivation in the three major channels. Picture the elderly client who wears a hearing aid, has glasses, and in whom the sense of touch is diminished. In addition, he or she might even have dentures, contributing to a gustatory loss.

Elderly clients can also assume the psychological characteristics of ill persons (Chapter 6); they often become more dependent and passive and experience greater anxiety, which results in a lowered feeling of self-worth. It is important for the nurse to pay attention to signs of depression and anxiety in older clients because these clients can be helped. In the primary care setting, the nurse may well be the only provider the older client sees. The nurse must be careful not to let his or her own fears of aging or stereotypes of the elderly interfere with the care that is given. Openly sharing concerns such as these with an understanding supervisor or colleague is an effective method of handling some of the discomfort primary care nurses feel with elderly clients.

A discussion of the use of the major channels—auditory, visual, and kinesthetic—in elderly clients and their relationship to communication in nurse-interaction follows.

AUDITORY LOSS. Deafness in varying degrees is common in the elderly. Approximately one-third of the elderly have minimal to serious hearing loss (Anwar, 1977; McNamee, 1978; Bozian and Clark, 1980). Hearing losses may be caused by a decrease in the overall sensitivity to sound or, even more commonly, to high-pitch sounds. There may be a greater loss in one ear than the other. Disturbances in sleep patterns and fatigue from concentration in order to hear are also characteristic of these clients (McNamee, 1978). Imagine yourself obtaining a health history from a client who has a moderate hearing loss. There are several things you can do:

1. If possible eliminate all background noise and find a quiet area or space to talk.
2. Speak slowly in low tones so the client has time to process the information. *Do not* make your voice "sing-song" (Bozian and Clark, 1980).
3. Face the client. Remember they are using the visual channel, providing the client's eyesight is all right. They will look at your lips, your facial expression, and your body language.
4. Check to see if the person has a hearing aid. If so, the hearing aid can be adjusted to your voice. It is also appropriate to check to see if the aid is switched on and the battery is working (Anwar, 1977).
5. Speak in a firm voice. There is a way to raise your voice without yelling. Yelling has an adverse effect on the elderly. How often do elderly clients

say, "Don't yell at me; I can hear you!" It is condescending to clients to be yelled at. Also, there is an incorrect tendency to generalize the hearing loss to *all* the elderly and thus to speak in a loud voice with all these clients.

VISUAL LOSS. The decline in the ability of the eye's lens to accommodate to lights of different intensity starts in the teen years and can result in serious consequences, with subsequent loss of vision in later years. The elderly client who has no visual problems is rare; it is safe to assume that your client will have some visual loss. However, with remedial steps and a prescription for glasses, clients can usually function effectively (Oyer and Oyer, 1976). The important thing to remember is that elderly clients usually *do not report* visual problems. They tend to assume poor vision or distorted visual images are part of being old. (Gardiner, 1977).

If the client has a visual loss, the nurse can communicate by using the auditory channel as the predominant channel (assuming there is minimal to no hearing loss). Because of this the nurse should be aware of what he or she is saying, as well as, *how* he or she is saying it: voice inflection, tone, volume. Despite some loss of higher pitched sounds, it is not uncommon for elderly clients to develop keen hearing and be able to hear even whispers at a distance. The feelings underneath verbal expressions are often detected by these clients with amazing clarity, and a direct and honest approach is best when communicating with them.

Some ways nurses can help clients with visual impairment are:

1. Make sure lighting is adequate.
2. Use large print for reading.
3. Use color coding for medications and treatments.
4. Watch for depth perception. Paint borders on steps.

KINESTHETIC LOSS. Older clients often do not respond to changes in temperature, either internally or externally, as younger persons do. Also, the speed of information decoding in the central nervous system may be slow, leading to the "foot-shuffling" seen in some older people. Nurses can:

1. Check the water temperature if the client is to have a bath or treatment to make sure it is not too hot (Bozian and Clark, 1980).
2. Make sure the carpet or tiles on floors are designed so that the client can see his or her feet on the floor, thus giving visual feedback.
3. Check the room temperature.

Another related kinesthetic "loss" is the lack of personal touch-contact many older people experience. The use of touch (holding hands, hugging, or an arm around a shoulder) is a powerful therapeutic tool that is difficult to overuse.

ISOLATION AND LONELINESS. Isolation and loneliness are two terms used to describe the elderly, although there is some question as to exactly how isolated and lonely most elderly people are (Lowenthal and Robinson, 1976).

The nurse who works in primary care settings is likely to encounter many elderly who live alone in neighborhoods with changing ethnic mixes. Because others have moved out or died, the older client may feel particularly isolated during illness, even though family are a local telephone call away.

There is a series of questions the nurse should keep in mind in working with older clients who complain of isolation:

1. What is the quality and amount of contact with the family?
2. What is the quality and amount of contact with informal social supports (friends, mailmen, bank tellers, etc.)?
3. Is the client lonely as opposed to depressed? (That is, is social contact or counseling needed?)
4. If the nurse is being identified as a substitute for a child ("You're so much like my daughter"), at what point does the identification become a problem in maintaining a therapeutic relationship? Also, at what point does the nurse feel uncomfortable about the relationship?

As was mentioned in Chapter 9, communicating with any older client will be most successful if the nurse imagines how he or she would want to be treated in the same situation. Empathy (as opposed to sympathy) and a congruent style (as opposed to blame, placating, superreasonableness, or irrelevance) should form the foundation of the therapeutic nurse-client relationship with older as well as younger clients.

Because the nurse may be the sole provider of services to the older client, the nurse's ability to link the client to appropriate programs and services *after* recovery from illness will influence the future course of the client's health status. Thus, the nurse must be able to communicate effectively and to obtain accurate information from the client, but he or she also must be able to communicate effectively with other services and agencies when taking on the role of advocate for the isolated or lonely client.

Nurses often have to *learn* to accept clients in primary care settings with respect and a positive attitude. It is natural that persons judge others using the value systems of their personal and professional role identities. Thus, novice nurses in primary care systems can fall into the pitfall of letting their subjective feelings determine how they view clients.

"He's old."
"She's poor."
"They are dirty."

The client can also feel put down and say to him or herself:

"I'm too old."
"I'm too poor."
"I'm too dirty."

The challenge is for the nurse to accept people as they are and not impose "conditions" of acceptance. Nurses do not have to approve of or accept the client's values, nor do they have to change their own values.

Terminally ill clients. To state that clients are terminal can lead to stereotype the client's role. We all have preconceived ideas as to what each of us thinks terminal means. It conjures up different pictures in our minds depending on what our past experiences have been. Clients can be terminal and continue to live anywhere from hours to years. Terminal means "end," and all of us face this end at some point in our lives. Nurses who are aware of their own attitudes towards death are better able to deal with clients who are facing imminent death.

The literature on death and dying is vast, and it is not our purpose to go into depth on this subject except to introduce you to the subject and reinforce two statements that might give you direction in a primary care nursing situation.

The first statement is: *"You do not have to say anything."* Inexperienced nurses after they have communicated with a client who is dying will often state: "I didn't know what to say." If terminal clients are able to share feelings with you, you can respond nonverbally through the therapeutic use of self, utilizing active listening, empathy, sharing your own feelings, or using caring touch. These concepts are presented in Chapter 4.

The second statement that is presented in relation to terminal clients is: *"Clients often know when they are dying."* (Kübler-Ross, 1969, 1974) Given this fact, what is important for you to communicate to the client in the primary care setting? There are two thoughts that are essential (Kubler-Ross, 1969):

1. You have not given up hope
2. You will not desert the client

Hope can be directed towards a cure (at beginning of the illness) or to prolongation of life (end of illness). Hope often changes during the course of the illness, becoming more focused on present events: "I hope I can make it until my son graduates from school in June." It is important for the nurse to listen and share the client's hopes. In experiencing this, the client begins to feel that the nurse has not given up hope.

Also, it is essential to let the client know you will return to visit. The nurse should indicate that he or she will not reject the client in spite of what the client is feeling. If the client is angry at the world or discusses his or her own death with the nurse, these feelings are OK with the nurse.

Most nurses feel they are able to cope with the emotions of dying clients but that often this type of interaction results in uncomfortable feelings (Popoff, 1975). If nurses are able to express their own feelings about death in a small-group situation, they are able to undertake the first step in developing mutual trust. If these feelings are accepted by the group, then they are able to express more revealing ones. Nurses who have been able to do this are able to communicate more effectively about death and dying with clients. All the key concepts presented in Chapter 4 are especially important in dealing with terminal clients.

Role Expectations for Nurses

The Nurse's Role. Role expectations of primary care nurses can be categorized into two major functions: the function of the nurse as an information taker and the function of the nurse as an information giver. Some essential tasks of primary care nurses involve the dual functions of eliciting information *from* the client and imparting information *to* the client. A discussion of each of the functions follows:

PRIMARY CARE NURSES AS INFORMATION TAKERS. The use of information-gathering skills is an essential part of the primary care nurse's role. The communication tool for information-gathering is the interview (Chapter 5), which may be structured or unstructured. Incorporated within the structured interview is the nursing history, which is often used by primary care nurses in outpatient settings. Nonstructured interviews are more often undertaken by the nurse in the client's home setting. In order for nurses to formulate nursing diagnoses, they must use effective information-gathering skills, and also be aware of the pitfalls in interviewing. It is important that nurses understand the nature of interpersonal techniques used in interviewing clients, in order to increase their ability to utilize congruent responses. This was demonstrated in a study in which nurses were given a course which presented basic techniques nurses need in responding to clients, and which also included a discussion of the attitudes these techniques express and how clients might react to each of them. The nurses showed a significant increase in the choice of congruent responses (Bernstein and Bernstein, 1980).

Oftentimes, primary care nurses lack certain pieces of information about a client. There is no chart readily at hand, such as in the hospital. Nurses are apt to have only half the essential information needed and must piece together the rest, either by consulting another health professional or by talking to the client. One piece of information that is not always available is the client's previous contacts with the health care system. Previous negative experiences in the health care system will impact on the present nurse-client interaction. Obviously, if a client has had a contact with a nurse who made no attempt to understand the client and the client felt put down, the next contact will be affected even though it is not with the same nurse. The client does not wish to be subjected to the same negative experience and will withhold trust.

Sociocultural Barriers. The communication barriers that are often encountered in nurse-client interactions in the primary care situation are of a sociocultural nature. The sociocultural barriers that influence communication include those due to cultural, language, and class and/or race differences.

CULTURAL DIFFERENCES. Nurses are often unaware of the power of culture in influencing a client's behavior until they find themselves in the strange environment of the client's home and neighborhood. Culture can be defined in numerous ways; for our purposes here, we chose the following definition: culture is the sum of "learned, shared and transmitted patterns of behavior that are totally directed toward the solving of some problem or problems experienced by human beings" (Jaeger and Simmons, 1970, p. 271).

It is hardly ever easy for nurses or others to interact with clients or other people who have totally different value systems and cultural backgrounds. The composite of attitudes and beliefs that make up one's value systems not only serves as a guide to one's behavior, but when shared, can also serve as a common bond between the client and the nurse. Differences or conflicts in values can often result in social distancing; that is, others become more distant because they are "different."

In communicating with clients, it is helpful for nurses to know the ways in which the client's cultural patterns influence perception of illness. Often, this can be ascertained by talking to the client and being open. Openness is the ability to understand the client—to listen and accept differences. It is interesting to note and be aware of the channels used to convey a message. Some clients, by virtue of their ethnic and cultural backgrounds, communicate more openly through auditory channels; they can be more expressive in their verbal response to pain, for example. The classic study by Zborowski (1969) demonstrated that there was a diversity of cultural patterns in attitudes towards and reactions to pain in four ethnic groups (Jews, Italians, Irish, and "Old American"). Other cultures are more visual. In some cultures, to look an older person in the eye, if one is young, is disrespectful (Indian and Puerto Rican) (Epstein, 1974). The nurse, in confronting a young person of such a culture who does not maintain eye contact, can misinterpret this behavior and think the young person is insecure. The tendency to label various ethnic groups in relation to the way they react and perceive illness is always present. One group might be termed "stoic," while yet another group might be seen as "sensitive and demanding." The client, regardless of ethnicity, should be looked at as a total person and as unique; in other words, no two clients will react to the same illness or stimuli exactly alike, regardless of their ethnicity. Their past experience, the type and length of illness, the amount of outside responsibility the client has (small children to take care of, for example) can be as *important as ethnicity* in terms of how they relate to their symptoms and how open or closed they are in relating symptomology to the nurse.

COMMUNICATION WITH MINORITY GROUPS. In primary care settings, nurses are likely to have contact with subcultures, that is, a group of persons within a culture who have an identity of their own but are related to the total culture (Murray and Zentner, 1975). Examples of subcultures include minority groups, e.g., blacks, Hispanics, Native Americans, and Asian Americans. Consider the following case situation:

> Debbie Jones, a 19-year-old black, unmarried mother has brought her three-month-old baby into the outpatient pediatric clinic because the baby has a fever. The nurse is filling out the record and taking the infant's temperature before the baby is seen by the physician. The nurse, who is white and also 19 years old, is finding it difficult to empathize with this client. She says to herself: "Why does this mother appear to love the baby so much? Perhaps the only reason she had it was to get the welfare payments."
>
> Ms. Jones notices the nurse's actions toward her and thinks to herself: "That nurse is treating me like dirt! She doesn't understand how much I wanted to have a baby of my own!"

Members of minority groups *can* have initial suspicion and fear of nurses because nurses are viewed as being powerful, one-up, and, if from a different racial group, nonempathic. However, this is *not* always the case. In addition, it *can* be the nurses who view the clients as powerless, one-down, and different. Of course, many nurses do not feel this way about the members of minority groups with whom they have contact.

While there is no question that some nurses have attitudes towards others that can be called stereotypic and that since minority group members have equally strong feelings about health professionals, the key issue for a communication text on nursing is:

"How can I (the nurse), with my values, perceptions, background and role, communicate effectively with a person from a different group with his or her values, perceptions, background, and role as a client?"

In discussing the issue of cross-racial communication there seems to be a tendency to try to figure out "who has the problem," that is, who is "at fault," when there is miscommunication, misunderstanding, or perceived prejudice on either side (client or nurse). While there is no question that prejudice has no place in professional nursing behavior, in terms of *improving* communication, deciding who is at fault is often a form of blaming that does not result in constructive changes, either for nurses or clients. Similarly, placating ("going along" or trying to appease the client), being superreasonable (rationalizing), or being irrelevant are not, in the long run, going to make things go well between nurse and client in a cross-racial situation. What is left is for the nurse to maintain a congruent communication style.

From a congruent standpoint, the nurse should be actively involved in maintaining the client's sense of self-worth. By respecting the individual client's dignity, the nurse can be an important therapeutic agent, even when the client is in dire social, economic, or health circumstances.

One part of respecting the client's sense of self-worth in cross-cultural situations is appreciating the other's cultural identity. This does not mean that the nurse in primary care has to read every book on cultural values. It is possible to ask for explanations and let the client be a cultural guide if it is done in a congruent manner, that is, nonblaming and nonpatronizing.

The nurse has to be sensitive to differences in cultural perceptions about many areas, including the sick role, the role of family, the roles of men and women, and even the symbolic importance of foods and diet. These and other cultural values become important when considering how to teach clients to comply with a medical regimen. Sensitivity to these is also crucial in developing trust. Again, they can be learned if the nurse is willing to be taught by the clients.

One of the most important aspects in cross-cultural communication between nurses and clients is the nature of the nurse-client relationship. The nurse needs to have a person-to-person relationship for trust to develop. Many of the values and skills presented in this book, including openness, appropriate self-disclosure, use of empathy, and a person, versus task, orientation are crucial in developing trust and effective communication. An impersonal, "distancing" manner will turn off many clients. The person-to-person connection is the beginning step in effective cross-cultural nursing. Just because two people are from different backgrounds does *not* mean that understanding, mutual respect, and caring relationships are automatically impossible. Rather than defining cross-cultural issues as barriers, they can be considered challenges and opportunities for learning and growth on both sides.

INABILITY TO UNDERSTAND THE LANGUAGE. Nowhere is the inability to communicate because clients are not able to speak or understand English more obvious than in the primary care setting. Clients find that because they are not able to speak English, they cannot express their needs or their feelings. Nurses are called upon to use their ingenuity if they too do not speak the client's native language. In some situations, nurses rely on interpreters to communicate effectively with clients who cannot speak or understand English. Sometimes the visits are planned around the presence of the interpreter. This again presents problems when talking about pregnancy or other sensitive issues. The inability to understand clients who are unable to speak English can be more the result of nurses *expecting not to understand* than really not having the ability to converse (Epstein, 1974). In situations where neither the client nor the nurse understands the other's language there can be a high level of anxiety. Try to imagine how one might feel in a foreign country where no one understood English. Often the anxiety level is so high that the words of the person with whom one is communicating do not make any sense at all. On the other hand, if one is comfortable in the situation, he or she can survive with relatively few words and observing nonverbal behaviors to make one's desires known.

There are situations in which children, acting as interpreters for a member of their family, communicate with the nurse in the primary care setting. In communicating with children, the nurse should be cautioned to ensure that the message communicated is adapted to the level of understanding of the child. Research has shown that while children (third through fifth grade) were able to name various parts of the anatomy in the human body, they were unable to relate these anatomical parts to each other. For example, children were able to name the heart, blood, and veins but did not understand their relationship in the circulatory system (Smith, 1977). Children (and others) will often indicate that they understand directions and explanations when in actuality they do not. They do this because they feel subordinate in the nurse-patient (child) communication interaction. The nurse is dependent on the child in order to communicate with the client, and it is necessary to establish a trust relationship with the child, one in which the child feels comfortable.

Obviously the most effective nurses in language barrier situations are bilingual nurses. The number of bilingual nurses of differing backgrounds continues to increase nationally. In looking at 37 families, Mayers (1975) found an interesting mix of whites, blacks, Mexican-Americans, Chinese, American Indians, and Filipinos. But when she looked at the nurses treating the families she found a similar mix: whites, blacks, Chinese, and Japanese. Certainly an overlap such as this between client and nurse will alleviate some of the language barriers, as well as the fear and anxieties that the nurses might have in the situation.

Primary Care Nurses as Information Givers. In assuming the role of a teacher, the nurse must start where the client is. It is unrealistic, for example, to teach a client to administer his or her own insulin injections if the client's hands are somewhat crippled with arthritis. If the nurse's objective is to teach a young mother about the importance of immunization shots for her baby, the feasibility of the mother's being able to obtain the shots must be considered.

Does the mother have to take a taxi across town and then wait for two hours in the outpatient clinic? The goal of the nurse is to give the client a sense of "want to do." Coercion does not work because the nurse is not always there. Clients must be internally motivated and able to perceive the health problem in order to carry out their own effective health care.

Both client and nurse have their own interpersonal style in the teaching situation. They bring to the situation their own internalized frames of reference. Nurses generally have an unchanging communication style. Thus, if a nurse tends to be a nondirective listener, she or he will probably use that communication style in every client situation (Mayers, 1975). Some nurses were identified in one study as "client-focused," that is, they pick up the clients cues; and others were "nurse-focused," that is, they responded to their own frame of reference. It is difficult for nurses to change these styles (Mayers, 1975).

In their role as information givers or teachers, nurses will often see clients who attempt to place a single causality on all health-related problems. The tendency to relate illness to one cause is called linear thinking. Examples of linear thinking are:

"I caught this cold because my feet got wet."
"My cancer was due to all that stress."

In actuality the cold might have been due to a number of factors: fatigue, lowered resistance, or exposure to others. The cancer also might have been influenced by more than one variable: a history of cancer in the family, repeated exposure to carcinogens in the environment, or age-related factors. The temptation is to say A (cause) $= X$ (illness), to attach a single variable to the cause of illness. Illness is usually multicausal: $A + B + C + D = X$. All the factors combined lead to the disease (X).

The tendency to linear thinking in today's world is very strong. Clients often choose unicausality because it best fits their needs:

"I had a heart attack because I didn't jog."
"I have emphysema because I smoked a lot."

While these causes for illness are partially true, clients often punish themselves by attributing their health problems to a single cause. In these instances, the nurse, through use of therapeutic communication, may have to reestablish the client's former sense of self-worth and change the client's patterns of thinking. If linear thinking is preventing the client from undertaking the proper health regimen, then the nurse must reinforce more complex thinking as opposed to linear explanations.

Effective teaching results in change. The presence of change is one way to indicate if learning has taken place. But change is not always easy: it tends to be threatening, and it is usually easier to maintain the status quo. Change also indicates learning and growth. The most effective way to bring about change is to find out what the client's values are and what *they* need to know about their health. The nurse might discover that what he or she thought was important was totally different from what the client perceived to be important. In other words, the client should be allowed to *choose* and *discover,* rather than be *compelled* and *judged,* in the learning situation. The client can then decide which of the options the nurse has presented that he or she wishes to take.

CONCLUSION

The content in this chapter has been focused on the nurse's role in primary care nursing practice and how the role influences communication. The primary care setting itself was described in relation to Lewis's three dimensions of structure. Although there is no prototype of a client in a primary care nursing practice, many clients are isolated and lonely, are elderly, and require terminal care.

The nurse in the primary care setting has a dual role of eliciting information *from* the client and imparting information *to* the client. In many instances, the nurse and client can actually switch roles, allowing the nurse to be the learner and the client the teacher. This is particularly true in nurse-client situations in which the client represents a different ethnic group and culture.

Sociocultural differences are sharpened in the primary care nursing setting, necessitating greater adaptability on the part of the nurse. In order to understand and empathize with clients, nurses have to know some of the idiosyncratic patterns of behavior that are normal in their own culture as well as those of other cultures. Nurses are cautioned against ethnocentricity, that is, the belief that the nurse's culture is *better* than the client's. This "ugly American" attitude only creates greater social distance in nurse–client interactions.

Primary care nursing provides an exciting challenge to nurses who choose to work in this setting. The nursing role is associated with greater autonomy and more independent decision making. Effective communication skills assume a large part of this role.

BIBLIOGRAPHY

Anwar, M. Communication difficulties with the elderly hard-of-hearing. *Nursing Mirror,* November 3, 1977.

Bernstein, L. & Bernstein, R. *Interviewing: a guide for health professionals* (3rd ed.). New York: Appleton-Century-Crofts, 1980.

Bozian, M. & Clark, H. Counteracting sensory changes in the aging. *American Journal of Nursing,* 1980, 8, 473–476.

Davis M., Kramer, M., & Strauss, A. (Eds.). *Nurses in practice. A perspective on work environments.* St. Louis: C.V. Mosby, 1975.

"Death and Dying Questionnaire," *Nursing 75,* August, 1975.

Epstein, C. *Effective interaction in contemporary nursing.* Englewood Cliffs, N.J.: Prentice-Hall, 1974.

Fagerhaugh, S. The work of the visiting nurse. In M. Davis, M. Kramer & A. Strauss (Eds.), *Nurses in practice. A perspective on work environments.* St. Louis: C.V. Mosby, 1975.

Gardiner, P.A. Failing vision in the elderly. *Nursing Mirror,* November 3, 1977.

Haase, P., Smith, M.H., & Reitt, B. A proposed system for nursing: theoretical framework, part 2. *Pathways to Practice* (Vol. 4). Atlanta: Southern Regional Education Board, 1976.

Harvey, et al., 1976. *The Principles and Practice of Medicine,* (20th ed.). New York: Appleton-Century-Crofts, 1980.

Jaeger, D. & Simmons, L. *The aged ill.* New York: Appleton-Century-Crofts, 1970.

Kelly, N. Taking the errors out of phone orders. *Nursing 78,* 1978, 19–20 and 28–29.

Kübler-Ross, E. *On death and dying.* New York: Macmillan, 1969.

Kübler-Ross, E. *Questions and answers on death and dying.* New York: Collier Books, 1974.

Lewis, J. Structural aspects of the delivery setting and nurse practitioner performance. *Nurse Practitioner,* 1975, Sept.-Oct., *1,* 16–20.

Lowenthal, M.F., & Robinson, B. Social networks and isolation. In Binstock, R.H., & Shanus, E. (Eds.), *Handbook of Aging and the Social Sciences.* New York: Van Nostrand Reinhold, 1976.

Lysaught, J. (Director), National Commission for the Study of Nursing and Nursing Education. *From abstract into action.* New York: McGraw-Hill, 1973.

Marram, G. *Primary nursing, a model for individualized care* (2nd ed.). St. Louis: C.V. Mosby, 1979.

Mayers, M. Home visit—ritual or therapy? In Spradley, B. (Ed.), *Contemporary Community Nursing.* Boston: Little, Brown, 1975.

NcNamee, C. Communicating. *Canadian Nurse,* 1978, March, 28–29.

Murray, R. & Zentner, J. *Nursing concepts for health promotion.* Englewood Cliffs, N.J.: Prentice-Hall, 1975.

Oyer, H. & Oyer, J. (Eds.). *Aging and communication.* Baltimore: University Park Press, 1976.

Popoff, D. "What are your feelings about death and dying?" Part I. *Nursing 75,* 1975, August, 16–24.

Schorr, T. Tunnel visionaries (editorial). *American Journal of Nursing,* 1976, 76 (4), 559.

Smith, E. Are you really communicating? (special feature). *American Journal of Nursing,* 1977, 77 (12), 1966–1968.

Strain, J. & Grossman, S. *Psychological care of the medically ill. A primer in liaison psychiatry.* New York: Appleton-Century-Crofts, 1975.

Yurick, A., Robb, S.S., Spier, B.E., & Ebert, N.J. *The aged person and the nursing process.* New York: Appleton-Century-Crofts, 1980.

Zborowski, M. *People in pain.* San Francisco: Jossey-Bass, 1969.

SECTION IV

COMMUNICATION IN INTERDISCIPLINARY TEAMS AND GROUPS

Working in an interdisciplinary team or group is a relatively new experience for many nurses. At times the student's introduction to team or group experiences can be a pleasant surprise. The following incident is true:

Nancy, a senior nursing student, arranged to work at St. Christopher's Hospice in London because she was interested in working with terminally ill clients. The first week she was asked in her role as a nursing assistant to attend an interdisciplinary team conference in which one specific client was to be discussed. After several minutes of discussion, the leader, who in this case happened to be a physician, turned to Nancy and asked,

"What do you think about this client, Nancy?" Nancy remembers her surprise at being completely included as a member of an interdisciplinary team.

It was stated earlier in this text that nurses communicate in a variety of professional settings, role relationships, and contexts. As their professional role continues to expand, nurses are beginning to lead groups in increasing numbers. The opportunity is there, since nursing has become a profession in which team and group work are common. There are numerous types of groups in which one can be either a leader or member. These groups and teams have formed in nursing for essentially two reasons; to provide mutual support for the client members of the group and to enable nurses to work collaboratively in a team context in carrying out nursing care.

In teams or groups several things can occur: (1) mutually agreed upon goals are set, (2) communication networks become established, and (3) leadership emerges in order to facilitate the goals and simplify the communication process. For the purposes of our discussion in the two succeeding chapters, groups will be considered as being composed of client members with a nurse leader, and teams will be considered as a "group" of health professionals working collaboratively on health problems.

Communication interactions among team and group members are complex. All groups can be thought of as systems; they are comprised of individuals interacting with each other to form a unified whole. A basic characteristic of any group is that the sum of the system is greater than the sum of its parts. In other words, the output of the group is potentially greater than each individual's output because of the interaction among its members. Put another way, the combination of individuals into groups or teams increases the output geometrically rather than arithmetically. The number of possible interactions with more than two people has been calculated by Hare*:

Size of Group	Potential Relationships
2	1
3	6
4	25
5	90
6	301
7	966

It can be well understood why group and team dynamics are so important and at the same time challenging!

*Hare, P. *Handbook of small group research.* Glencoe, Illinois: Free Press, 1965.

Working with groups or on teams can be fraught with difficulties, many of which are centered around communication between the members of the team or group.

Nursing is on the threshold of expansion into group and team work to solve client problems. This can be seen in community clinic settings, extended-care facilities, and occasionally in private practice, and is in the early stages of being introduced in the hospital settings. Self-care groups and therapeutic health education groups, an outgrowth of the consumerism movement in health, are also beginning to form. Chapters 12 and 13 present some of the basic theory about communication patterns in teams and groups.

Chapter 12
Interdisciplinary teams and communication

BEHAVIORAL OBJECTIVES

By reading this chapter students will be able to:

1. Define the interdisciplinary team concept and know the rationale and history of interdisciplinary health teams
2. Understand how the complexities of small-group communication behaviors can affect team situations
3. Identify context for team communication
4. Assess team communication in terms of three dimensions; openness-closedness, implied relationships, and "intent" of communication
5. Relate six communication patterns to group behavior
6. Describe six games team members play
7. Examine team dynamics by analyzing team communication patterns in five areas: goal setting, role negotiation, decision making, conflict resolution, and work atmosphere
8. Review communication skills as they relate to teamwork.

One of the most exciting concepts to emerge in health care in the last 20 years is that of the interdisciplinary health team. While there have been "teams" in medical and mental health settings for many years, the current trends in interdisciplinary collaboration between doctors, nurses, and other health professionals suggest changes in roles and communication patterns that warrant particular attention in a text such as this one.

Two types of team exist in nursing today; one is the *intra*disciplinary team discussed in Chapter 9. Intradisciplinary nursing teams consist of nurses working in health care settings and usually have at least three levels: registered nurses, licensed practical nurses, and nurse's aides. *Inter*disciplinary teams are relatively new to nursing. These health teams consist of nurses, doctors, social workers, nutritionists, psychologists, and many other categories of health care professionals working together *with* the client. They represent one future trend in nursing care.

The possibility exists that nurses might not have the experience of working on an interdisciplinary team early in their nursing careers. The purpose of introducing this concept at this point is to enable nurses to acquire a knowledge of basic communication dimensions existing in interdisciplinary teams in order that they might be able to analyze this approach as they observe teams in action during the course of their work.

DEFINITION, HISTORY AND RATIONALE OF TEAMS

Definition

Teamwork implies that people involved are working towards a common goal. Yet, presumably, all health professionals are working for a common goal, namely, to reestablish or maintain an optimum state of health for the client. What, then, makes a team different?

There are several key aspects of an interdisciplinary health team that make it a unique situation. First, professionals from several disciplines are working in the same organizational unit, as opposed to being organized as disciplines. Second, there is a greater tendency for health professionals to work collaboratively rather than competitively. This means that teamwork implies working together, with trust and open communication as ideals. Third, in many health teams, decision making and leadership are ideally shared by members according to client need or individual expertise, not necessarily by role. That is, the nurse or physician are not always the leaders.

These three points lead up to a working definition of the health team: a group of professionally trained individuals working interdependently on a common task (Kindig, 1974). This definition implies that the members of the disciplines involved are communicating with each other.

History

In the health field, the term "team" has traditionally meant a group of health professionals under the guidance and leadership of a physician (Kindig, 1974). With the advent of the interdisciplinary approach starting in the late 1940s (post–World War II) and its implied democratic values, health professionals began to explore alternate models for working together (e.g., Silver and Stiber, 1957; Leininger, 1973). In addition, it was felt that increasing medical costs, lack of trained personnel, and other changes in health care warranted new approaches to client–provider interaction (Wise, 1974; Thornton, 1976).

One of the first examples of a team approach to health care in nursing was started at the Loeb Center for Nursing and Rehabilitation (located in the Montifiore Medical Center) in 1963. At this hospital center, which is totally staffed and administered by professional nurses, each nurse is involved as the primary planner for the client and supervises the "carers" (the other member of the health team). The physicians, as well as all ancillary workers, report to the nurse, who has the primary responsibility for the client. In this case, the nurse assumes the leadership role within the interdisciplinary health team (Englert, 1971).

Over the past 10 years, the concept of interdisciplinary health team has become more of a reality in nursing, with members of several health disciplines working together to solve the multiple complex health problems that are seen in clients today. Two areas in which the interdisciplinary health team is becoming more visible are the acute coronary care setting and the geriatric setting. The multidisciplinary approach to client care in both these settings can involve physicians, nurses, physical therapists, mental health specialists, clinical psychologists, dieticians, respiratory and occupational therapists, as well as others.

As Kane (1975) has pointed out, teams have functioned in such areas as rehabilitation, mental health, and educational settings. Nursing has been slow to respond to the concept of teams for many reasons, some of which are role ambiguity, unequal status between nursing and other health disciplines, sexism, protection of professional identities, unequal power distribution, differences in terminology, competitiveness between members of different disciplines, and differences in legal responsibilities among health professions (Given and Simmons, 1977).

Rationale for Teams

Given these issues, why even bother to have teams? Why make people work together when it seems difficult to accomplish? Kane (1975) has summarized the rationale for teamwork as follows: (1) coordination of service; (2) efficient management of interdependent problems; (3) integration of services by providers; (4) improved communication among professions; (5) easier access among professionals; and (6) better linkages between providers and ancillary health care providers. From the client's perspective, the advantages of a team approach to health care include obtaining services at one location, a sense of continuity of care, and a focus on the whole client rather than just one aspect of the client's functioning. In other words, if nurses are members of a team which has the opportunity of meeting together in a spirit of collaboration, there is a greater likelihood that the advantages listed will take place than if each discipline worked separately.

Of course, simply putting health providers together and saying, "You're a team," does not insure that teamwork will occur. The present nature of professional training in this country tends to separate the various health professions and make them suspicious of each other. Professionals are generally socialized into a competitive model of achievement. Thus, asking nurses, doctors, psychologists, social workers, speech therapists, and other possible members of a team to work together runs counter to their personal and professional socialization.

Teamwork can, however, be rewarding. Wise (1974), Eichorn (1973), Edinberg et al., (1978), and Baldwin et al. (1980) have written on some of the exciting aspects of teamwork. The implication behind all of this is that teamwork takes work and practice—it can be considered a skill or a goal to achieve. It can be professionally rewarding and of benefit to the client.

The following two sections on communication and team maintenance issues are included to give nurses the skills and concepts to be effective team members. Their purpose is to serve as ancillary tools to help with the hard work and continuing attempts to create trust and build good communication between nurses and the other team members.

COMMUNICATION IN TEAMS

The communication that takes place in team settings can roughly be categorized into two components, communication with the client and communication among team members. While the major emphasis of this section is on team member communication, the team format has several implications for client communication that should be noted.

First of all, the team approach implies that several health providers will be working with each client. A fundamental question for communication with the client is then, "Will one person or several serve as primary communicator?" Another related question, which reflects how well the team is communicating internally, is, "Will the messages from health providers be consistent or not?" A third questions is, "How does the concept of team get communicated to the client?"

The answers to these three questions serve as a description for client-team communication. One way of assessing the effectiveness of communication between the team and the client is to find out how consistent the messages are between team and client, as well as how accurate the client's understanding is of how the team delivers health care.

In traditional health settings, there is often minimal communication among health professionals, which results in the client receiving messages independently from each health provider. One of the major issues in team communications is whether team members can understand each other's language (jargon) or can obtain clarification when a point is not understood. It is assumed that health professionals are able to communicate effectively before entering a team situation. This is often *not* the case. In addition, the newness of teams and the complexities of small-group dynamics and communication can make team communication difficult, as shown in the following scenario with a nurse, physician, social worker, and speech therapist in an extended-care facility such as a nursing home.

SOCIAL WORKER: I'm glad you could make it today. I feel that since I'm running the meetings this month, you're showing support for me.
NURSE: Good. We need to talk about Ms. Johnson, who had a stroke two weeks ago. Who has information on her?
SOCIAL WORKER: How is she doing in therapy?
PHYSICIAN: I think we need a little medical background before we get up to the therapy. Do you have it?
SPEECH THERAPIST (to social worker): Which question should I answer first?
NURSE: I think we should get our communication straight and get our case presentations organized; at least we should be consistent.
PHYSICIAN: Right, otherwise these meetings become tedious and waste time.
SPEECH THERAPIST: I still don't know which question to answer.

A conversation like the one above can mean that the team is having severe problems or that they are not listening to each other very well. One thing is certain, the communication is confusing, and collaboration will be quite difficult if these communication patterns continue.

The interaction of personalities, professions, team/group dynamics, and communication styles of the people involved can make or break teamwork. This is particularly true at this point in the history of health teams, because they are new and are often touted as the "wave of the future"; yet we do not have enough experience with or related knowledge about them to ensure their success or to put together efficient models for trouble shooting when team problems occur. For these reasons, the communication among health professionals on teams is both a key indicator of team process and a key ingredient to their success in providing health care (e.g., Eichorn, 1973).

Contexts for Team Communication

Most authors writing about team functioning focus on team communication in face-to-face meetings (e.g., Thornton, 1976). In terms of overall team functioning, there are two contexts in which team communication takes place—formal team meetings and informal exchanges between pairs or small subgroups of team members. Each context lends itself to different types of communication or to transmission of different kinds of information.

Formal team meetings (for either the whole team or a subgroup) are defined by virtue of their being planned and by having a designated convener, one member who sets up the meeting. Team meetings are usually convened on a regular basis to review client care and handle administrative issues.

A well-functioning team will also spend scheduled time working on improving communication, as well as on processing other team dynamics (decision making, role negotiation, and conflict resolution). Spending time on team development is difficult for many nurses who want to focus on the task of care. However, nurses can use their time more efficiently when part of the time is spent on "maintenance" as well as "task." In addition, some teams can make efficient use of an outside consultant to help them with their development (see Edinberg et al., 1978).

The communication that takes place in formal team meetings is public and "a matter of record," if notes are kept. Team members have a right to know what was said if they were not present. Team meetings are also the place where communication problems can be dealt with in the open, that is, some teams will operate with a norm of settling differences "publicly."

Informal meetings are those that just happen or take place without a specific agenda. While formal team decisions should not be made in these more private meetings, much of the information exchanged affects team functioning. Alliances can be made, and strategies for team development can be discussed in what is perhaps an easier or safer context for the team members involved than the formal meetings. Informal meetings may also occur when one member needs advice or help from another. A third reason for informal meetings is that an emergency can occur and only a few team members are available for a "team discussion." One of the facts of team life is that everyone is not always available for meetings. Informal communication and time for catching up in team meetings is one way of handling the communication gaps that will occur on any health team.

Obviously, one danger of overreliance on private and informal communication is that the formal team meetings can be undermined. This is especially true when there is low trust and when team members withhold relevant information or feelings and then influence others outside of the team meetings.

One way to think about assessing communication in teams is to compare communication in the informal to formal contexts. Does information or a view expressed informally resurface at team meetings? Are reports of team discussions accurately transmitted to absent team members? In general, do team members express opinions as easily in team meetings as in informal discussions with other team members? In a team that is functioning fairly well, one would expect there to be similarities in formal and informal communication, the one exception being the team in which no one talks to anyone either formally or informally.

Types of Communication in Teams

As a team member, the nurse needs to be an effective communicator as well as assessor of others' communication. One way to improve assessment of others' communication is to develop the ability to think about what is said and done in team meetings in terms of three crucial dimensions: (1) "openness-closedness," (2) "implied relationship" (e.g., symmetry-complementarity) and (3) "intent" (e.g., requesting information, giving information, and clarifying).

These three dimensions can be used to categorize any communication in teams and have in part been used in researching how teams communicate (Thornton, 1976).

Openness-Closedness. This first dimension was previously introduced in Chapter 2 as a way of categorizing a communication style. It is reintroduced here because the degree to which a given team member is open in her or his communication will affect the manner in which others respond as well as the content of their response. Openness means the degree to which the communication leaves others with opportunities to respond, make comments, or ask for clarification. For example, if, in a team meeting, a team member said, "I don't like what's going on and I don't want to talk about it," this statement could be described as being closed, especially if it were accompanied by crossed arms and legs ("closed" body language) and a scowl on the sender's face.

However, if a team member said, "I do not like what is going on here. I find it hard to say this and need to think some more before I can be specific or listen to the rest of you," this statement could be described as being neutral or slightly open, depending on the body language and voice tone.

Or, if a team member said, "I do not like what is going on. It is hard for me to say more at this moment, but I want to hear your responses in hopes that I can say more," this statement could be described as an "open" statement. The following exercise should help you sharpen your ability to categorize team communication for its openness.

Exercise in Assessment of Team Communication

Categorize each statement in the following team meeting as "open," "neutral," or "closed." In the case of a closed statement, think of a way to make it more open. Answers and transformations of closed statements are given on the right side of the page. Keep them covered until you have given your answer. The team members are a nurse, physician, psychologist, and social worker.

Communication	Type
PHYSICIAN: Did we get the lab work on Mr. White?	Neutral
SOCIAL WORKER: I have the chart. I think it's in it.	Neutral
PSYCHOLOGIST: I don't understand why we have to bother reviewing it here. Let's get on with business.	Closed. Transformation: I feel impatient and do not understand why we are reviewing lab data.
PHYSICIAN: You are generally impatient with nonpsychological stuff. Give us a minute. (Laughs)	Open
PSYCHOLOGIST: You're right, go on.	Open
NURSE: Let me see the chart. The lab work is here. His blood is OK. I think the main problems are hypertension and anxiety. What is his personal life like?	Neutral
SOCIAL WORKER (crosses legs, arms): Well, I already mentioned in the chart: he works too hard, spends no time with the family, and seems uptight.	Closed. Transformation: I think it's there, but I'll summarize for the rest of you. He works hard, is away from home, seems uptight at clinic.
PSYCHOLOGIST: Yes, but everyone is uptight at a clinic. Anyway, what will we do about him?	Closed. Transformation: We don't know how much of his behavior in the clinic is duplicated outside. What do you think?
NURSE: I think I can be of some help here.	Open
SOCIAL WORKER: Are you sure you can help?	Closed. Transformation: What are your ideas?

Interdisciplinary Teams and Communication

NURSE: Look, I have a lot of experience.	Closed. Transformation: It seems like you're uncertain about what I can do.
PHYSICIAN: I think we have some things to work on.	Open
SOCIAL WORKER: I'm sorry. I think I was out of place.	Open

Implied Relationship. Implied relationship is the second dimension that nurses can use to assess the communication of others in a team situation. Watzlawick et al. (1967) pointed out that any communication has at least two messages, one arising from the content and the other a statement about the implied relationship between the sender and receiver. Watzlawick talked about two types of communication, in terms of implied relationship: complementary, in which the sender and receiver are in a one-up, one-down situation, and symmetrical, in which the sender and receiver are of equal status. For example, if the physician were to say to the nurse, "Now pay attention," it is clear that a complementary message is given, that the nurse is of lower status than the physician. Similarly, if the physician were to say, "I'm so sorry to bother you, I know you're terribly busy...," it is also complementary, but this time the nurse is being put in a one-up position and has higher status than the physician. A more symmetrical or even status message might be, "I need you to listen to this," although the voice tone, body posture, and gestures of the sender could imply a complementary role relationship.

Although Watzlawick et al. talked about the two types of relationship messages, it is useful to practice categorizing the team statements in *three* categories:

Symmetrical (sender and receiver are of equal status)
Complementary (sender one-up)
Complementary (receiver one-up).

In an ambiguous role situation like the primary health team, implied messages about status can become part of a team norm by default. That is, if team members imply that one member has higher status consistently by the nature of their communication, that team member will be able to exert influence on decisions that may not reflect that team member's expertise or ability. Also, implied higher status can allow the senders to not take responsibility for their own actions on the team. Similarly, continually implying lower status to a team member will decrease the other's influence and is likely to encourage disengagement, sabotage, or "resistant" behavior. We all respond strongly to implied messages about our status, which we hear as statements about our self-worth.

Exercise in Symmetrical–Complementary Team Communication Identification

For each statement in the following team script, classify it into one of the three categories:

Symmetrical (sender and receiver have equal status)
Complementary sender one-up: (sender has higher status than receiver)
Complementary sender one-down: (receiver has higher status).

If the message is complementary, think about how it could be rephrased into a symmetrical message. We have included categorizations and rephrasings of complementary messages into symmetrical messages on the right side of the page. Cover them until you have made your own decision. The team is composed of a male physician, female social worker, male psychologist, and female nurse.

Communication	Category
PHYSICIAN: Does anyone have anything to discuss?	Symmetrical
SOCIAL WORKER: I'm not sure if this is the right time, I mean, you're all so busy.	Complementary, sender one-down. Rephrase: I feel uncertain raising this now.
PSYCHOLOGIST (laughs): Just like a woman...I'm only kidding.	Complementary, sender one-up (even if "only kidding").
NURSE (slightly blaming): Keep your jokes to yourself.	Complementary, sender one-up. Rephrase: That's not called for.
PSYCHOLOGIST: I'm sorry.	Symmetrical
SOCIAL WORKER: That's OK, I shouldn't have said it; it's in part my fault. What I wanted to say is that it seems as if our team recommendations on client care focus only on health or mental illness. There isn't really much you all have to say on social or family factors. Now, I know that you're all coming from a more scientific basis than social work, but I mean, shouldn't families be mentioned in the reports?	Complementary, sender one-down. Rephrase: Apology accepted. Symmetrical Complementary, sender one-down. Rephrase: Social work has a different view from the rest of you, which is why it belongs on the team.
PHYSICIAN (patronizing): Now look, we spend a lot of valuable time discussing these matters. Of course we all appreciate your value. After all, you do home visits and see the families. If you want to add some-	Complementary, sender one-up. Rephrase: I believe you have value. Your point is well taken.

thing on that to our reports, it's all
right with me.

    SOCIAL WORKER: Really? — Complementary, sender one-down.

    NURSE: Wait a minute. I'm not sure if you support her or not. — Symmetrical

    PHYSICIAN (puzzled): I do. What's the problem? — Symmetrical

    NURSE: No problem. I hear you. — Symmetrical

    PSYCHOLOGIST: Anyway, I have a similar question. You two (nurse and physician) are so gung-ho about problem-oriented records. How come you haven't helped us figure out how to get our information in? — Complementary, either sender one-up or one-down depending on emphasis on words, gestures, etc. Rephrase: I think I still need help in problem-oriented recording.

    NURSE: I didn't know you had trouble. — Symmetrical

    PHYSICIAN: You never asked. — Symmetrical or complementary, sender one-up, depending on tone.

    SOCIAL WORKER (overly sweet): Oh, are you having problems with that? — Complementary, sender one-up. Rephrase: That's not the issue for me.

    PSYCHOLOGIST: I really am. I think the record system is more difficult for social or psychological recording. — Symmetrical

    NURSE: If you would like, I can help you. I had to use it in a psych rotation, and it *was* difficult. — Symmetrical

    SOCIAL WORKER: But you all are ignoring my point! — Borderline—could be complementary, sender one-down. Rephrase: There's more to it than the records.

    PHYSICIAN: Which is? — Symmetrical

    SOCIAL WORKER: That the family problems are never discussed together; that we do not include socioeconomic and cultural considerations in planning patient care. — Symmetrical

    NURSE: I think you're partially right. We have been a bit too much disease-oriented. — Symmetrical

Responses to One-up or One-down Messages. In the previous exercise, you were asked to consider what you might say or do in response to a sender one-up or sender one-down message. The first step in determining an effective response is to be able to identify the "problem" aspect of the message (which is done by being able to classify the implied relationship in the message). As in any communication choice, there is an infinite number of possible responses;

that is, wordings, word emphasis, facial expression, body language, etc. For purposes of clarity responses have been classified into the following six categories:

Ignoring it
Sender one-up
Sender one-down
Meta-commenting
Giving feedback
Turning the dyadic into a team communication

IGNORING IT.   When nurses receive the sender one-up or sender one-down message, they can act as if there was no such message implied. This is a useful temporary strategy but will leave the door open for other similar comments.

SENDER ONE-UP.   In this instance, the response is such that nurses imply that they are of higher status than the person who originally sent them a one-up or one-down message. For example, if a team member said, "Oh, why don't you take care of that, you're good at that sort of thing" in a slightly condescending manner (sender one-up) a sender one-up response would be, "I'll be happy to do it since you can't."

This interaction sequence could be considered hostile on both sides and it is not recommended as trust-building or healthy for a team.

SENDER ONE-DOWN.   A third type of response to sender one-up or sender one-down messages is to respond in such a way that the other is assumed to be of higher status than the nurse. In the case of having just received a sender one-up message (that is, the nurse is one-down) this type of response can be viewed as compliance:

For example, if the other team member said, "You nurses don't seem to pay as much attention to the whole person as we do."
NURSE (meekly): Nursing is trying to become more holistic but hasn't done it as well as some other disciplines.

In this instance, the nurse goes along with the implied inferior status. This is an ineffective strategy both from the perspective of changing professional roles and from collaboration on a team. While it may be true that nursing is trying to become more holistic in its approach to health care, there is no evidence that other disciplines have made more progress with this approach. Furthermore, in this particular instance, the message is unclear. What is meant by "pay *as much* attention" or "as we do"?

META-COMMENTING. Another type of communication strategy in response to a one-up or one-down message is making a comment about the communication, or meta-commenting. For example, if as in the previous situation, another team member said, "You nurses don't seem to pay as much attention to the whole person as we do." A meta-comment would be, "You're implying that nursing is an inferior profession. Is that your intent?"; or, "That sounds like you're putting yourself one-up on nursing."

Meta-comments are useful in that they bring the implied relationship aspects of communication into the open. At the same time, the team may not be ready to deal with them, either due to its stage of development (i.e., not enough trust or open communication) or because of felt pressure to work on the task (e.g., there are 10 cases to review in an hour). Unfortunately, there are no automatic, magic communication strategies that always are effective in health teams.

GIVING FEEDBACK. Giving feedback is closely related to meta-commenting and, in the right context, can be effective in surfacing relationship issues and other communication problems in teams. This important skill is discussed in detail in another section of this chapter.

Feedback has been defined as "information sent by the receiver back to the source of a message, allowing the original sender to gauge the effect of his message" (Schmuck et al., 1972, p. 35). For our purposes, feedback can be differentiated from meta-commenting in that a feedback response: (1) is directed to the source (sender) and (2) gives a direct statement of the receiver's affective reaction to the message.

For example, when the team member in the previous example said, "You nurses don't seem to pay as much attention to the whole person as we do." Feedback responses would include, "That type of comment makes me feel defensive."; or, "That comment sounds like a put down. I feel angry about that." Note that meta-commenting can be a part of feedback.

TURNING THE DYADIC INTO A TEAM COMMUNICATION. Another way of responding to a sender one-up or sender one-down message from a team member is to respond in such a manner that other team members are drawn into the communication. Drawing other team members in can be done in conjunction with meta-comments, feedback, or even ignoring, with appropriate eye contact with other members plus a suitable gesture such as a shrug of the shoulders.

Usually, a direct request to another team member or to the team as a whole for feedback, perceptions, or information will succeed in changing a dyadic interaction into a team interaction. While this strategy is useful for many areas of team functioning, it can be quite effective in having the team deal with one-up or one-down relationships and communication.

As an example, the following are ways the dyadic exchange could be turned into team communication when the teammate says: "You nurses don't seem to pay as much attention to the whole person as we do."

"I have trouble understanding what you mean by that. Does anyone else?"

"I feel you're putting me down. Is this something we all need to talk about?"

"Intent" of Communication. The third dimension, intent of communication, provides another useful way to analyze team communication, that is, to attend to the "purpose" of the statement (Thornton, 1976). What is the sender doing by saying whatever is said? Based on work by Thornton, the following categories are useful to consider:

Requests information
Gives information
Clarifies previous statement
Attempts to manage tension
Focuses on team dynamics (process)
Addresses role relationship

REQUESTING INFORMATION. This refers to any question or implied request for factual data or opinions from other team members; the following are examples:

"What do you think about this?"
"I was wondering if Ms. Jones had her pap smear."
"Why were you late today?"

GIVING INFORMATION. Any comment that adds to the information available to the team is obviously giving information. So is any statement that expresses personal feelings, beliefs, or values. Examples would include the following:

"I think a second opinion is needed."
"Mr. Bell's blood pressure was 140/90/80."
"Yes, Ms. Jones had her pap smear."
"My car didn't start. Sorry I was late."

CLARIFICATION. Clarification refers to any attempt to give a better explanation of a previous statement. This can be done in several ways; for example:

"Did you mean you don't trust the doctor?"
"I meant to say I was unsure."
"You offered two opposing solutions. Which one do you prefer?"

ATTEMPTS TO MANAGE TENSION. Some team communication seems to be intended to make a situation less tense. At times, these comments will be meta-comments (comments about what is going on). At other times they can be humorous or irrelevant. The following are examples:

"Do I hear the sound of a fight starting?"
"Time out—get back in your corners."
"The team that hates together, relates together."
"Let's take a second and cool off. It's not the end of the world."

FOCUSES ON TEAM DYNAMICS. Some team communication directly addresses how the team is functioning. These "process" statements are intended to draw attention to team dynamics (refer to the section on team dynamics in this chapter for a full explanation). Examples of statements that focus on team dynamics include:

"I think there's a role conflict here."
"Is this in line with our goals?"
"This conflict has to be resolved."
"You two are controlling too many decisions without input from the others."

ADDRESSES ROLE RELATIONSHIP. Certain kinds of communication on teams focus on the role relationship between two members, usually in reference to equal or unequal status. Statements that address role relationship can be either direct or indirect:

"Boy, you doctors think you're gods compared to nurses."
"What can your discipline possibly offer that we don't already do?"
"Now she wants to be the boss."

These categories of "intent" may overlap a bit. In addition, they are conceptual in nature and may not be of immediate help to the nurse as a team member until they are tied into communication patterns, dynamics, power, and leadership in teams. For example, if it turned out that the only person who made process comments was the social worker and the nurse and physician made only informal statements, we could begin to paint a picture of a team with a rift between the social scientist and the medical personnel.

As a general guide, nurses working on a team should keep track of who makes what kinds of statements and how the team accepts, rejects, or handles what each member says. This rough assessment should begin to allow them to uncover some elementary communication patterns in their team and could also serve as a springboard to important nursing research.

Communication Patterns in Teams

Communication patterns in teams are somewhat more difficult to decipher than the categorization of a single statement (by openness/closedness, inferred relationship, or intent). A communication pattern is any sequence of communication that takes place consistently on a team. To discover what the patterns are, as well as to determine their effects (i.e., are they efficient, trust-building, destructive, etc.), is quite difficult for a team member, who has to participate, give care to clients, and pay attention to his or her own communication.

At the same time, there are seven general configurations for determining flow of communication that, in turn, can be used to pinpoint individual or discipline influence, power, and function in communications in a team setting. The seven patterns are shown in Figure 12.1.

Centralized Pattern. This refers to communication patterns in which one member is the "conduit" of communication, that is, the member is the one to whom all information or questions are addressed. The conduit also controls which questions are asked of other members. An example of this kind of communication pattern would be one member asking each other member in turn what he or she thinks about a particular problem.

Peripheral Pattern. In a peripheral pattern, each member has one or two others with whom he or she communicates, and there is no member who is the focus of communication. You might find peripheral communication patterns taking place before a formal meeting starts, where members are talking to the persons sitting near them.

Hybrid: Central plus Peripheral Pattern. In certain circumstances, the communication pattern may be one where the pattern includes both a central team member and some side communication. We have labeled this pattern as a hybrid. Obviously, if both are going on simultaneously, there is competition for attention, and the team cannot fully understand both sets of communication. Another example of the hybrid pattern would be where the meeting leader asks group questions, which are followed by somewhat random dialogue among members.

Interdisciplinary Teams and Communication

Hierarchical Pattern. A hierarchical pattern implies that a high-status individual communicates only with one or two members, who then relay the information to others who are assumed to be of even lower status. Although it is unlikely that this pattern would emerge in formal face-to-face meetings, it certainly could emerge as an informal or written communication pattern on a team. For example, if the physician continually transmitted his orders to the social worker via the nurse, a hierarchical communication pattern would be operating.

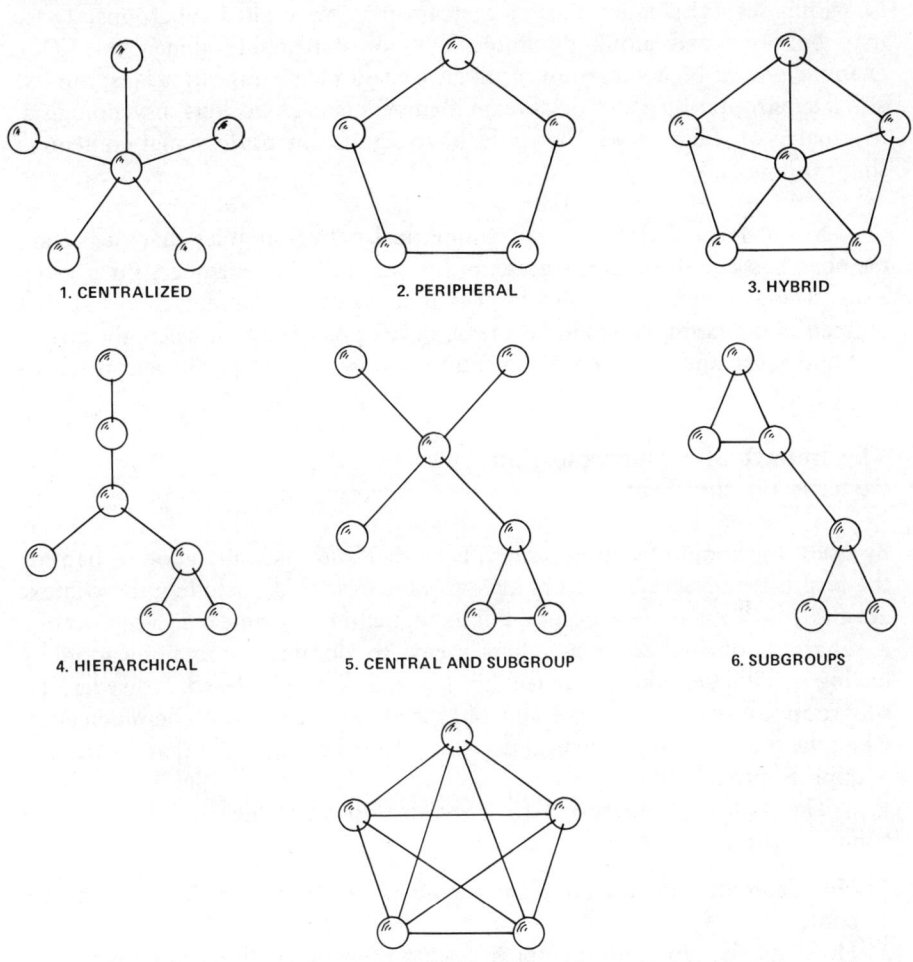

1. CENTRALIZED
2. PERIPHERAL
3. HYBRID
4. HIERARCHICAL
5. CENTRAL AND SUBGROUP
6. SUBGROUPS
7. SYMMETRY

FIGURE 12-1. Communication patterns in teams.

Central plus Subgroup Pattern. At times, there seems to be a subgroup of team members who have a high-level of communication among themselves. This could be found on a team where two nurses and a social worker, all women, exchange knowing glances and little smiles when the team physician, a male, makes sexist comments. It should be noted that the subgrouping pattern can be helpful, a source of survival for its members, or destructive to the team.

Subgroup Pattern. At other times, communication on teams seems to be within several smaller clusters of team members called subgroups. These may be organized along discipline, sex, or personality dimensions. One example would be a subgroup of medical team members (physicians, nurses) and a subgroup of psychosocial team members (social workers, psychologists, psychiatrists), each of which would have significant professional content to share on cases.

Symmetrical Pattern. The symmetrical pattern implies that each team member has equal impact, status, and access to other members on a given issue. The symmetrical pattern implies that no one is running things at that moment. One example would be a team development session where the goal is to build trust and good communication through equal participation.

The Impact of Communication Patterns on the Team

By itself, the communication pattern is neither automatically good or bad for the health team. Several factors have to be considered, including the context around which the pattern occurs. For example, if every time a decision occurs, a subgroup of two team members seems to dominate communication by having a dialogue, others may feel left out and disenfranchised. However, if a subgroup consisting of nurse and physician dominated the communication when the focus was on a medical decision, the team might feel that the pattern is appropriate.

The kinds of questions to be asked in assessing the impact of a communication pattern on a team are:

1. How comfortable do all team members feel with this pattern in this context?
2. How openly can team members discuss their perceptions of the pattern?
3. Does the pattern help or hinder the exchange of information relevant to the matter at hand?

Different communication patterns will emerge on a team for different

Interdisciplinary Teams and Communication

issues, dynamics, and aspects of communication. For example, it is possible for one team to have a hierarchical pattern for medical decisions, a more symmetrical pattern for administrative decisions and a subgroup pattern for written communication (where the person sending the memo consults with a small subgroup before sending it). It is natural to expect different patterns to emerge for formal meetings, informal meetings, and different team dynamic issues (see below for description), as well as different topic areas that come up in the team's work.

It has been stated previously that communication patterns are difficult to decipher. The ones presented here should provide a point of reference for nurses as they participate in team experiences. By presenting them visually to others, the nurse can help a team uncover communication blocks or problems.

Communication Games Team Members Play

Another way of thinking about communication patterns in teams is to consider the "games team members play." At times, a complicated series of interactions can take place between two or more members that appears to be consistent and "gamelike." "Gamelike" means that each member acts as if there are rules governing his or her communication in terms of what can be said, what kind of role can be played (usually one-up or one-down), and even who can talk to whom about what. Some of the more common games can be labeled as follows:

1. The doctor–nurse game
2. The social scientist–medical personnel game
3. Silent go along
4. We're (I'm) open
5. The doctor is different
6. Two-way but one-way communication.

While all of these games are used on teams, each one serves to prevent open and effective communication, as well as to hinder shared decision making, two of the reasons for having health teams.

Games will be prevalent in a low-trust team situation where members are attempting to survive psychologically. In a high-trust context, there will be less game playing, which is time- and energy-consuming. The result is improved communication and information exchange, which should lead to better client care.

The Doctor–Nurse Game. The doctor-nurse game (Stein, 1967) has been discussed in Chapters 7 and 11. For purposes of review, the main characteristics of the game are as follows:

1. The goal is for the nurse to suggest what the doctor should do, with the doctor assuming "responsibility," that is, not directly seeking or acknowledging the nurse's suggestion.
2. The doctor is dominant (one-up).
3. The nurse is submissive (one-down).
4. The nurse's suggestions are embedded, "hidden," in questions or statements.
5. The penalties for not playing the game for the nurse are
   a. being labeled "aggressive" or
   b. being labeled a "bad nurse."

Maintaining the doctor-nurse game can be a comfortable position for both parties. If, however, nursing is to move toward symmetrical and collaborative relationships with medicine (and other disciplines), then this game inhibits those goals. The interdisciplinary health team is one arena in which the new role of the nurse is congruent with the philosophy of professional relationships.

The Social Scientist–Medical Personnel Game. Another game that can be played on health teams is one that goes on between the social scientists (e.g., social worker, psychologist, communications expert) and the more medically oriented team members (e.g., physician, nurse, physician's assistant). The game comes from a perceived inequality of status by the social scientists: that is, they may feel left out or one-down because the focus of the team's deliberations is on health care, and because the medical staff has some knowledge about mental health and social problems, but the social scientists are generally in the dark about physical health.

One result of these factors is that social scientists may feel pressured to find a role on the team. What is it that is uniquely their "territory?" What can they add that is not already covered by another discipline?

What can happen in this instance is that the social scientists become the in-house "experts" on team process, which then gives them a role on the team. However, by taking this role, the social scientist can be inadvertently coerced into having to live by the rules of *only* communicating openly, even if others do not. Another rule that can become part of the game is that the social scientist has to *act* as if everyone else is also communicating openly. That is, there is no option for disbelief (and possible disagreement) because of the idea that this is a "team" and that "team" implies that its members are open and honest. The social scientist who plays this game thus has a limited repertoire of communication options (always being open is limiting), and he or she may feel hurt (and one-down) if others do not "play fair."

One of the outcomes of this game is that the social scientist, by being the team expert, can prevent others from taking appropriate responsibility in developing team trust and effective communication. That is, the social scientist becomes the judge of good communication, openness, and trust. Others may accede to this, with the result that a hierarchical pattern emerges with the team members who argue the strongest for collaboration assuming the one-up role.

We're (I'm) Open. Another communication game played by teams is "we're open" or, if played by an individual, "I'm open." As is the case in all games, more than one player is needed. The game has the following rules:

1. One team member is allowed to comment on how "open" he or she is while not actually being so.
2. Other players must either believe player 1 *or* not directly confront 1 with discrepancies in behavior and words.
3. If by chance, a discrepancy is noted (by a client, a teammate breaking the rules, or an outsider), the discrepancy is denied or rationalized.
4. If another team member confronts the player, the confrontation gets turned around so it is the confronter's problem, misunderstanding, etc.

Needless to say, this game blocks open communication. When it is being played, and other team members are going along, attempting to end the game is difficult for a single member to accomplish (especially since the rules identify anyone who openly confronts the discrepancies as having the problem). One way to approach changing the game is to affect how the rest of the team responds to the player.

The Silent Go-along. Another type of communication game on health teams has to do with implied but not real compliance to team decisions. We call this game the "silent go-along." A brief description of the game is as follows:

1. A decision is proposed by one or two team members.
2. The others "go along" silently, even though they disagree.
3. But they do not follow through on the decision or sabotage its implementation without directly saying so.

One sign of the silent go-along is that reservations are only voiced in informal communication, not in team meetings. One way to counter this game is to ensure that objections to decisions are voiced without fear of being put down and that time is given to think important issues through before a decision is made.

The Doctor is Different. Another communication game that gets played on teams is a variation of the doctor–nurse game. In "the doctor is different," the physician, by virtue of high status and important responsibilities, is "excused" for behavior for which other team members would receive criticism. The usual forms of the behavior are being late for meetings and clients, participating actively only in team discussions that focus on medical care (as opposed to team development, communication, etc.), or not following through on busy work, such as preparing minutes, arranging meetings, or sending out correspondence.

"The doctor is different" comes from the traditionally high status that physicians have in the health system. Any physician who joins a team is already risking a loss of power. One way of tacitly acknowledging this is for other team members to excuse his or her behavior that might be bothersome.

This game can also be played by other team members if they are sick, overworked, or undergoing a personal crisis. While some consideration of a team member's personal life is appropriate, if matters get to the point where anger is developing but cannot be expressed because of team "norms," then the game is being played.

Two-way but One-way. There are times in a team's life when it seems that communication between teammates is two-way, that is, that there is an opportunity to respond to the communication of the others. However, in some of these instances, subsequent events indicate that the communication was really one-way and that the responses and feedback did not affect a team member's original stance or communication. This pattern or game is called "two-way but one-way communication."

There is a built-in problem in assessing whether or not "two-way but one-way" is being played. The problem is that the communication seems to be open, honest, and clear while it is going on, i.e., that it is, effective two-way communication. It is only later, after the fact, that one indirectly finds out that another team member was sending but not receiving.

For example, a health team member might start off a discussion of referrals by saying he or she would never make a referral without the doctor's prior permission. The physician and others on the team might then reassure this team member that a prior OK was not necessary. The member nods his or her head and everyone concludes that the communication was two-way. However, about a week later, in a chart review, a team member finds that the only referrals being made by the originator of the referral discussion were those approved by the physician. That is, while the communication seemed to be two-way, subsequent events indicated it was really one-way.

Because this game is only uncovered after the fact, and usually not during a formal meeting, it becomes a bit tricky to figure out how to stop it. This game is a fairly sure sign that the team needs some work on its communication and development.

As was mentioned earlier, these games are complicated. They are also indicators that communication is not open or accurate and that (usually) a hierarchical set of relationships is being assumed despite the goal that team members are supposed to be collaborating. The results of the game include lowered self-worth for participants, unclear communication, and lowered trust. On the other hand, the games provide a structure and some stability for the game players. One of the tasks of health teams is to promote the necessary risk taking to break down the games so that more efficient communication and health care will take place.

TEAM DYNAMICS

As is the case in any group setting, there are dynamics and stages of development that teams encounter. It is not unreasonable to assume that the team develops as other groups do, with beginning, honeymoon, leadership, individual relations, and work phases like those proposed by Bennis and Sheppard (1956) or like Tuckman's (1965) forming, storming, norming, and performing stages. In addition, Eichorn (1973) has proposed that the key to a health team's success is getting to the point where the team is able to communicate differences which are usually overlooked.

However, the health team is more than a group of individuals. The health team at times functions as a group, a task team, and as an organizational entity, with different pressures and concerns arising from each aspect of the team's functioning. There is a set of issues that becomes increasingly important in assessing the team's functioning, since the concept of the team is not simply as a voluntaristic group but as a health service unit or task team, the aim of which is the provision of health care to individuals or families. These areas are not unlike those used in examining the functioning of other small organizational groups (e.g., Schmuck et al., 1972). An extensive self-development training program for teams based on similar concepts has been developed by Rubin et al. (1975).

Team dynamics can be defined as underlying processes or patterns in an area of team functioning. Dynamics are inferred from the behavior (usually communication) of the team. They are therefore conceptualizations of "what is going on."

The major areas in which team dynamics are found are:

Goal setting
Role negotiation
Decision making
Conflict resolution
Work atmosphere

Each of these areas can be examined by analyzing the communication that takes place around related issues.

Goal Setting

Every team has to set objectives for health care, based on some philosophy (even if not explicit) of what health care is. Certain parameters of the goals may be structurally defined by the setting. For example, a pediatric health care team knows it will be working with children and parents and that its goals will have to be formed around pediatric care. However, a team set up to staff a neighborhood health clinic will probably have to devote considerable time determining what client group they should be seeing, as well as the limits of what can be provided by the clinic.

All questions about what the team is supposed to be doing are related to goals. When statements such as "I'm not sure what we're doing" or questions about the appropriateness of various team services arise, there is uncertainty about team goals.

Team goals may have to change as the team itself develops. Also, team members may not all have the same understanding of the goals, even if these are static or unchanging. Thus, time will have to be spent periodically on goal setting if team functioning is to be effective.

Role Negotiation

There is an overlapping of the skills that different members such as nurse–physician and psychologist–social worker bring to the team. In addition, the implied collaborative value of teamwork brings with it new kinds of working relationships wherein traditional roles such as the physician-leader, nurse-follower, and social worker-ancillary support are not the only way of functioning. For example, in a health team at the University of Nevada Reno's School of Medical Sciences in the late 1970s, the team psychologist and social worker did intake and history taking as a negotiated part of their team duties.

Ideally these new roles are decided upon through a communication sequence that allows the skills and interests of team members to be combined with client needs in a way that results in effective health care delivery. The process by which team members decide who will do what is called role negotiation.

Obviously, there are certain legal and professional restrictions on which aspects of roles can be negotiated in a team. For example, drug prescription by a nonphysician is illegal. Similarly, from a common sense perspective it would be inappropriate if the social worker spent 100 percent of his or her time taking health histories, preparing clients for physical exams, and discussing medication while the nurse only did counseling. However, since counseling is considered an important part of nursing and social work, there is room for negotiation as to who should do it for which clients.

Even without formal role negotiation, this issue (who does what) can be decided by team members simply assuming roles and functions. In this case, there will be very little team time spent communicating about who does what. If roles are negotiated "silently," however, there is an increased likelihood that the decision will be based on status or traditional discipline areas of expertise than on the basis of the individual team member's skills and the client needs. Furthermore, there is a good chance that in areas of overlap—such as counseling, some health education functions and health assessment—distrust will occur if roles are decided *without* negotiation.

Decision Making

Another area of team functioning that is strongly related to communication patterns is decision making, that is, the process by which decisions are made. There is a variety of decisions that are made on a team, including staffing, hours, evening call, work schedules, clinical procedures, referral procedures, and client follow-up.

The kinds of questions one can ask to assess how effective decision making and related communication are include:

Are all appropriate team members involved in decisions?
Which decisions are made arbitrarily?
Which decisions are made collaboratively?
How do decisions get made? (What kind of team communication patterns are used?)
Who has influence in swaying various decisions?

The last question addresses an important issue for several areas of team functioning, namely influence. Some team members will have more influence on decisions than others by virtue of their status, personal style, or perceived power. Generally, those with strong influence will either do much of the talking, be asked for opinions, or be listened to carefully when they do speak in team meetings. By addressing the influence issue openly, teams can make sure that influence does not inappropriately affect team decisions.

Conflict Resolution

Conflict resolution is defined as how differences of opinion get settled on a team. Conflict can range from mild to serious, when it can be uncomfortable for all members.

There are a variety of ways in which conflict gets resolved. At the closed end of the conflict-solving continuum, the conflicts are hidden (team members pretend there is no conflict) or are resolved arbitrarily by either the team member with the greater status or an outside authority. At the open end of the continuum, conflict is shared with appropriate team members, the issues are mutually understood, and the resultant collaborative resolution is accepted by all team members involved in the conflict.

Open conflict resolution takes time, trust, and a willingness to share on all sides. If the conflict resolution processes of a team include much game playing or many arbitrary decisions, the same problems will continue to emerge, although they may be camouflaged and disguised.

Team Atmosphere

Team atmosphere refers to the subjective feelings team members have about belonging to their team. The kinds of questions that can be asked about team atmosphere include:

"How does it feel to be a member of the team?"
"How comfortable do you feel during team meetings?"
"Do you enjoy coming into work in the morning?"
"Do you have headaches, stomachaches or feel uptight during team meetings?"

If the team atmosphere is unpleasant, that is, people feel bad about working together, then it is likely that there are problems with goal setting, role negotiation, decision making, conflict resolution, and the communication that goes on in each of these areas. Problems can also be due to external difficulties such as funding cuts, but team atmosphere and other team processes are tightly intertwined. When one is not going well, the other is usually affected.

EFFECTIVE COMMUNICATION SKILLS FOR TEAMS

A portion of this chapter has focused on how miscommunication can take place on teams. While the opportunities for miscommunication are great in an interdisciplinary setting, so are the possibilities for effective communication. The kinds of effective communication skills that are useful on teams include virtually everything discussed in the first section of this book: effective use of communication channels, congruency of style, empathy, and the ability to obtain needed information from another and to comment on underlying

Interdisciplinary Teams and Communication

group/team dynamics are all excellent attributes for the nurse communicator on the team. We now review several communication skill areas as they relate to teamwork so that nurses can understand how they might be used in a team context. Most of them have been covered in more depth in previous chapters on therapeutic communication (Chapter 4), interviewing (Chapter 5), and roles (Chapters 6–8). The areas are:

- Meta-commenting
- Paraphrasing
- Giving feedback
- Being congruent
- Using empathy
- Listening
- Reflecting
- Asking for clarification
- Summarizing
- Using humor

Meta-commenting

Meta-commenting refers to making statements about the process by which things happen. An appropriate meta-comment can help a team uncover communication patterns that are blocking effective team work. For example:

NURSE: I think we have conflicting goals. (meta-comment)
PHYSICIAN: You might be right. Let's spend time on this.

Meta-comments can also be used to avoid doing the task. In addition, they may not be well received:

NURSE: I think we have a goal conflict. (meta-comment)
PHYSICIAN (OR OTHER TEAMMATE): We don't have time for that.

How well the comment is received will depend on the way in which it is sent (is the sender anxious or unclear?), the team atmosphere (relaxed, uptight), the stage of team development (are such comments part of the team norms?), and the matter at hand (is this a business meeting with a packed agenda, are there 20 cases to be reviewed, is this an emergency meeting because several decisions have to be made by tomorrow?). The effective nurse communicator should be able to time meta-comments so they will have maximum impact, although there is no sure-fire way to guarantee success.

Paraphrasing

The ability to paraphrase, to give back your understanding of another's message in your own words, is extremely important in an interdisciplinary team setting, where the language of different disciplines can create misunderstanding about the crucial issue, the health care of the client. One of the main reasons for teams is to *decrease* misunderstanding between disciplines. Paraphrasing is an important skill to use for this purpose.

For example, in a team conference focusing on a care plan for discharge of an elderly client, the social worker might say: "I don't think we should not let Ms. Johnson go to the senior center unless she's resistant." This double negative is difficult to understand, and the term resistant is also potentially confusing. The nurse can aid everyone on the team by paraphrasing (without blame). "You mean she should decide herself whether or not she should go?" Double negatives, jargon, terminology, or long explanations from other teammates are all worthy of being paraphrased.

Exercise in Paraphrasing

1. Form into triads. *A* will be a physician, *B* will be a nurse, and *C* a social worker. You can all pretend you are learning about teams together.
2. *A* will start the conversation by making a statement he or she believes to be true about teams, the functions, and so forth.
3. Before *B* or *C* respond to *A*'s statement, they must paraphrase it and check out their interpretation with *A*. After the previous statement has been paraphrased, either *B* or *C* can respond. The general topic is, "What I know or believe about health teams."
4. The next person to speak must paraphrase the statement that was just said.

It is obvious that no team would use this exercise for ordinary communication, but exercises like this can be useful in helping teams with problems to communicate more effectively.

Giving Feedback

Feedback, as has been mentioned in several places in this text, refers to information given to a message sender about the impact of the message. Generally, feedback is thought to be most desirable when it is "well-timed, direct and given with emotion" (Reddy and Lippert, 1980).

The general characteristics of feedback that seem to make it useful to others are that it be nonjudgmental and descriptive of recent behavior. Some research (Jacobs, 1974) suggests that sharing feelings and behavioral descriptions is useful for positive feedback, but describing behavior without affect is better received if the feedback is negative.

For example, on one team the psychologist may have been feeling ambivalent about the need for a client to receive psychotherapy and finally verbalizes it: "Despite the fact that I feel I need more to do on the team, I am not convinced Ms. Wilkins needs therapy." This is an opportunity for positive feedback (affective plus behavior description) by the nurse: "I appreciate your saying that—you're able to voice ambivalence. I can understand what you are going through."

As another example, on another team, the pharmacist might only show up for meetings he feels are important without sharing this decision with others. An example of how the nurse could give negative feedback with low affect and high behavioral description is: "I notice you have been missing some team meetings. You've missed three in the last two weeks. I'd like to know what's going on, since you're an integral team member."

Negative feedback is tricky, in part because teammates are generally unaware of what they are doing that is disturbing to others. Also, receiving negative feeling feedback is unpleasant. If a confrontation is necessary, we suggest that the feeling part be handled first or separately from the behavior description.

Exercise in Feedback

1. Form into triads. One member will be *A*, one will be *B*, and one *C*.
2. In each triad ("team"), discuss how the semester, course, or workshop in which you are reading this text has been (five minutes time limit).
3. At the end of the five minutes, think of what kinds of things you can say to each of your partners that would be positive and negative feedback, that is, the feedback should be nonjudgmental, recent (related to what was said), and descriptive of behavior.
4. Then give each other the feedback. Give feedback that is both positive (what you like) and negative (what you do not like) to each "teammate," *remembering* that an affectively neutral description of behavior seems to be received better when the feedback is negative. Positive feedback is well received with appropriate feeling.
5. Discuss in the large group how it feels to give and receive positive and negative feedback. Also, how is it to observe others giving and receiving feedback?

Using Empathy

While the use of empathy is generally thought of as a therapeutic skill, it can be quite helpful in building trust, morale, and cohesion on a team. There will be times when the work load, personal problems, or team conflict creates a sense of despair for any health professional. Being able to be emotionally supportive and feeling supported in the team are two of the benefits of good teamwork.

Listening

Along with empathy, the ability to listen to others' communication is a positive skill that team members should have. By listening we mean that what is said is received and that implied messages (about relationships, personal feelings, etc.) are noted. Paying attention to others on a team takes energy and concentration.

Reflecting

Reflection is a team skill that is related to listening, the use of empathy, and giving feedback. Reflection refers to the ability to paraphrase feelings. It also represents a source of emotional support for other teammates. The use of reflection is important in times of conflict, decision making, or role negotiation. It serves to project an image of openness and respect for others, which can make conflict resolution and decision making easier.

Asking for Clarification

A skill that is particularly useful along with paraphrasing is the ability to ask for clarification without implying the original message sender is dumb or stupid. That is, team members need to be able to ask for further explanation of unfamiliar concepts or unclear communication in a way that implies symmetrical, as opposed to complementary, relationships. For example, if the physician said: "I'm not sure if we should keep Mr. Jackson's medication consistent." It would be possible to respond by asking for clarification *using the same* words in both symmetrical and complementary (sender one-up or one-down) ways by varying the tone of voice and other nonverbal aspects of the communication:

> NURSE (blaming): What do you mean by consistent?
> NURSE (clarifying): what do you mean by consistent?

Exercise in Clarification

---

1. Pair up. One partner will be *A* (team member), the other *B* (nurse).
2. *A* will say the unclear statements in List 1 below. After each statement, *B* will ask

Interdisciplinary Teams and Communication

for clarification two ways, first by sending a one-up or one-down message with the request for clarification, followed by a request that implies a symmetrical relationship and respect for A.
Example:

A: Well, you can say what you want, but I know how I feel.
B (complementary): If you're so sure, why don't you share your view? You think you're so hot? (puts A in one-down)
B (clarifies): Exactly how do you feel?

Note: Remember to use appropriate voice tone and gestures to accompany each message.

List 1
1. "I don't think we shouldn't consider letting her have more medication."
2. "Well, you know that boys will be boys."
3. "Don't worry, I'll take care of this problem." (But to B: find out *how*.)
4. "Don't you think someone should be in charge of everything?"
5. "These things are not worth it."

3. Now switch roles so B reads each statement on List 2 as a team member and A responds to each statement by asking for clarification two ways, one complementary and the other symmetrical.

List 2
1. "Don't you think some of us work too hard?"
2. "I'm not at all convinced that we should not rotate hours so some won't have to work harder than others."
3. "After all, these things will happen."
4. "If you didn't care so much, we wouldn't have to spend so much time not doing the important work."
5. "Is this person a neurotic neurasthenic personality with paranoid tendencies at times of situational stress or does he have a basic inadequate personality with schizoid tendencies?"

4. Discuss in the large group your reactions to receiving the two kinds of requests for clarification.

Summarizing

Being able to summarize succinctly what has been said is a useful skill for team meetings, where conversations may wander and decisions can be forgotten easily. Also, being able to summarize several points of view can help move a team into effective decision making. There is no exercise for this skill, since it has to be practiced in the team context.

Using Humor

The use of humor is a subject which is often glossed over in discussions of communication. Yet, from our personal experience on health teams, an appropriate sense of humor is invaluable in thrashing out the complicated issues that arise in a team's existence. At its best, humor can provide a release from tension, a shared laugh, and a sense of perspective that may have been temporarily lost.

However, humor can easily be used in a negative way. Many jokes or humorous comments have an underlying hostile or put-down message that has a negative effect on listeners. *Most* jokes about older people, minorities, and sexual issues (usually about women or homosexuals) put down the group the joke is about. This message of "one-down" will come across even if it is not intended or the joke teller says, "Now look, I know you women won't take this personally." Humor has the power to wound as well as to heal. Also, being able to appreciate a humorous comment is just as valuable a skill on a team as being able to make one.

CONCLUSION

This chapter was designed to give nurses an overview of the growth of interdisciplinary health teams and to acquaint them with the issues and communication patterns and skills used in team collaboration. As new types of health care and professional roles develop in all health professions, nurses will have an integral role to play in collaborative health care ventures. It is hoped that they will take the skills and concepts from this chapter with them and share them, in conjunction with other literature (e.g., Rubin et al., 1975), with fellow health professionals who may not have as much background in this area as they now have.

BIBLIOGRAPHY

Baldwin, D.C., Baldwin, M.A., Edinberg, M.A., & Rowley, B.D. A model for recruitment and service—the University of Nevada's Summer Preceptorships in Indian Communities. *Public Health Reports*, 1980, Jan.-Feb., 19–22.

Bennis, W.F., & Sheppard, H.A. A theory of group development. *Human Relations*, 1956, 9, 415–437.

Brunetto, E., & Birk, P. The primary care nurse—the generalist in a structured health care team. *American Journal of Public Health*, 1972, 62, 785-794.

Domer, L.R. The skills of a manager in a team practice. *Dental Clinics of North America*, 1974, *18*, 755–769.

Edinberg, M.A., & Baldwin, D., Jr. Levels of interaction—group, team, and organization. In D.C. Baldwin, B.D. Rowley, & V.H. Williams (Eds.), *Interdisciplinary health care teams in teaching and practice*. Reno: University of Nevada, 1980.

Edinberg, M.A., Tsuda, M.K., & Gallagher, E.S. Training interdisciplinary student health teams in a gerontological setting. *Educational Gerontology*, 1978, *3*, 203-213.

Eichhorn, S. *Becoming: the evolution of five student health teams*. New York: Institute for Health Team Development, 1973.

Englert, B. How a staff nurse perceives her role at Loeb Center. *Nursing Clinics of North America*, 1971, *6*, 281–292.

Given, B. & Simmons, S. The interdisciplinary health care team: fact or fiction. *Nursing Forum*, 1977, *16*, 165–184.

Jacobs, A. The use of feedback in groups. In A. Jacobs and W. Spradlin (Eds.), *The group as agent of change*. New York: Behavioral Publications, 1974.

Kane, R.A. *Interprofessional teamwork*. (Manpower Monograph No. 8). Syracuse, N.Y.: Division of Continuing Education and Manpower Development, Syracuse University, 1975.

Kindig, D.A. Primary health care teams: issue for team delivery and interdisciplinary education. Speech delivered AAMC Institute on Primary Care, October 7, 1974.

Leininger, M. An open health care system model. *Nursing Outlook*, 1973, *21* (3), 171–175.

Reddy, B.R., & Lippert, K.M. The processes and dynamics within experiential groups. In P. Smith (Ed.), *Small groups and personal change*. London: Methuen, 1980.

Rubin, I.M., Plovnick, M.A., & Fry, R.E. *Improving the coordination of care: a program for health team development*. Cambridge, Massachusetts: Ballinger Publishing, 1975.

Schmuck, R.A., Runkel, P.J., Saturen, S.W., Martell, R.T., & Derr, C.B. *Handbook of organization development in schools*. Palo Alto: National Press Books, 1972.

Silver, G. *Family health care*. New York: Ballinger Press, 1973.

Silver, G.A., & Stiber, C. The social worker and the physician—daily practice of a health team. *Journal of Medical Education*, 1957, *32* (5), 324-330.

Stein, I. The doctor-nurse game. *Archives of General Psychiatry*, 1967, *16*, 699–703.

Thornton, B.C. Communication and health care teams: a multimethodological approach. Unpublished dissertation, University of Utah, Salt Lake City, 1976.

Tuckman, B.W. Developmental sequence in small groups. *Psychological Bulletin*, 1965, *63*, 384–399.

Watzlawick, P., Beavin, J.H., & Jackson, D.D. *Pragmatics of human communication: a study of interactional patterns, pathologies and paradoxes*. New York: W.W. Norton, 1967.

Wise, H., Beckhard, R., Rubin, I., & Kyte, A. *Making health teams work*. Cambridge, Massachusetts: Ballinger Publishing, 1974.

Chapter 13 Communication and groups

BEHAVIORAL OBJECTIVES

By reading this chapter, students will be able to:

1. Describe reasons for and against the use of group work
2. Describe common group dynamics and stages of development
3. Describe parameters that affect group communication (degree of participation, influence, style of influence, decision-making style, task functions, morale maintenance atmosphere, membership, expression of feelings and group norms)
4. Describe the forces affecting the nurse–leader's communication with the group (member concerns, stage of group development, ongoing dynamics, relationship of members to the leader and leader's style)
5. Distinguish between major group goals (information exchange, focused problems, social skills, learning about group dynamics, therapy, and self growth)
6. Distinguish between type of groups.

References to group dynamics in nursing have traditionally emphasized such areas as interactions between the members of a group, the cohesiveness of the group, or the size of the group and its effect on group dynamics. In this chapter, the emphasis is on the nurse as a leader or facilitator of a group of clients. The material presented provides nurses with information on leading client groups; the psychosocial needs of clients are stressed.

A group is defined, for our purposes here, as two or more clients who are interdependent; they have a common task (Loomis, 1979). The number of client groups that have emerged within the total health care system in recent years is staggering! Many of these groups have different tasks; some are therapeutic, for example, "stroke" groups or groups of diabetics or "ostomy" clients. Others are self-help groups, for example, Alcoholics Anonymous, Weight Watchers, and drug abuser groups. Still others are groups whose purpose is to promote growth and development or self-actualization. Examples are *T*-groups, encounter groups, or groups of elderly clients who are trying to become more assertive or to gain a healthier attitude about themselves through positive reminiscing.

Nurses are assuming much of the responsibility in health care settings in leading these groups. Communication in groups is one of the most complex, demanding, and yet often misunderstood areas for all health professionals. Why should this be true? What makes groups different from individuals? After all, communication patterns should be similar among individuals in terms of channels, styles, patterns, and goals, regardless if it takes place in a group setting.

The answers to these questions constitute the content of this chapter on group settings and communication. The nature of groups, their dynamics, the specific type of group and its goals, structural factors, the communication patterns characteristic of groups, the attributes of the leader, and the leader's function are the aspects that continually interact to affect the group's functioning (Burnside, 1978). It is the interaction of these factors that makes group work difficult yet exciting. These factors are outlined below.

Before each aspect of group functioning is discussed, a word of caution is given. The content presented on the following pages is intended to be an *introduction* to group work, as well as an examination of communication in groups. It is not intended to take the place of a course in group leadership. However, it can serve as a basis for further reading and learning about group process.

REASONS FOR GROUP WORK AND CAUTIONS TO CONSIDER

As was mentioned, nurses are moving toward group work in increasing numbers. A logical question to ask is, "How come?" Why see a number of

Communication and Groups

clients together rather than separately? There seems to be a variety of reasons nurses are choosing to do some of their work in a group context, as outlined in the following list:

1. Cohesion—clients obtain a sense of identity (Yalom, 1970).
2. Mutual emotional support—clients feel valued by peers.
3. Therapeutic value of the group—certain issues and/or problems seem best handled in group setting.
4. The group is a "laboratory" in which clients can learn about their own behavior in group settings and practice new behavior.
5. Relationships—clients can develop meaningful relationships or make new friends.
6. Interpersonal learning—clients can learn from each other.
7. Options for participation—clients can have high or low participation and play a variety of "roles."
8. Status—being in a group can be seen as high status by outsiders (Burnside, 1978).
9. Socialization.
10. Cost-effectiveness—many clients can be worked with in a short period of time at a lower cost per client hour.
11. Impact on systems—both the leader's visibility and the number of clients seen can have positive impact on the host system.

While all of these reasons are valid, some will not make sense in a given group setting. However, a nurse should consider using a group approach whenever several of the reasons for doing so seem to fit the nursing context and the nurse has appropriate skills and supervision for the type of group (discussed below).

Cohesion. Yalom (1970) defines cohesiveness as "the attractiveness of a group for its members" (p. 37). While he does not feel that cohesion is in and of itself a "curative" process, he sees it as a precondition for therapy, and distinguishes between group and individual cohesiveness, the former roughly being an "addition" of all the individuals' sense of cohesiveness.

We consider the sense of cohesion slightly differently than Yalom, in part because we are writing about all of the kinds of group settings in which nurses might work. The sense of cohesiveness, that is, the sense of belonging or having an identity as a group member, is an important psychological asset. In our society, people obtain some pleasure from belonging to organizations, clubs, honor societies, colleges, and so on. At a *personal* level, group membership can be rewarding in and of itself, especially when the clients have few other positive social identifications, which can be the case for single parents, both institutionalized and community elderly, or adolescents. Thus, under the right circumstances, being a group member in and of itself will have value and can enhance the self-worth of the client.

Mutual Emotional Support. Along with a sense of belonging, another advantage of the group is that members can provide emotional support for each other in ways the nurse cannot. For example, a nurse working with a group of diabetics will be seen as "not understanding how it is" unless the nurse, too, is a diabetic. Empathy may be more acceptable from a peer than from a health provider, both because peers know "how it is" (at least in the client's eyes) and because support may be easier to accept from an equal than from an "authority figure" such as a nurse.

Therapeutic Value of the Group. The group experience carries with it the potential of being therapeutic (Yalom, 1970). That is, the experience of being in a group can help clients solve some of their own life problems, conflicts, and decisions by making a commitment and participating in group activities or sessions, depending on the goals of the group. In addition, some types of personal problems seem best handled in a group context, such as socialization or exchange of ideas. One notable example is Alcoholics Anonymous (the most effective treatment to date for alcoholism), which uses large group meetings as its work format.

The group is a laboratory in which clients can learn about their own behavior. Groups have both "real world" and "non-real-world" aspects. The real world aspect is that there are other people present who can observe the client and give their reactions and perceptions of the client's behavior, as well as giving emotional support. The non-real-world aspect of the group is that it is time-bound, has a non-work focus, and a defined leader. These "laboratory" aspects mean that things that usually do not get communicated between people (like sharing observations about what each other just did and how it felt) can be emphasized and promoted by the group leader. Similarly, clients can try new behavior either in simulation (e.g., role playing with another client) or for real (e.g., making an explicit contract with other group members to use "I" statements for a session) in a context (the group) that is less risky than trying these things at home, on the job, or with friends. Thus, the group can become a relatively safe place to try new behavior before venturing out into the real world. The new behavior will still feel risky even in a safe and supportive group context.

Relationships. Group settings can provide the basis of personal relationships that can go beyond the time span of the group. A self-help group in a Senior Day Care Center, a group of coronary clients, or a health education group at a church can create or strengthen relationships between group members. This issue is quite important when the group is a major source of socialization for the clients (e.g., in a nursing home) and is time-limited. In fact, the relationships may be more important than the work done by the leader!

Interpersonal Learning. A group setting offers group members the opportunity to learn from each other as well as receive emotional support. Depending on the focus of the group, clients' experience in dealing with the issues can provide useful options, e.g., a nutrition group on ways to save money at the grocery store, or how to include exercise in a daily routine.

Options for Participation. In an individual setting, the client is expected to be an active participant in the communication process. In a group setting, there are opportunities to be a highly active participant, a moderately active participant, or even more of an observer. In addition, there are a variety of roles clients can take in group sessions, including gate-keeper, joker, leader's helper, voice of reason, passive, dominant, and others. While some may be more beneficial to the client and group than others, the opportunity to try new roles is a distinctive advantage of group settings.

Status. In certain settings, being a member of a group can be viewed as a sign of status. This has been observed in nursing homes (Burnside, 1978) and in senior citizen centers and is likely to take place in situations where the social environment is limited.

Socialization. A group setting can provide socialization for isolated individuals. Certain groups are designed specifically for this goal. In others, it is a byproduct.

Cost-effectiveness. Groups allow one nurse to be in contact with many clients at the same time. With an appropriate focus, the group setting costs less per client hour than individual sessions. Often, nurses who have to work with large numbers of clients who are geographically close and have shared psychosocial or health education problems will use groups for this reason.

Impact on Systems. The nurse who is running groups in an institutional setting becomes highly visible because of the need to schedule rooms and time for group meetings. Also, if clients are responding positively to the group experience, word can get out to that effect. This kind of notice and "good press" can have an impact on the host system, even if it is only noted by staff comments like, "What are you doing?" The nurse who is interested in being an agent of change in the system could begin to use this success as a springboard to make changes, such as having staff groups around communication issues. A successful group or two can give the leader higher credibility in the system.

It should be noted that while each of the above reasons is an incentive for nurses to work with groups, it is rare that all of them will make sense in a specific setting. Similarly, there will usually be reasons for the nurse *not* to use group work. Several are listed below. The final decision on implementing a group approach will include a weighing of pros and cons, some assessment of the possibility of having groups in a particular setting, and a self-appraisal as to whether one has the prerequisite skills to undertake such a venture.

Cautions to be Considered in Group Work

The following cautions should be viewed as concerns to be raised when groups are being considered. While the authors advocate the use of group methods by nurses, we feel that the educated nurse will also know the potential problems of group work and be able to minimize their impact on the group process.

1. *The nurse may be unprepared or inadequately trained to work with the group.* There are no hard and fast guidelines for how to be prepared to work with groups. Different types of groups require different levels and types of skills from nurse leaders. For example, a health education class may require that the nurse know the cognitive material and be able to facilitate a discussion. On the other hand, working with a group of teenage drug abusers requires a knowledge of drugs, drug culture, and adolescent development, as well as skills in dealing with hostility, suspicion, low trust, low self-worth, and severe psychological problems.

    The usual ways in which the nurse receives experience in group work is to be a member of several types of groups (with acquaintances and/or friends), take some training in leading groups, and participate as a co-leader (or occasionally a leader) in a supervised setting. Even with appropriate background, it is always appropriate for the nurse to ask, "Do I have the skills and knowledge necessary to run this particular group?" before taking on the responsibility of being a group leader.

2. *The screening and selection processes for group membership can be inadequate.* Reddy (1972) presents a thorough review of issues involved in screening clients for group experiences. There are several issues involved in deciding on group membership. At one end of the spectrum, some "growth centers" have no screening for their group sessions. Their argument is that individuals must take responsibility for their own behavior and that screening is either arbitrary or unfair or an unnecessary control by the group leader(s). Screening is considered to be an important aspect of group

work for the group and the individual group members. The kinds of questions a nurse should ask before setting up a group include:

"What is the purpose of the group?"
"What are the characteristics of people who will benefit from the group?"
"What are the characteristics of potential members that will either not benefit or cause problems for other group members that would be detrimental to the group's goals?"
"How can I get information from prospective clients that ensures that the group members are likely to benefit from the experience?"
"How will clients be informed and give full consent to participate in the group?"

By answering these questions in light of the type of group and situational context (hospital, community center, clinic, nursing home, day-care center, etc.), the nurse should be able to come up with appropriate screening procedures (questionnaires, informed consent forms, interviews) for any group.

3. *The heterogeneity of group members can leave some feeling left out; others may drop out.* Even with adequate screening, any group will represent a range of personalities, life styles, and health and emotional problems. Without careful monitoring by the leader, some clients may feel that the group is not for them, not verbalize it, and become passive members. Others may drop out, that is, attend infrequently or not at all.

It may take personal contact via telephone or an individual interview to regain contact with a client who has dropped out of a group. This can be done as an "exit interview," which can be stipulated as a condition for joining the group.

4. *Some group members can dominate at the expense of others: the most psychologically needy could take over.* This consideration is also related to certain group dynamics described below. Domination of "air time" in a group can be interpreted as the client's expression of a need for attention or control. If the focus of the group is on interpersonal relationships, then the leader can use the behavior as a source of group learning. If, however, the focus is on health problems, the exchange of ideas, or a focused group (weight loss, smoking, etc.), the "needy" person who dominates may have to be confronted or counseled out of the group setting, which requires a fair amount of assertion on the part of the nurse leader.

5. *Some clients would derive more benefit from individual sessions.* One of the cautions in choosing group formats is that clients who can benefit from individual sessions may not receive the attention they need. These clients would include individuals who are not ready for a group setting or for

whom the benefits of a group (cohesion, support) are not important in light of their health and psychosocial problems.
6. *Some clients will be scapegoated.* One of the themes that can emerge in the life of a group is the scapegoating (blaming or putting down) of certain clients. The nurse has to be alert for scapegoating and must be able to provide some protection for the victim as well as have the skills required to use the process for the group's learning (if this fits the group's goals).
7. *Negative status can be given to group members by others.* Although, as was mentioned earlier, positive status can be given to clients in certain group settings, it is just as easy for a negative status to be given to group membership by others, either out of ignorance, jealousy, or their own fears. Because the source of this labeling comes from outside the group, the nurse may only have indirect evidence, such as comments from staff in the halls before or after the group meetings. This is an issue that may have to be dealt with both at a group and organizational level.
8. *A dependency relationship between the client and the nurse can develop and may not be worked through.* The issues of leadership are an integral part of group dynamics and are discussed later in this chapter. One precaution that goes with the power of being the leader is that clients may become dependent on the nurse as a source of validation of their behavior, feelings, and thoughts. While such dependency is an expected process in the life of many groups, it is important for nurses to be aware of the need for clients to work it through to the point where the nurse is no longer the powerful validating figure by the time the group's life is over. It is beyond the scope of this chapter to suggest how clients can be guided to work through dependency. The references at the end of this chapter provide further reading in this area.

GROUP DEVELOPMENT, PROCESSES, AND COMMUNICATION

In order to make sense out of the communication that takes place in groups, group leaders and researchers have developed several models for understanding *group development* and *group processes*. Group development means that the communication in groups varies in systematic ways or patterns throughout the group's life and that the systematic variations symbolize what can be called stages or phases of the group's life. Group processes (or group dynamics) refers to the implied relationships between group members at a moment in time in the group's life (Yalom, 1970). Group processes can be related to a series of conceptualizations or themes such as power and issues of leadership. Many of these themes are tied to stages of group development. As a way of introducing you to group processes, several major theories of group development are reviewed and group processes that occur in various stages are described, with examples of related communication.

One word of caution should be noted before launching into this subject. Group processes and development are difficult to unravel from immediate experience. That is, they are conceptualizations drawn out of a bewildering array of comments and gestures. (Think for a moment of all the things that go on in a classroom or seminar. Then try to distill the major underlying themes about how your group develops!) A succinct statement of the issues in uncovering process in therapy groups was made by Yalom (1970):

> We search not only for the process behind a simple statement but for the process behind a sequence of statements made by a patient or by a number of patients. What does this sequence tell us about the relationship between one patient and the other group members, or between clusters or cliques of members, or between the members and the leader, or, finally, between the group as a whole and its primary task? (p. 110)

The main theoretical frameworks that are commonly used to analyze group development are Bennis and Sheppard's (1956) stages of group development, Bion's (1961) concepts about "work-groups" and "basic assumption groups," the "focal conflict" model of group development (Whitaker and Lieberman, 1964), and Tuckman's phases of development (1965). As Reddy and Lippert (1980) point out, there is significant overlap among these theories. A brief summary of each and a discussion of related dynamics follows.

Bennis and Sheppard's Model

Bennis and Sheppard (1956) suggested that there are two major issues that influence the development of any group, authority relationships (relations with the group leader) and personal relationships (relations among group members). They state that there are two general phases in the development of any group, the first phase being one of dependence (focusing on authority issues) and the second being interdependence (focusing on interpersonal issues). Each phase has its own subphases. In phase I, the subphases are submission, rebellion, and resolution of dependence. In phase II, the subphases are enchantment with member identification, disenchantment, and resolution of the interdependence problem. In addition, the movement between phases is uneven, with cycles of several steps forward, one backward, and so on.

One of the major contributions of this theory is to point out how different personalities in the group can be dominant at different stages of development. For example, if the group is in the counterdependent subphase (one of the subphases of dependency), it is expected that the people who are most counterdependent (either hostile to the leader or least tied emotionally to the leader) will exert the most influence.

Thus, in examining communication and influence of group members, the nurse should remember that at different times in the group's experience, various group members will be dominant. Also, dominance will shift as the group goes through different stages of development.

Bion's Concepts of "Basic Assumption" and "Work Groups"

As opposed to Bennis and Sheppard, Bion was less concerned with the sequence of group development than with the symbolic issues with which groups seem to deal. Bion made a distinction between two kinds of groups (or two basic stages of the same group). The key to the distinction is whether or not the group is dealing fully with the "real" issues at hand or is acting (communicating) as if an unspoken yet controlling assumption is determining how the group functions. This implies that the internal processes of the group take up its time and that it does not fully focus on "the task." The former group is called the "work group." The latter group is called a "basic assumption group." According to Bion, work groups are rare and usually come about after a group has "worked through" its basic assumption issues.

Bion posed three basic assumption groups: the dependency group, the fight-flight group, and the pairing group. The basic assumption of the dependency group is that the group is formed to receive security from the leader. The leader is supposed to protect the group member's comfort. The basic assumption of the fight-flight group is that the group meets to protect its members from the outside world. The choices are symbolic: whether to fight the world or flee. The pairing group meets with the basic assumption that it is to produce a savior, usually through a (symbolic) pairing of two group members.

The description of these three basic assumption groups may seem a little overdrawn. Remember, the three assumptions are conceptualizations that the group seems to be acting on, as deduced from what is communicated in the group. For example, on a given day, the group members may make comments like:

"Well, you're the leader, so you should take care of Bill."
"We can't hide anything from you!"
"You're the only one who can do anything for us."

According to Bion's theory, these would indicate that the group is in a dependency state.

One could suspect that the group was acting in a fight-flight mode, if the statements being communicated were similar to:

"I don't trust any of this introspective stuff."
"I think everyone outside of this group thinks it's dumb."
"We should all get together and protest."

Finally, the expression of either hope or pairing suggests that the group is in a pairing phase if the communications could run along these lines:

"Things will improve when winter is over."
"Everyone ought to have marriage therapy."
"Bill and Sally here could really teach everyone a thing or two."

Bion's work has been used in many settings. It also includes guides for group leaders on how to help groups get through their assumption stages so they can become work groups. You are encouraged to read his book *Experiences in Groups* (1961) for a more in-depth presentation of this material.

The Focal Conflict Model

Whitaker and Lieberman (1964) proposed a variation on the themes given in Bion's work to describe how therapeutic change takes place in groups, although their concepts are useful in describing the dynamics of nontherapy groups as well. Their basic concepts include the following processes:

1. Individual behavior and communication in the group is collectively related to a singular unspoken concern about what is currently happening in the group.
2. All events that occur can be thought of as the expression of a hidden or covert conflict, which is the result of a wish that is opposed by a fear. Both parts are related to "here-and-now" issues.
3. When this "focal conflict" occurs, a solution is sought that will both satisfy the wish (as much as possible) and alleviate the fears.

What this simplified set of concepts implies is that the communication that goes on in groups can only be understood by trying to figure out the fear, the wish, and the "solution." All three have to be deduced from the overt communication.

As a simple example, consider the following statements that could be made by group members:

A: I'm tired. Maybe we could go home early tonight.
B: Me too, but weren't we told the sessions would last the full two hours?
C: Enough of this, let's get down to business.

Taking a focal conflict perspective, one could interpret A's statement as an expression of an underlying wish for independence (leaving early); B's agreement in being tired as a sign that the wish was shared; B's question about "being told" as a sign of fear or criticism by the leader; C's implied suggestion to drop the issue as a solution, and, if the others then changed the subject, acceptance of the solution. Obviously, the solution would be more direct if group members asked the leader about ending early, but in this group that "solution" would probably have been too threatening at that point. One would hope that the group would, over time, be able to deal with the independence issue through a series of "solutions" that become more and more direct.

Focal conflict theory is a useful set of concepts to use in understanding indirect communication in groups. It also alerts the leader to the fact that issues are continually being resolved and "re-resolved." Whitaker and Lieberman's book, *Psychotherapy Through the Group Process* (1964), explains the theory in detail.

Tuckman's Phases of Development

Tuckman (1965) proposed that groups go through four stages of development:

>   Forming
>   Storming
>   Norming
>   Performing.

"Forming" refers to the initial interaction among group members and with the leader. There is a lot of initial testing of boundaries (limits of acceptable behavior), as well as the formation of dependency relationships with the leader.

Examples of communication that can be indicative of forming include:

>   "Will we meet for the full hour every week?"
>   "Is it OK to smoke in here?"
>   "Is anyone here married?"

"Storming" refers to a stage of conflict and side-taking (polarization). Tempers may flare, and if the group has a defined task, it will be avoided or resisted. Examples of the kind of communication that is expected during the storming phase include:

"I think you're all picking on Jerry."
"Why do we have to do this, anyway?"
"You're not listening to what I say!"
"You three are all wrong. We just think alike, we're not against you."

In the "norming" stage, a sense of group cohesion occurs, there is some shift in roles as the group is no longer polarized, and new standards (or norms) for group communication emerge. It now may be possible to disagree without polarization or escalation of feelings:

"You know, I never thought I'd be able to say this to you, but I admire your brassiness."
"It seems like we disagree on this and that's OK."
"I'm tired of keeping the peace. Someone else can do it."

The last stage Tuckman proposes is "performing." When a group is in a performing stage, it is able to use the resources of group members productively and creatively for the matter at hand. Group tasks can now be accomplished efficiently. Communication will focus more on task than on interpersonal or dynamic issues, although ideally, these issues will be dealt with openly if they arise.

The forming-storming-norming-performing sequence is easy to remember. It may also be a sequence that gets repeated in the same group over time, especially if a new member joins, the task is changed, or other factors significantly alter the group's life.

Other Aspects of Group Functioning That Affect Communication

Along with attending to the stage of the group's development, the group leader can also analyze the group's communication along the following dimensions. The description and dimensions are adapted from the 1972 Annual Handbook of Group Facilitators entitled *What to Look for in Groups*.

Degree of Participation. Some group members will participate a great deal. Some will keep relatively quiet. Some members will help facilitate communication. Some will block it. Participation patterns may be a key to a "hidden" issue.

Influence. It is possible for a group member to have much influence but participate infrequently. Influence may be divided into two or more "camps," which would suggest that rivalry is going on.

Styles of Influence. Styles of influence are related to styles of communication. Needless to say, the style (or "how") of influence will affect its impact. Four styles from the 1972 Handbook for Group Facilitators (pp. 21–22) include:

Autocratic—pushes to get own way
Peacemaker—avoids conflict, agrees
Laissez-faire—apparent lack of involvement
Democratic—tries to include everyone in decisions.

Decision-making Style. How does the group make decisions? Some groups allow one member to make decisions unilaterally, without including others. Some groups vote. Some use consensus (all have to accept the solution, whereas in voting, all do not). In some groups, certain members make suggestions that have no impact, whereas other members' suggestions are implemented.

Task Functions. How does the group go about doing its task or solving a problem? Who gives feedback, who summarizes? Also, how does the group stay with the task as opposed to being tangential?

Morale Maintenance. Communication that is aimed at producing good working relationships among group members can be considered as serving the function of maintaining morale. This can be done by helping silent members participate (gate-keeping), stopping "over-talkers" (gate-closing), and supporting other group members' self-worth, even when there is disagreement with their ideas.

Group Atmosphere. The communication in a group will have a general feeling sense that is called group atmosphere. Groups can be friendly, warm, cool, intellectual, hostile, playful, and so forth. There may even be conflicting preferences in members' wishes for type of atmosphere.

Membership. This dimension refers to inclusion or exclusion as a group member. Some members may become part of an "in-group" or "out-group." Individuals may express feelings or concerns about being a "real member."

Expression of Feelings. The whole question of how feelings are communicated in groups is an important one. Most of the feelings generated by group experience are not verbalized, especially in the early stages of the group's development. The leader has to look for visual and auditory cues for how members are feeling (e.g., body language, gestures, tone of voice).

Group Norms. Both what is communicated and what is not give clues as to what is acceptable behavior in the group. The rules of behavior may include which topics are acceptable, which are taboo; what kinds of confrontations are acceptable, which are not; and other behavioral dimensions such as attendance, taking a break, or leaving the session early.

THE NURSE LEADER'S COMMUNICATION WITH THE GROUP

Given all of the previous ways of interpreting group communication, the nurse leader has to be aware that there are at least three levels of group communication reflecting several issues at any moment in time: individual concerns, "stage development" issues, and possibly other group dynamic questions (e.g., membership, decision making). Initially, it is difficult for a leader to decide how to respond to the different levels, even if the nurse is sure of her own perception of what is going on.

Suppose that in an initial group meeting, it becomes obvious that the group is testing your limits as a leader. They seem to be in a dependency state (similar to the stages noted by Bion, Tuckman and Bennis and Sheppard). One group member is nonverbally hostile to you for the whole session. Finally, she says somewhat sarcastically, "So how can you help us?" You would probably be torn between putting her in her place, defending your role, and also wanting to encourage participation and perhaps modeling good communication skills. Also, if the goal of the group was for the group to learn to solve its own problems, you would eventually want the group to handle this member's hostility in a way that kept her as a group member. (In this instance, a nondefensive "in any way I can" is enough of a reply in an initial session's reply.)

A further complication for the nurse leader is that everything he or she says is responded to not only as communication, but as communication *from the leader*. The role relationship between leader and group has all sorts of nuances, one of which is that the group responds differently to the leader at various moments in time. Another is that the group members respond individually to the leader. It also seems that the group members do not realize that they respond differently to leaders than to other members of the group. It may be denied. Leaders do not necessarily have an accurate perception of how group members feel about them (Lundgren, 1975).

Your own personal style will also affect how groups respond to you. For example, one review of group work research (Reddy and Lippert, 1980) concludes that the precise effect of the leader's style is still uncertain. However, leaders who are warm, supportive, and active seem to bring about positive changes in group members. Other stylistic characteristics that seem beneficial in facilitating positive changes in group members are being active (Russell, 1978), being able to accept direct hostility from group members (O'Day, 1976), and liking the individual group member (Babad and Melnick, 1976). Nurses can develop their own leadership styles by getting feedback from peers, supervisors, and clients about how they come across in the spirit of discovery rather than self-blame or judgment. Also, the material in Chapter 3 may be helpful in discovering more about communication style as it applies to leadership.

An additional issue to consider in figuring out how leaders communicate with the group is that different types of communication may be effective at different stages of the group's development. That is, the group may be able to respond to direct feedback (either positive or negative) at some points but not at others. Similarly, while being active in general was noted as being related to positive changes in group members, there will be times when the group "needs" the leader to be silent so the group can do its own work.

The hardest part of all of this discussion comes when a student asks, "Well, what do I do when Ms. Peterson gets uppity in the self-help group?" In part, the answer is, "It depends." What it depends on is how Ms. Peterson gets uppity (what she communicates), what others say in response (a focal conflict?), how long the group has been meeting (stage of development), the communication role Ms. Peterson and others seem to play in this issue, the leader's style, the leader's skills, the context in which the group meets, and its goals. Also, the group members may intervene effectively and be more helpful at one moment than the leader. By knowing that each of these issues exists conceptually, the group leader will be able to come up with effective communication strategies for handling Ms. Peterson and helping the group, as a whole and individually, to develop and do its task.

The Nurse-leader in the Nursing Context

Along with paying attention to group development and to the benefits of the group to its members, the nurse should also be aware of the role of the group leader within the nursing context. Nurses and nursing students can be asked to lead groups in a wide range of settings, although most groups will be run in secondary care settings. Furthermore, there are several roles the nurse may play in the group: these include:

a. Process observer—watches and listens, takes notes
b. Junior leader—leading the group along with a more experienced leader

Communication and Groups

c. Co-leader—leading the group as an equal partner with another person
d. Leader—in charge of the group; may have a co-leader, junior leader, or process observer present

Each of these four roles requires increasingly advanced skills and knowledge. Before undertaking the leadership of a group, the nurse should assess the type of group, the constraints and supports within the system, and the degree of skill required by the role the nurse is expected to play. Too often, nurses are requested to lead groups when they should be junior leaders. A second danger is that the nurse is in over his or her head as far as the type of clientele. A third danger is the lack of support from the setting, including adequate supervision and back-up if clients develop problems that the group setting is not conducive to handling.

TYPES OF GROUPS

There are a bewildering number of group treatment modalities. You probably have heard of therapy groups, encounter groups, *T*-groups, and growth groups. The list could go on and on. We have chosen to organize the various group modalities into six general categories based on the goals of the group: information exchange, learning how to cope with a specific problem, learning an area of social skills, learning about group dynamics, therapeutic change, and personal growth. Many of the groups to be discussed overlap categories. We have chosen them as a rough way of organizing what otherwise is an unmanageable array of names, types, and forms of group work.

The categories of goals, types of group within each category, prerequisite leader needs and leader role are presented in Chart 13–1. The following discussion is an expansion of the information presented there.

Information Exchange Groups

The first category of group is one in which the primary goal is for participants to gain information about problems, health care, referral sources, etc. The nurse who runs these groups should have substantive knowledge about the topic and be able to guide a group discussion on the topic area. The nurse is generally active, guides the questions and answers, and serves as a source of information as well as being the leader.

Health Education Groups. A health education group is run for the purpose of promoting client knowledge about health and related life-style

CHART 13–1
Types of Group Work, Goals of Group Work, Prerequisite Leader Knowledge and Leader's Role

Goal	Example of type of group	Leader's knowledge	Leader's role
Information exchange	Health education, discussion group, seminars/inservice	Knows information, how to promote participation, basic knowledge of group dynamics	Active, guides discussion
Coping with or changing a focused and identified problem	Weight loss, smoking, parents without Partners, Alcoholics Anonymous	Knows problem area, as well as psychosocial aspects; some knowledge about group dynamics	Active, varies on directness, guides learning experience
Learning-support in a social skill area	Assertion, parenting skills, widowhood groups, reality orientation, (remotivation, resocialization) reminiscence groups, social competency groups	Knows problem area, how to teach the skills, group dynamics	Active, direct at times, allows group to go its own way
Learning about group dynamics, group functioning	Tavistock groups, T-groups, leadership training	Excellent understanding of group dynamics	Not active, provides interpretation, allows group to develop, and guides in the process
Therapeutic change, clients identified by psychological dysfunction	Psychotherapy group (focal conflict), art therapy, music therapy, gestalt therapy, movement-dance therapy	Excellent understanding of psychopathology, psychotherapy modality in group setting	Varies; can be interpretive, confrontive, active, passive, depending on client-group needs
Self-growth and development	Encounter group, sensitivity training, marathon group, movement, psychodrama, meditation, consciousness-raising, interracial, intercultural groups	Excellent understanding of the modality, principles underlying the format (human behavior, growth models, etc.); good understanding of group dynamics	Generally active, controls the format, style of group; can push clients to limits; also maintains "safety"

326

factors. Information on smoking, nutrition, exercise, compliance, and other aspects of consumer health can be effectively presented in a group format, which should include time for clients to discuss and integrate the information.

Discussion Group. Discussion groups are often run as part of a recreational or social activity program. Topics can be chosen by the leader or group. If the discussion group is formed to be an open-ended "bull session," the format will be looser. Discussion groups are an excellent way for nurses to get used to leading a group. They can also serve as an entree into client social systems, such as at senior citizen centers, community centers, or schools.

Seminars and In-service Training. Seminars and in-service training do not necessarily have to be taught in a group format. Both are generally regarded as topic-oriented. That is, seminars and in-service sessions usually have a pre-arranged agenda. However, the nurse who has some group work skills can make many seminars and in-service sessions into group discussion sessions fairly easily.

Groups for Coping with a Focused and Identified Problem

Some kinds of problems seem to be handled well in a group setting. The cohesiveness and support by other group members, while secondary, is useful, because there are other clients who "understand." Also, these groups allow for clients to learn while watching or listening to others. That is, peer modeling can go on.

The kinds of group included in this category are weight loss groups, groups for stopping smoking, and peer groups such as Alcoholics Anonymous. All of these groups are formed for people with the same problem so there is likely to be a fair degree of homogeneity among the group members in terms of personality, although not necessarily in terms of race or socioeconomic class. This type of group also usually has targeted goals that are easily measured (weight loss, decrease in smoking).

In working with a focused problem group, the nurse needs to have substantive knowledge about the problem area (obesity, nutrition, smoking, etc.) and understand the psychological aspects of the problem (anxiety, sexual aspects of obesity, body image, etc.). The nurse should also have some background in and understanding of group dynamics. Finally, the nurse should have skill and knowledge in the mode of treatment (behavior monitoring for weight loss or smoking, etc.).

The nurse's role in the focused problem group is twofold. One role is that of group facilitator, one who aids the group to develop cohesion and peer support. The other role is that of instructor for the form of treatment (if one is being used, since focused problem groups are sometimes more for mutual support than behavior or health changes).

Learning and Support Groups in Social Skill Areas

Along with focused problem groups, nurses have worked with groups that are organized to help clients on a more general level but still with a problem focus. One term used to describe this kind of group is a group for "social skills."

The groups that fall into this category include: *assertion groups* (e.g., Edinberg, 1975), designed to help participants be able to state their wishes and needs in a way that is respectful of the rights of others and the client; *parenting skill groups* (e.g., Gordon, 1975), designed to help parents learn effective communication and problem-solving skills for child-rearing; *widow groups* (Burnside, 1978), generally run for the support to the recently bereaved; *reality orientation, remotivation, and resocialization groups* (e.g., Dennis, 1978, Taulbee, 1978), generally following specific reinforcement procedures based on behavioral principles and used to increase reality testing and extinguish signs of confusion with older clients suffering from organic brain syndrome; *reminiscence groups* (e.g., Ebersole, 1978), which use memories guided by pictures, sounds, or feelings to provide life review and a source of group interaction for the elderly; and *social competency groups* (e.g., Maney and Edinberg, 1976), designed to work on any coping problem a member may have.

The nurse's role in a social skills group is both active and directive. Many social skills training programs require the leader to coach, direct, and lead exercises or role-played situations to help clients develop desired behavior.

Groups to Learn About Group Dynamics

Although not a treatment modality, groups are often formed for health professionals to learn about group dynamics and their own behavior in groups at an experimental level. Many of these groups are based on early work done by Lewin and his followers, who started National Training Laboratories (NTL), an organization that runs groups and is highly involved in organizational development. Another constituency within the "learning about groups" movement are those who use the "Tavistock method," based originally on work of Bion. The type of group associated with each of the above "thrusts" is the *T*-group (NTL) and the Tavistock group. The leader often assumes a relatively inactive role, providing interpretive comments to facilitate development of the group and group member learning.

Therapeutic Change Groups for Clients Identified by Psychological Dysfunction

In an attempt to separate this category of group work from the one that follows, we have defined it by two criteria: (a) the goal is therapeutic change, and (b) the clients are defined (labeled) as having some sort of psychological dysfunction. Some nurses and other group leaders will argue that growth groups and therapy groups are the same and that to distinguish between groups for "normals" and groups for "psychologically distressed" is inaccurate, unfair, and based on an unproven model of mental illness. At the same time, there are aspects of therapy groups (homogeneity of clients, their being so labeled by an institution or society) and prerequisite group leader knowledge (psychopathology and psychotherapy) that warrant some distinction, even if just for academic purposes.

As was mentioned above, the nurse's role as leader of a therapy group is to facilitate the therapeutic process for each client. This assumes a knowledge of psychopathology and the techniques of the therapeutic modality, as well as an understanding of group dynamics. In each of the treatments briefly described below, groups have been used as a therapeutic treatment modality.

Group Psychotherapy (Yalom or Focal Conflict). A traditional group psychotherapy approach is described in Yalom (1970). After client selection and screening, some sort of contract is set for members as to goals, expectations for attendance, and ground rules. The group meets with the "task" of working on individuals' problems. The group's development aids members in working through their individual problems as those problems are symbolically worked through by the group.

Psychodrama. Psychodrama was pioneered by Moerno (Yablonsky, 1972). It involves having group members "become" and act as significant others for each other. Scenes from a member's life can be played out by the group.

Art Therapy. Art therapy groups use self-expression through art media, such as painting, drawing, or collage work. Here, the group is used to share feelings and artistic creations. Art is one approach to "unlock" nonverbal clients (Naumberg, 1966).

Music Therapy. Music therapy groups are of two types, either listening to songs and responding to the words and feelings brought up by the music or participation in musical expression through instruments, singing, or chanting. The group can react to or perform a piece of music together. The goal is to encourage verbalization of feelings through music. Appropriate musical selections are very useful with adolescents and the elderly (Hennessey, 1978).

Gestalt Therapy. Based on the work of Perls and others, gestalt therapy groups are quite similar to gestalt "growth" groups as far as the application of gestalt techniques (Fagen and Shepherd, 1970). The general approach is to focus on feelings in "the here and now" to learn how to express them and to resolve a person's dichotomies, which Perls referred to as the "top-dog" and "underdog." Clients at times role-play with themselves by sequentially taking the "top-dog" and "underdog" roles in two chairs that face each other.

It should be noted that there is a wide range of therapeutic and growth groups called "gestalt" these days, sometimes to the point where the term "gestalt" has no useful meaning as a type of group.

Dance-movement Therapy. One of the newer group treatment modalities is movement therapy. The goal of dance therapy is to help clients explore their feelings and emotional problems through movement, either to music or in response to a structured exercise (e.g., "give a movement that shows your depression") (Schoop, 1974). Movement groups have been run for a wide range of clients, including the young and the institutionalized elderly (Sandel, 1978). The group provides a safe place where clients can express themselves in new ways.

This brief description of therapeutic groups is not intended to review every kind of therapy group. It should, however, serve as an introduction to the variety of treatments used in group work.

Groups for Self-Growth and Development

Much of the publicity the "group movement" received in the late 1960s and early 1970s focused on growth groups. The human potential movement can be traced back to the work of Lewin and his colleagues, the writings of Rogers and Maslow (Rogers, 1970), and, we believe, to the climate of "hope" in the United States expressed during the "New Frontier" of the Kennedy presidency in such ways as the civil rights movement, the war on poverty, and the Peace Corps and VISTA, in which young Americans volunteered to work to "make the world a better place." Primarily on the West Coast, group leaders started running group sessions for "normals," since their definition of mental health did not focus on illness but rather on well-being and self-actualization.

Esalen, perhaps the best known of the growth centers, came into being at this time. Other growth centers have since developed across the United States and in other countries, and to this day they offer group experiences in a variety of modalities for anyone willing to participate and pay for it.

The underlying philosophy of many growth groups is that the participant is responsible for his or her own behavior, the individual can thereby gain a knowledge of the limits to which he or she can go, psychologically, without risking personal safety. The leader should understand the modality, principles, or theory behind such group work. The leader's role is generally active, since the client's limits can be "pushed" or stretched given the assumption that the client is responsible for his or her own safety. At the same time, the leader has significant influence on group norms and can facilitate an atmosphere in which clients can take or refuse risks.

Several of the types of groups for self-growth have been discussed earlier, such as *gestalt* and *dance-movement groups*. Other kinds of growth groups include: *encounter groups,* in which participants (the term "client" is inappropriate in a growth group) develop self-awareness by encountering other members of the group on a "here-and-now basis"; *sensitivity training,* which overlaps with encounter groups but the focus of which is more on individual awareness, with more exercises done individually than as a group; *marathon groups,* in which participants stay together for an extended period of time, usually 24 to 48 hours; and *consciousness raising groups,* designed around a specific issue such as feminism, race, or sex role identity.

The leader's role in growth groups varies considerably. Generally, the leader sets the format for sessions. Also, the leader can work with individuals and challenge them. The leader has a responsibility to insure some sense of psychological safety to group members. In all of the growth groups, leaders will have "exercises" or structured experiences that may be used to "warm-up" the participants. All of the communication exercises for pairs or triads that are in this book are also applicable to the appropriate group setting.

The group's life will be influenced by the leader's style, the exercises used, the personalities of the group participants, and the events that transpire in the group. It is difficult to summarize how a typical growth group might take place, as the factors mentioned will vary. The leader has many choices in structuring the experience. Many growth groups are more eclectic than single "type," that is, the leader may use aspects of gestalt, movement, encounter, and even therapeutic modalities to promote participant growth and development.

CONCLUSION

It becomes obvious from reading this chapter, communication and group behavior are intertwined. The effective nurse communicator needs to have a knowledge of group dynamics and the roles of a group leader in order to be effective. He or she will also benefit by having group dynamics background when working as a group member in task group or health team.

REFERENCES

Babad, E.Y., & Melnick, I. Effects of a T-group as a function of trainers' linking and members' participation, involvement, quantity and quality of received feedback. *Journal of Applied Behavioral Science,* 1976, 12, 543–562.

Bennis, W.F. & Sheppard, H.A. A theory of group development. *Human Relations,* 1956, 9, 415–437.

Bion, W.R. *Experiences in groups.* New York: Basic Books, 1961.

Burnside, I.M. *Working with the elderly: group processes and techniques.* North Scituate, Massachusetts: Duxbury Press, 1978.

Dennis, H. Remotivation therapy groups. In I. Burnside (Ed.), *Working with the elderly: group processes and techniques.* North Scituate, Massachusetts: Duxbury Press, 1978, Chap. 14.

Ebersole, P. A theoretical approach to the use of reminiscence. In I. Burnside (Ed.), *Working with the elderly: group processes and techniques.* North Scituate, Massachusetts: Duxbury Press, 1978, Chap. 9.

Edinberg, M.A. Behavioral assessment and assertion training of the elderly. Unpublished Doctoral Dissertation, University of Cincinnati, 1975.

Egan, G. *Encounter: group processes for interpersonal growth.* Belmont, California: Brooks/Cole Publishing, 1970.

Fagen, S., & Shepherd, I.L., (Eds.). *Gestalt therapy now: theory techniques applications.* New York: Harper & Row, 1970.

Gordon, T. *Parent effectiveness training.* New York: Plume Books, 1975.

Hennessey, J.J. Music and music therapy groups. In I. Burnside (Ed.), *Working with the elderly: group processes and techniques.* North Scituate, Massachusetts: Duxbury Press, 1978, Chap. 16.

Loomis, M. *Group processes for nurses* St. Louis: C.V. Mosby, 1979.

Lundgren, D.C. Interpersonal needs and member attitudes toward trainer and group. *Small Group Behavior,* 1975, 6, 371–388.

Maney, J., & Edinberg, M. Social competency groups: a training and teaching modality for the gerontological nurse practitioner. *Journal of Gerontological Nursing,* 1976, 2, 31–33.

Naumberg, M. *Dynamically oriented art therapy: its principles and practices.* New York: Grune & Stratton, 1966.

O'Day, R. Individual training styles: an empirically derived typology. *Small Group Behavior,* 1976, 7, 147–182.

Reddy, W.B. Screening and selection of participants. In Solomon L.N., & Berzon B., (Eds.), *New perspectives encounter groups.* San Francisco: Jossey Bass, 1972.

Reddy, W.B. Screening and selection of participants. In Solomon L.N., & Berzon B., groups. In P. Smith (Ed.), *Small groups and personal change.* London: Methuen, 1980.

Rogers, C.R. *On encounter groups.* New York: Harper & Row, 1970.

Russell, E., The facts about encounter groups: first facts. *Journal of Clinical Psychology,* 1978, 34, 130–137.

Sandel, S. Movement therapy with geriatric patients in a convalescent hospital. *Hospital and Community Psychiatry,* 1978, *29,* 738–741.

Schoop, T. *Won't you join the dance?* Palo Alto, California: National Press Books, 1974.

Solomon, L.N., & Berzon, B. (Eds.). *New perspectives on encounter groups.* San Francisco: Jossey Bass, 1972.

Taulbee, L.R. Reality orientation: a therapeutic group activity for elderly persons. In I. Burnside (Ed.), *Working with the elderly: group processes and techniques.* North Scituate, Massachusetts: Duxbury Press, 1978, Chap. 13.

Tuckman, B.W. Developmental sequence in small groups. *Psychological Bulletin,* 1965, *3,* 384–399.

What to look for in groups (The 1972 Annual Handbook for Group Facilitators) University Associates.

Whitaker, D.S., & Lieberman, M.A. *Psychotherapy through the group process.* Chicago: Aldine Publishing, 1964.

Yablonsky, L. Psychodrama and role training. In L.N. Solomon & B. Berzon (Eds.), *New perspectives on encounter groups.* San Francisco: Jossey Bass, 1972, Chap. 16.

Yalom, I.D. *The theory and practice of group psychotherapy.* New York: Basic Books, 1970.

Glossary

Academic school of thought. The conceptualization of the nurse's role as a professional, which arose when nursing programs moved to academic settings.

Acceptance. Allowing others the freedom of their own beliefs and feelings without giving up the right to disagree; also having positive regard for others.

Active listening. The ability to understand fully what another is communicating and in turn communicating that the content and feelings are understood and accepted.

Administrative school of thought. A post-World War II conceptualization of nursing's role involving a shift away from the client and towards administration of health care.

Advice giving. The presentation of an opinion to the client by the nurse, who acts as the "authority"; usually considered a pitfall in communication.

Affect dimension. A measure of reciprocity in communication relationships that relates to the feelings health care providers have toward each other.

Aggression. The ability to stand up for one's rights, often done in such a way that the rights of others are violated.

Analogical communication. All aspects of verbal communication that are not related to the grammatical meaning of the words spoken (e.g., tone, volume, pitch, rate of speech).

Art therapy. The use of artwork to help individuals unlock feelings and conflict: a psychotherapeutic modality.

Assertion. The ability to put forth one's wishes, desires, and needs in a manner that respects the rights of the other and one's self.

Assertion groups. Groups that focus on teaching members how to express their wants, wishes and needs accurately but without disregarding either their rights or the rights of others.

Assessment. The initial phase in the nursing process in which the nurse obtains information about the client.

Attending behavior. Nonverbal behavior that implies that the nurse is paying close attention to the client, e.g., eye contact, posture, and proximity.

Auditory channel. Refers to sensory input and symbolic language that has to do with hearing. Thus, groans, sounds, noise, and words like *hear, say, speak* are auditory.

Authority dimension. A measure of reciprocity in communication relationships that relates to how much power each health care provider has in relation to other health professionals.

Autocratic. Insistence on have one's way; one style of influence in a group.

Basic assumption group. Developed by Bion, this refers to stages in a group's development where the members act and communicate as if there is a shared and unspoken assumption about the nature of the group; these assumptions block effective work on the group's task.

Blaming. One of Satir's categories for communication style, characterized by low self-worth, disagreement, and use of phrases such as "you always" and "it's your fault." A blaming stance is symbolized by standing with one hand on the hip, the other arm extended with a pointing finger.

Body language. A person's communication activities through body movements, for example, how one stands or looks with eyes. This will vary with sex, race, and culture.

Bureaucracy. The way in which a health care system is organized. Four major bureaucratic characteristics are specialization, hierarchy of authority, an explicit set of policies, and an impersonal attitude.

Care-giver. A role in primary nursing in which the nurse administers direct care to the client.

Care Orientation. An emphasis on those health activities related to the psychological and emotional needs of clients.

Care planning. A role in primary nursing in which the nurse assumes 24-hour responsibility for client care.

Caring touch. The use of touch to communicate empathy and concern for the client.

Centralized team communication. A communication pattern within a team in which all communication goes through one member.

Channel. The medium through which a message is transmitted in a communication sequence, namely, the visual, auditory, or kinesthetic channel.

Clarification. The use of questions or statements to help the other communicate a confusing point or issue more clearly.

Clinical school of thought. A current conceptualization of nursing's role, which includes direct client care and the emergence of nurse practitioners.

Close-ended question. Any question or implied question that limits the possible response to usually one or two words, such as a "yes" or "no."

Closed system. A system that allows little or no information to pass between itself and the external environment.

Closing. At the end of an interview, giving the client the sense that the interview is over.

Glossary

Cohesion. The sense and degree of identity or belonging that exists in a group.

Communication. The process by which information is transmitted. This includes the verbal and nonverbal aspects of information transmission.

Communication channels. Refers to the sensory channel to which aspects of communication are literally or symbolically (in the case of language) related: visual, auditory, kinesthetic, olfactory, or gustatory.

Communication style. In general, a consistent manner in how one communicates. Aspects of communication style include openness, person-task orientation, self-disclosure, acceptance, defensiveness, and congruence.

Complementary relationships. A communication interaction in which the partners are unequal; one partner assumes a superior one-up position with regard to the other.

Conflict resolution. The way in which a team goes about resolving differences of opinion, an important aspect of team dynamics.

Congruence. One of Satir's categories of communication styles, in which the internal feelings, words, and body language in a message are consistent and self-worth is high.

Consciousness-raising groups. Groups run for a single constituency (such as women, men, singles, or a particular ethnic group) intended to help members learn about psychological issues especially relevant to that reference group.

Consensus. An agreement reached that is acceptable to all group or team members.

Context. The setting in which communication takes place, including the content or focus of the communication.

Cure orientation. An emphasis on those health activities related to the disease and pathology of the client's illness.

Dance therapy. A treatment modality using body movement as a way to uncover and represent feelings and emotional conflicts.

Decision making. The way in which a team goes about determining the various issues that arise for the team, including staffing, hours, referral and follow-up; an important aspect of team dynamics.

Decoder. In a communication sequence, the receiver of a message who attempts to figure out its meaning.

Defense mechanism. Any of several ways individuals have of defending against anxiety. Defense mechanisms are learned, automatic patterns of communication and include denial, projection, rationalization, reaction formation, and repression.

Defensiveness. Responding to a situation as if it were an attack on self-worth: usually involves a defense mechanism (e.g., denial, projection) of an incongruent communication style (blaming, placating, superreasonableness or irrelevance).

Deference dimension. A measure of reciprocity in communication relationships that relates to whose needs take preference, the client's or the health care provider's.

Degree of participation. The amount of interaction of a group or team member.

Degree of visibility. Refers to how observable a nursing function is to others.

Democratic. Acting to include all group members in decisions; one style of influence in a group.

Denial. A defense mechanism in which the communicator rejects an uncomfortable impulse or truth by saying it is not so or not admitting to it.

Digital communication. The denotative meanings of the words used in a communication.

Dyadic communication. A face-to-face communication between two people.

Empathy. The ability to understand fully how another experiences the world; an essential ingredient in therapeutic communication.

Encounter groups. A group whose purpose is the development of the self-awareness of its members through intense emotional interaction with the others in the group.

Evaluation. The fourth phase of the nursing process in which the nurse determines the success of nursing intervention.

Expectation of participants. One of three dimensions of a health care system's structure; refers to how the members of the system view each other relative to their roles.

Facial expression. The way a face looks that conveys a message about internal feelings. The position of lips, jaws, eyebrows, nostrils, and facial muscles all contribute to facial expressions, the internal meaning of which can vary by culture, race, and sex.

False reassurance. Reassuring the client in a way that is insincere or implies denial of a real concern or problem, as in, "Don't worry, it will be all right"; a common pitfall in interviewing.

Feedback. The information a message sender receives from others about the impact of the message. Feedback is usually thought of as being either positive or negative.

Focal conflict. In group work, the underlying conflict between a wish and opposing fear that dominates group communication at a moment in time. One theoretical way of understanding group dynamics.

Focused question. A question that limits the area to which an individual can respond but still gives the individual a range of responses (as opposed to asking for a single-word answer); for example, "How has your family reacted to this?"

Formal team meetings. In a health team, any meeting that is called ahead of time, has a designated convener, and is usually held on a regularly scheduled basis.

Forming. In Tuckman's developmental sequence of groups, the initial interaction and stage of a group's life, including boundary testing.

Functional nursing. A system of delivery of nursing care in which nurses perform specialized duties for clients in a hospital unit; for example, one nurse gives medications while another performs treatments.

Gestalt therapy. Pioneered by Frederick Perls, a type of psychotherapy in which group members focus on feelings in the "here and now"; generally a treatment modality with a high degree of confrontation and a wide range of related techniques.

Gestures. Movements of hands and arms during communication that emphasize statements or convey specific meanings.

Goal setting. The process by which a team decides its objectives and philosophy of health care; an important aspect of team dynamics.

"Good nurse." A nursing role that involves a task-orientation to the point of ignoring relevant client needs.

"Good patient." A role sometimes taken on by clients in which they become stoic and do not complain or make any requests of nursing staff, even if help is needed.

Group atmosphere. The general emotional tone of a group, how it feels to be a member of the group.

Group dynamics. Concepts and ideas that explain recurring behavior and communication patterns in a group's functioning, usually related to themes such as power, leadership, authority, and interdependence.

Group norms. Rules that develop in a group regarding acceptable and nonacceptable behavior and communication.

Group psychotherapy. Treatment of clients' psychological problems in a group setting.

Health team. A group of health professionals working interdependently and collaboratively on providing health care to clients.

Hearing. The reception of auditory information, as opposed to "listening" or perceiving.

Helping professionals. Refers to all health professions that provide help to clients, such as dentistry, medicine, nursing, psychology, and social work.

Hierarchical team communication. A team communication pattern in which one high-status member initiates communication that is then passed on through "subordinates."

High visibility. Nursing tasks that can be observed easily by others and that require psychomotor skill.

"Hostile patient." A label attached to clients who appear not to cooperate with the hospital system and who are demanding and difficult for nurses.

Hybrid team communication. A team communication pattern with both centralized and peripheral communication.

"I" statements. The use of the word "I" in therapeutic communication by the helper.

Implementation. The action phase of the nursing process in which care is carried out.

"Implied" relationship. How the sender and receiver perceive each other in a communication relationship, either one-up, one-down, or as equals.

Influence. The amount of power one team or group member has over others; related to the amount of time spent talking in meetings and how often one's suggestions are implemented.

Informal meeting. A meeting that is not planned ahead with regard to time and agenda.

"Intent" of communication. The purpose of the statement; for example, giving or requesting information.

Interdisciplinary health team. A group of professionals from various health disciplines who work collaboratively on clients' health problems.

Interview. Any communication sequence in which one of the people involved either elicits information or helps the other person.

Irrelevance. One of Satir's incongruent communication styles in which the communicator responds to stress by changing the topic, distracting others, and ignoring the matter and feelings at hand.

Judging the client. Communication in which the nurse or helping professional evaluates the client in terms of "good" or "bad" behavior; considered a communication pitfall.

Kinesthetic channel. All communication or symbolic language related to feeling. These feelings, touch, physiological reactions to others, and words such as *feel, hard,* and *tough* can be conceptualized as being in the kinesthetic channel.

Laissez-faire. Acting as if one were uninvolved; one style of influence in a group.

Leading statements. Communication that indirectly "puts words in a client's mouth"; for example, "You're tired because you're depressed, right?"

Linear thinking. One's tendency to see a single causality in a health-related problem rather than acknowledge that illness is caused by many factors.

Listening. Accurately hearing and making meaning of digital (words) and analogical (nuances, other aspects of auditory information) communication through the auditory channel.

Low visibility. Nursing interventions that are not easily observed or measured, such as counseling the client.

Maintenance functions. In groups, teams, or meetings, conceptual issues that relate to how the group does its work; similar to group or team dynamics and processes.

Marathon groups. Growth groups run for an extended, continuous period of time, usually 24 to 48 hours.

Message. Verbal (words) and nonverbal (cues) stimuli that are transmitted by the sender for the receiver.

Meta-comments. Comments about how the communication process is going; explicit meta-communication.

Meta-communication. Communication that focuses on how the communication is being carried out, i.e., communication about the communication.

Moralizing. A form of judging the client in which the client is implied to be guilty of violating the nurse's code; for example, "How can you smoke at your age?"; a pitfall in communication.

Multiple questions. A series of questions, asked rapidly, without giving the client an opportunity to respond to each one. Often this is done by asking a series of "or...or..." questions; a pitfall in communication.

Music therapy. The use of either reactions to music or participation in musical experiences to elicit emotional responses and work therapeutically with associated feelings.

Non-verbal reassurance. One of several ways in which the nurse can demonstrate care and concern for the client, including appropriate body posture, head nodding, and use of "um-hmm."

Norming. In Tuckman's developmental sequence in groups, the third stage in which group cohesion and standards for group communication are noted.

Nurse-client peer practice. An approach to health care in which the nurse and client function as peers or equals in goal setting and decision making in the management of clients' health care.

Nursing history. Data obtained by the nurse about a client's past and present as they relate to the client's health status.

Observing. An intermediary step between seeing and perceiving. When a nurse is observing, certain limited judgments are made, e.g., "client slept well."

One-way communication. Any communication sequences in which the flow of information is in one direction; there is no opportunity for feedback or response in one-way communication.

Open-ended question. Any question or implied question that gives the other a wide range of possible response, such as, "Tell me about yourself."

Openness. One's ability to listen and accept clarification or criticism from others.

Open system. A system that allows free exchange of information between itself and the external environment.

Organization of activities. One of three dimensions of a health care system's structure. Refers to the daily routine and the bureaucratic nature of the setting.

Orientation phase. The most superficial stage of a nurse-client relationship, in which roles begin to be clarified by an exchange of information.

Paraphrasing. Restating another's communication in one's own words.

Parenting skill groups. Groups designed to help parents learn communication skills and concepts that will help them be effective in rearing children.

Parroting. Continually repeating phrases the client says in an attempt to be reflective; a pitfall in communicating with clients.

Passive behavior. Actions that allow one's rights to be violated by ignoring these rights or by letting others infringe on them.

Patronizing the client. Any communication that "talks down" to the client while attempting to be comforting; often used with children and elderly. A pitfall in communication.

Peacemaker. One who adopts placating and avoidance of conflict as a style of influence in a group.

Perceiving. The highest cognitive and conceptual reaction to information. This can include diagnosis or a statement of prognosis and may utilize information from visual, auditory, or kinesthetic channels.

Performing. The fourth stage in Tuckman's developmental sequence for small groups, in which the group is able to make use of its resources productively and creatively.

Peripheral team communication. A communication pattern in teams in which communication occurs randomly among individuals.

Person-task orientation. The degree to which a communicator focuses on personal relationships or the task at hand.

Personal role identity. The facet of one's individualilty that has been shaped by such forces as family, school, and friends.

Personal space. The abstract sense of territorial boundaries that surrounds one's body. Intrusion into this territory by another person can cause discomfort and anxiety.

Physical setting. One of three dimensions of a health care system's structure. Refers to medical equipment, space, and means of communication.

Physiological nursing actions. Those nursing activities that relate to the physical needs of clients.

Placating. One of Satir's incongruent communication styles in which the communicator automatically agrees, takes the blame for everything, and puts self one-down to all others.

Plan. The second phase of the nursing process in which priorities and goals are set.

Posture. How the individual stands or sits. Nuances in posture can reflect and communicate internal feelings and sense of self-worth.

Primary nursing. A system of delivery of nursing care in which one nurse assumes total 24-hour responsibility for a limited number of clients. This nurse also directs other nurses and health personnel in the overall care of these clients.

Primary system of nursing practice. Nursing care directed toward clients who are well or in the nonacute stages of an illness in outpatient or community settings.

Probe. Any question or statement used to inquire for further detail about an area during an interview.

Problem solving. A step-by-step process of inquiry to facilitate the solution of a problem.

Procedural touch. The use of touch when administering nursing care; not necessarily a therapeutic intervention.

Process observer. In a group, a nonmember (often a student) who takes continuous notes on what is happening in the group with some description of emerging dynamics.

Professional role identity. The facet of one's individuality that has been shaped by one's profession, such as nursing.

Projection. A defense mechanism in which the communicator puts his or her internal conflicts on others or aspects of the external world.

Psychodrama. A group technique in which group members act out significant events and relationships in a member's life.

Psychological aspects of illness. A client's mental characteristics as expressed in association with physical illness states; for example, fear or self-rejection.

Psychological nursing actions. Any nursing activity that affects the emotional well-being of the client.

Rapport. A feeling of mutual trust between client and nurse.

Rationalization. A defense mechanism in which the communicator makes up inaccurate excuses or "reasons" to justify behavior.

Reaction formation. A defense mechanism in which the communicator acts contrary to how he or she really feels.

Reality orientation. A continual reinforcement of awareness of person, place, and time used systematically with clients with organic brain syndrome, generally as a first step in their treatment.

Receiver. The individual who receives the message in a communication sequence.

Reflection. Giving the other the affective parts of his or her message by paraphrasing, repeating, or focusing communication on the other's feelings.

Reminiscence groups. Groups designed to give psychological help to older people through life review and use of memories of past events.

Remotivation. A second "step" in treating organic brain syndrome clients, in which the client is reinforced to relate to the physical environment through structured group discussion.

Repression. A defense mechanism in which the communicator denies uncomfortable thoughts, desires, or feelings by becoming aware of them.

Resocialization. A third "step" in treating clients with organic brain syndrome, in which the client learns to interact in a social environment.

Role negotiation. The way in which a team decides who will perform various tasks in the care of the client; an important aspect of team dynamics.

Secondary system of nursing practice. Nursing care directed toward clients with common and well-defined illnesses in community hospital settings.

Seeing. The act of visually taking in information. The communicator is more cameralike at a seeing level than when observing or perceiving.

Self-care. A health concept in which one assumes the major responsibility for one's health by taking an assertive stance in decision making and planning for one's health care.

Self-disclosure. Sharing personal information and feelings.

Self-worth. One's evaluation of one's self, usually in terms of how "good" or "bad" one is in relation to particular thoughts or behavior.

Sender. The person who initiates a message in a communication sequence.

Sender one-down message. Any communication that implies that the sender is inferior to the receiver.

Sender one-up message. Any communication that implies that the sender is superior to the receiver.

Sensitivity training. Group work focusing on individual growth and development using a wide range of structured or unstructured exercises; widely used term to define many types of growth groups.

Glossary

Service school of thought. An early concept of the nurse's role, i.e., that the nurse was supposed to serve clients in a hospital milieu.

Social competency groups. Groups designed to help clients with any coping problems they have.

Socioeconomic nursing actions. Those functions of nursing relating the client to the larger environment, e.g., discharge planning, referrals.

Source encoder. The sender of the message in a communication sequence.

Storming. In Tuckman's developmental sequence of groups, the stage in which there is conflict and polarization among the group members.

Stress. The physical and mental reactions to an event that is perceived to be a threat to self-worth.

"Stumped" silence. A silence during an interview in which both the client and nurse are uncertain what to do or say.

Subgroup team communication. A communication pattern in teams in which smaller sections or subgroups of team members share information among themselves.

Summarizing. In interviewing, the drawing together of major points and issues in a verbal statement to the client.

Superreasonable. One of Satir's incongruent communication styles in which the communicator ignores feelings and focuses only on the content of the message through rationalization.

Symmetrical relationship. A communication interaction in which the partners are equal and mirror each other's behavior.

Symmetrical team communication. A team communication pattern in which any team member can communicate with any other.

Sympathy. Feeling sorry or taking pity on another; usually the nurse reacts subjectively to the client's emotional and physical needs.

Task dimension. A measure of reciprocity in communication relationships that relates to the division of activities delegated to the particular health care provider.

Team atmosphere. The general emotional climate of a team; how it feels to be a team member.

Team dynamics. Underlying processes inferred from communication patterns in teams. These processes are generally thought to be crucial in affecting team functioning and include goal setting, conflict resolution, role negotiation, team atmosphere, and decision making.

Team nursing. A system of delivery of nursing care in which nurses are assigned to specific groups of clients under the direction of a team leader.

Termination phase. In nurse-client relationships, the stage in which the relationship is ending.

Tertiary system of nursing practice. Nursing care directed toward clients with rare and complex illness in university or research institutions.

Therapeutic communication. Any communication designed to increase self-worth of the client or alleviate psychological distress; implies unconditional positive regard for the client from the nurse and is done in a caring, concerned, and empathic manner.

Therapeutic skill information exchange groups. A category of groups in which the purpose is to learn facts or ideas.

Therapeutic touch. A healing modality based on the laying on of hands, in which nurses assist clients in the repatterning of energies to enable them to cope more effectively with illness.

Therapeutic use of self. The full use of one's personal skills, knowledge, resources, understanding, and compassion to provide comfort and care for another individual.

"Traditional" role of the nurse. One in which the nurse "does" for the ill client; the client assumes a dependent role in the nurse-client relationship.

Triadic communication. Interactions involving three people in a face-to-face situation.

Trust. An underlying aspect of therapeutic communication, the expectation that another is reliable, has integrity and is accepting.

Unconditional positive regard. In Rogerian counseling, how the counselor views the clients; a nonjudgemental and empathic approach.

Verbal reassurance. The use of words to help the client know he or she is being listened to and that the nurse cares.

Visual channel. All aspects of communication that are seen and language that symbolically represents vision are categorized as "visual." Thus, body language as seen by others and words such as *view, look,* and *review* are visual.

Voice pitch. The highness or lowness of sound, in terms of frequency, of an individual's voice when talking.

Voice tone. The quality of the sound of a voice; usually important in reflecting feelings and meanings.

Volume. The degree of loudness of sound or speech.

Working phase. An in-depth phase of a nurse-client relationship in which the client trusts the nurse and shares true feelings and concerns.

Index

Acceptance, 57
Active listening, 96
Advice, giving, 125
Affect dimension, 168
Alcoholics Anonymous, 310, 312, 327
Analogical communication, 31
Anatomy of an Illness, 35–36
Appearance, 29–30
Art therapy, 329
Assertion groups, 328
Assertion training, 181
Assertive behavior, 181–183
  types of, 183–185
Assessment phase of nursing process, 13
Assumed similarity, 225
Attending to client, 86–87
Auditory language, 43–44
Auditory thinking, 39–40
Authority dimension, 168

Basic assumption group, 318
Bennis and Sheppard's model of group development, 317–318
Bion's concepts of "Basic Assumption" and "Work Groups," 318–319
Blaming, 64–67
Blaming client, 126
Body language, 28–30

Boundaries, 220
Bureaucracy 217, 234
  explicit set of policies, 219–220, 256–257
  hierarchy of authority, 218–219, 228, 255–256
  impersonal attitude, 220–221, 257
  specialization, 217–218, 254
  in tertiary care setting, 242–243
Busy atmosphere, as communication barrier, 214

Care-giver, 145
Care-planner, 145
Caring touch, 102–104
Channel, 6
Channel identification, 48–50
Channels, three primary, 6
Clarification, 116–117, 304–305
Client, changing role of, 154
  and nurse–client peer practice, 154
  and problem-solving model, 155–156
  self-care, 154
Client groups, 309–310
  types of, 325–331
Closed-ended questions, 133–134
Closing interviews, 123–124
Coalition triad, 244

Cohesion, in group, 311–312
Communication, 3–5
  barriers to nurse–client, 157–161
  between nurse and client's family, 244–245
  dyadic, 146, 226
  five elements of, 6–7
  in high- and low-visibility tasks, 17–19
  one-way and two-way, 9–12
  sociocultural barriers to, 263–268
  three principles of, 8–9
Communication, in community hospital setting, 222
  multichannel, 224–226
  stereotyping of client role, 223–224
  triadic, 226–230
Communication, in team setting, 278–279
  contexts for, 280–281
  effective skills for, 300–306
  games team members play, 293–296
  impact of, 292–293
  intent of, 288–289
  patterns, 290–292
  types of, 281–288
Communication channels, 24
  auditory, 31–33
  identification of, 48–50
  kinesthetic, 34–36
  speaking in, 41–47
  specific and nonspecific language in, 46–47
  thinking in, 38–40
  three general categories of, 25
  three primary, 25–27, 37–38
    auditory, 31–33
    kinesthetic, 34–36
    speaking in, 41–46
    thinking in, 38–40
    visual, 26–30
  use of, 37–38
  visual, 26–30
Communication levels, 25
Communication models, 5–7
Communication of Ideas, The, 6
Communication patterns, in teams, 290–292
  impact of, 292–293
Communication sequence, 4
Communication skills, 81–82, 106
  development of trust, 82–84, 253
  for health teams, 300–306
  four techniques in, 95–105
  and plan of care, 105–106
  therapeutic, 86–95
Communication styles, 53–54, 80
  acceptance, 57

Communication styles (*cont.*)
  blaming, 64–67
  categorizing, 61
  congruence, 60–61, 77–79
  defensiveness, 58–59
  interpersonal incongruency, 76–77
  irrelevance, 74–76
  noncongruent, 63–64
  openness, 54–55
  person-task orientation, 55–56
  placating, 68–70
  self-disclosure in, 56
  self-worth, 61–62
  stress, 62–63
  superreasonable, 71–72
Communication triad, 227, 229, 252
Conflict, 200–201
Congruence, in communication, 60–61, 77–79
Consciousness raising groups, 331
Cost-effectiveness, of group, 313
Critical care, 241
Culture
  definition of, 263
  as influence in client's behavior, 263–264
Cure vs. care, 173, 175
Cycle of shifts, 247

Dance-movement therapy, 330
Decoder, 6
Defense mechanisms, 58
Defensiveness, 58–59, 127–128
Deference dimension, 168
Denial, 58
  of all aspects of communication, 74
  of "self" and "others," 71
Dependency group, 318
Digital communication, 31
Doctor in different game, 295–296
Doctor–nurse game, 293–294
Dyadic communication, 146, 226
Dyads, 146
  complementary relationship in, 146–147
  issue of symmetry-complementarity, 148
  nurse–client, 150–162
  nurse/co-worker, 166–186
  nurse–nurse, 189–203
  symmetrical relationship in, 146

Ehmann's model for empathetic process, 99
Elderly, five truths about, 224

Index

Elderly clients, 257–258
  auditory loss, 258–259
  isolation and loneliness, 260–261
  kinesthetic loss, 259
  visual loss, 259
Empathetic process, model for, 99
Empathy
  in communication interaction, 97–100, 245, 260, 303–304
  vs. sympathy, 98
Encounter groups, 331
Environmental factors in health problems, 250, 251
Esalen, 330
Evaluation, in nursing process, 13
Experiences in Groups, 319
Exploring personal issues, in interviews, 119–121
Eye contact, 28–29

Facial expression, 28
False reassurance, 128–129
Feedback, 7, 302–303
Fight-flight group, 318
Focal conflict group model, 319–320
Focused problem groups, 327
  nurse's role in, 327–328
Focusing, in interviews, 112–113
Forming–storming–norming–performing sequence, 320–321
Functional nursing, 219

Generalists, 212
Geriatric clients, 223–224
Gestalt therapy, 330
"Golden Helping Rule," 100
Group(s)
  defensive behaviors, 246
  dynamics, 328
  impact on systems, 313–314
  psychotherapy, 329
  as laboratory, 312
  socialization, 313
  for self-growth and development, 330–331
    leader's role in, 331
  stress, 246–247
Groups, client. *See* Client groups
Group work, 310, 325
  development, 316–321
  nurse–leader in nursing context, 324–325

Group work (*cont.*)
  other aspects of functioning, 321–324
  potential problems of, 314–316
  processes, 316–317
  reasons for, 311–314
  six general categories of, 325–331

Health care system, 206
Health team dynamics, 297
  conflict resolution, 299–300
  decision making, 299
  goal setting, 298
  role negotiation, 298–299
  work atmosphere, 300
Hearing, 31–32
Helping relationship, 81–82
High- and low-visibility actions, characteristics of, 16
History taking, 18–19, 208
Human potential movement, 330
Humor, 306

ICU syndrome, 236
Illness, 156
  labeling as barrier to effective communication, 156–161
  psychological aspects of, 156–157
  sociological aspects of, 157
Implementation in nursing process, 13
Implied relationship, 283–288
Information exchange groups, 325
  discussion, 327
  health education, 325–327
  seminars and in-service training, 327
Information-gathering techniques, 109
  interview, 110–123
  pitfalls, 124–139
  techniques used, 111
Interactive communication, 4
Interdisciplinary group
  definition of, 272
Interdisciplinary health team, 275, 306
  communication in, 278–289, 300–306
  communication patterns in, 290–292
  definition of, 272, 276
  dynamics in, 297–300
  games team members play, 293–296
  history of, 277
  rationale for, 277–278
Interdisciplinary teams and groups, 271–273
Interpersonal incongruency, 76–77
Interpersonal learning, in group, 313

Interviews and interviewing, 110, 262
  asking open-ended questions, 111–112
  clarifying, 116–117
  closing, 123–124
  exploring personal issues, 119–121
  focusing, 112–113
  integrating skills and avoiding pitfalls, 139–143
  paraphrasing, 114–116
  pitfalls, 124–139
  probing, 113–114
  summarizing, 122–123
  testing discrepancies, 117–118
Intradisciplinary team, 276
Intraprofessional behaviors, 192
Irrelevance, in communication, 74–76, 127
"I" statements, 87–88

Judging client, 129–130

Kinesthetic language, 44–45
Kinesthetic thinking, 40

Labeling, as limit to effective communication, 157–161
Language of caring, 193
Laswell's communication model, 6
Leading statements, 131–132
Learning and support groups, in social skill areas, 328
Levels of nursing practice, 208
Limited two-way communication, 12
Linear thinking, 267
Listening, 32–33, 304
Loeb Center for Nursing and Rehabilitation, 277

Making Contact, 61
Marathon groups, 331
Message, 6
Meta-commenting, 287, 301
Metacommunication, 9, 59, 61
Model for nursing, 206
Montefiore Medical Center, 277
Moralizing, 132
Mrs. Reynolds Needs a Nurse, 158
Multidisciplinary approach to client care, 277
Multiple questions, 132–133
Music therapy, 329–330
Mutual emotional support, in group, 312

National Training Laboratories (NTL), 328
Negative feedback, 303
Noise level, as communication barrier, 213, 237
Nonspecific language, 46–47
Nonverbal reassurance, 92–93
Nurse
  bilingual, 266
  changing role of, 150–154
  communications with physician, 255–256
  definition of professional, 191–192
  four behaviors characteristic of, 192–193
  in tertiary care setting, 241–247
Nurse–aide relationship, 175
  three barriers to effective communication between, 176–178
Nurse–client dyad, 149–150, 162
  barriers to effective communication in, 157–162
  changing role of client in, 154–155
  changing role of nurse in, 150–152, 162
  development of trust in, 253
  importance of communication in, 150, 152
  and problem-solving model, 155–156
  role of illness in, 156–157
  and self-awareness, 152–154
  sense of self-awareness in, 152–154
  Szasz-Hollender model of, 151
  three phases of, 151
Nurse/co-worker relationships, 166, 178–179, 186
  communication skills in, 179–180
  four dimensions of, 167–168
  four schools of thought influencing, 166–167
  nurse and aide, 175–178
  nurse and physician, 171–175
Nurse–nurse dyad, 189–190, 199–200, 202
  dealing with conflict, 200–202
  dealing with stress, 200
  personal vs. professional identity, 190–193
  student-student communication, 193–194
Nurse-physician relationship, 171
  conditions for collegiality, 172
  differences in orientation, 173–174
  and nurse practitioner, 174–175
Nurse practitioner, 174–175

Index

Nursing, 20–21
  definition of, 150
  four schools of thought influencing, 166–167
  two settings of, 205
Nursing actions
  degree of visibility in, 15–17
  three major groups of, 14–15
Nursing history, 110–111
Nursing practice
  levels of, 208
  systems of, 205–208
Nursing process, four phases of, 1, 12–13
Nursing systems, 206
  identifying, 208
  open and closed, 207
  three kinds of, 207–209
Nursing systems model, 206

Observing, 27–28
Olfactory language, 45–46
One-up, one-down messages, 284–285
  responses to, 285–288
One-way communication, 9–11
  vs. two-way communication, 11, 12
Open-ended questions, in interviews, 111–112
Openness, concept of, 54–55, 263, 281, 282
Openness-closedness, in team communication, 281–282
Options for participation in group, 313

Pairing group, 318
Paraphrasing
  in interdisciplinary team setting, 302
  in interviews, 114–116
Parenting skill groups, 328
Parroting, 135
Patronizing client, 135–136
Peer practice, 154–155
Peoplemaking, 61
Perception, 25
Personal identity, 190–191
Personal space, 215–226, 236–237
Person-task orientation, 55–56, 243–244
Physical space, 237
Physiological nursing actions, 14
Physiological reactions, 35–36
Pitfalls of interviewing, 124
  blaming client, 126–127
  changing topic, 127
  defensiveness, 127–128
  false reassurance, 128–129

Pitfalls of interviewing (cont.)
  giving advice, 125
  judging client, 129–130
  leading statements, 131
  moralizing, 132
  multiple questions, 132–133
  overuse of closed-ended questions 133–134
  parroting, 135
  patronizing client, 135–136
  placating client, 136
  rationalizing feelings, 137
  stumped silence, 138
  "why" questions, 138–139
Placater's denial of "self," 68
Placating, 68–70, 136
Planning phase of nursing process, 13
Posture, 29
Primary care, 250
  definition of, 207–208
Primary care nurse, 207–208, 249–251, 268
  as information giver, 266–267
  as information taker, 262–263
Primary channels, 6
Primary nursing, definition of, 208, 220–221, 250
Primary system of nursing practice, 207–208, 249–251, 268
  client's role in, 257–262
  nurse's role in, 262–268
  organization of activities, 254–257
  physical setting of, 251–253
  sociocultural barriers to communication, 263–268
Probing, in interviews, 113–114
Problem definition, 155–156
Problem-solving, 155
Procedural touch, 102
Professional identity, 191–192
Projection, 58
Psychodrama, 329
Psychological aspects of illness, 156–157, 263
Psychological nursing actions, 14
Psychotherapy through the Group Process, 320

Radio, as one-way communication, 10
Rationalization, 58
Rationalizing feelings, 137
Reaction formation, 58
Reality orientation, 240
Reality orientation, remotivation, and resocialization groups, 328

Receiver, 6
Reciprocal nurse/co-worker relations, 167–168
Reflection, as a skill, 88–90, 304
Relationships, in group, 312–313
Reminiscence groups, 328
Repression, 58
Response patterns, 183
Rigid routine, as communication barrier, 213
Role ambiguity, 243
Role relationships, 145, 162
   barriers to nurse-client communication, 157–161
   changing role of client, 154–155
   changing role of nurse, 150–152
   complementary, 146–147
   issue of symmetry–complementarity, 148
   symmetrical, 146
Ross's model of communication, 7

Satir's categories, in communication, 61–64
Secondary system, of nursing practice, 207–208, 212, 230
   communication barriers in, 212–214
   communication patterns in, 222–230
   expectations of participants, 221–222
   organization of activities, 217–221
   physical setting of, 212, 215–216
Seeing, 27
Self-therapeutic use of, 84–86
Self-awareness, 152–154, 201
Self-care, 154
Self-disclosure, 56
Self-worth, 61–62, 168–169, 170
Sender, 6
Sensitivity training, 331
Sensory loss, 257–258
Sensory overload, 245
   and defense mechanisms, 246
Sex distribution between nursing and medicine, 173–174
Shared feelings, in communication, 100–101
Silence, therapeutic uses of, 94
Silent go-along game, 295
Social competency groups, 328
Social scientist–medical personnel game, 294–295
Sociocultural barriers in communication, 263
   cultural, 263–264

Sociocultural barriers (*cont.*)
   inability to understand the language, 265–266
   minority groups, 264–265
Socioeconomic nursing actions, 15
Sociological aspects of illness, 157
Source-encoder, 6
Space, concept of, 215–216
Status, in group, 313
Stereotyping, 223–224
Stress, 62–64, 200, 202, 241–247
Student–nurse relationships, 194
   external factors in, 196–198
   four perceptions in, 195
   three common difficulties in, 199
Student–student communication, 193–194
Stumped silence, 138
Summarizing, 122–123, 305
Superreasonable communication, 71–73
Supervisory role, in community health agency, 255
Sympathy vs. empathy, 97, 98
Szasz–Hollender model of nursing process, 151

Tactile communication, 240
Task dimension, 168
Tavistock method, 328
Team nursing, 218–219
Technical language, 193
   as communication barrier, 213
Television, as one-way communication, 10
Terminally ill clients, 261–262
Tertiary system of nursing practice, 207–208, 233–234, 247
   clients in critical-care setting, 235–238
   communication barriers in, 237
   communication channels in, 238–241
   expectations of participants, 234–235
   organization of activities in, 234
   physical setting of, 234
   stress and stressors in, 241–247
Testing discrepancies, in interviews, 117–118
Therapeutic change groups, 329–330
Therapeutic communication, 19, 168
Therapeutic communication skills, 86–95
Therapeutic touch (TT), 104
Therapeutic Touch, The, 105
Therapeutic use of self, 84–85
Therapeutic value of group, 312
Thinking in the auditory channel, 39–40
Time, as external factor, 196–198

Index

Touch and touching, 34–35, 93
  new areas of health care based on, 104–105
  use of, in nonverbal communication, 102–104
"Touch for Health," 105
Transforming an incongruent style into a congruent response, 79
Triadic communication, 226–230
Trust
  development of, 82
  three levels of, 83–84
Tuckman's phases of development, 320–321
Two-way but one-way game, 296–297
Two-way communication, 11–12

Uniforms, as communication inhibitor, 213–214

Verbal reassurance, as communication skill, 91–92
Visibility of nursing actions, 15–17
  and communication, 17–20
Visual hallucinations, 240
Visual language, 41–43
Visual thinking, 38–39

Watzlawick's principles, 8–9
Weight Watchers, 310
Wellness, 156
We're open game, 295
What to Look for in Groups, 321
"Why" questions, 138–139
Widow groups, 328
Work group, 318